To
my mother Olinda
and
my father Francisco whose great
love for medicine and history has
influenced me

HEALTH AND HYGIENE IN COLONIAL GOA
(1510 – 1961)

XCHR STUDIES SERIES

No. 1   Joa De Barros : Portuguese Humanist and Historian of Asia
        – C.R. Boxer
No. 2   Coastal Western India : Studies from the Portuguese Records
        – M.N. Pearson
No. 3   The Black Legend of Portuguese India : Diogo Couto, His Contribution to the Study of Political Corruption in the Empires of Early Modern Europe (XCHR)
        – George Davison Winius
No. 4   Health and Hygiene in Colonial Goa (1510-1961)
        – Fatima da Silva Gracias
No. 5   Trade and Finance in Portuguese India : A Study of the Portuguese Country-Trade, 1770-1840
        Celsa Pinto

About the Author

Dr. Fatima da Silva Gracias, joined the Department of History of Dhempe College of Arts and Science, Panjim-Goa in 1975. She has previously contributed on Health and Hygiene in Goa in publications and at research seminars in Goa and Portugal. Currently a Fellow of Fundação Oriente, Lisboa-Portugal, Dr. Gracias is working on a post-doctoral research project on *Women in Goan Society 1510-1961*.

XCHR Studies Series No. 4

HEALTH AND HYGIENE IN COLONIAL GOA
(1510–1961)

FATIMA DA SILVA GRACIAS

CONCEPT PUBLISHING COMPANY, NEW DELHI-110059

All rights reserved. No part of this work may be reproduced, stored in a retrieval system, or transmitted in any form or by any means, electronic, mechanical, photocopying, recording or otherwise, without the prior written permission of the copyright owner and the publishers.

ISBN 81-7022-506-X

First Published 1994

© Fatima da Silva **Gracias**

Published and Printed by
Ashok Kumar Mittal
Concept Publishing Company
A/15-16, Commercial Block, Mohan Garden
NEW DELHI-110059 (India)

Lasertypeset by
Printing Express
H-13, Bali Nagar
NEW DELHI-110015

FOREWORD

The publication of this research monograph by Dr. Fatima Gracias on *Health and Hygiene in Goa, 1510-1961* in the *XCHR Studies Series* (No. 4) is specially significant for the Xavier Centre of Historical Research. It is the revised version of the first Ph. D. thesis submitted through this Institute to the Goa University.

This book is not an exercise in antiquarian research, but seeks to reconstruct the past of the Goan people in their struggle to achieve a better quality of life. It has direct bearing on the present-day social concerns and continued struggle for the same goals. It is the kind of resarch orientation that the Xavier Centre of Historical seeks to promote, making historical research as relevant as possible to the people living today and to the generations to come.

The author deserves credit for drawing on scattered archival evidence and oral tradition to present a connected picture of the problems and solutions relating to Goa's health and hygiene during the whole period of the Portuguese colonial presence, bringing us to the times when it is left to us to work out our salvation with greater autonomy and freedom.

11th August 1993 TEOTONIO R. DE SOUZA
Xavier Centre of Historical Research *Director*
Alto Porvorim, Goa

CONTENTS

Foreword	7
Abbreviations	11
Glossary	13
Preface	17
Introduction	19

1. Living Standards in Goa — 23
2. Population Trends and Health Implications — 46
3. Personal Care and Environmental Sanitation — 64
4. Diseases and Epidemics — 86
5. Hospitals and Extension Services — 116
6. Indigenous Medicine and Traditions — 152
7. Western Medicine : Training Facilities and Trained Doctors — 175
8. An Overview — 204

Bibliographical Essay	211
Chronological Index of Health Legislation	227
Statistical and Documentary Appendices	249
Bibliography	283
Index	296

ABBREVIATIONS

APO	Archivo Portuguez-Oriental
ARSJ	Archivum Romanum Societatis Jesu, Rome
BNL	Bibloteca National, Lisboa
BG	Boletim do Governo do Estado da India
BO	Boletim Oficial
CD	Correspondencia Diversa
CLP	Central Library, Panjim
DI	Documenta Indica
EPB	Encyclopedia Portuguesa Brasileira
HAG	Historical Archives of Goa
LREI	Legislação Relativa ao Estado da India
MR	Monçoes do Reino
PAR	Provisoes, Alvaras e Regimentos
PP	Patriarchal Palace
RC	Rois de Christandade
Re.	Rupee
VP	Visita Pastoral
XCHR	Xavier Centre of Historical Research

GLOSSARY

(+) The cross-mark indicates words of Portuguese origin. The remaining words are of local vernacular derivation.

Alvara+	A decree issued either by King, Viceroy or Government official and valid for one year without the royal confirmation
Almude+	A measure equal to 16.8 litre
Arratel+	A pound of weight
Arroba+	A fourteen and a half kilograms
Arroz preto+	Black rice
Asilo dos Alienados+	Mental Asylum
Bailadeira+	Temple dancer
Baili-pidda	Foreign disease
Bakri	Rice bread
Bindul	Copper vessel used to draw and carry water from the well
Boia	Palanquin bearer
Bonguis	Scavengers
Boticario+	Apothecary, pharmacist
Bajus	Dress worn by women of upper strata
Cabayas	A kind of overcoat worn by Christian middle class men in Goa
Canarins	Native Christians of Goa
Cartazes+	Safe-conduct issued to non-Portuguese ships
Casados+	Portuguese married settlers in the city of Goa
Codel	Chair (an item of Goan furniture)
Choli	Tight fitting blouse worn on saree by women
Comprador+	Purchaser

Confrarias+	Pious confraternity
Curandeiros+	Quacks
Dai	Native midwife
Delegado de Saude+	Health Officer
Delegacia de Saude+	Health Office
Dobo	Disease of the liver
Dolim	Means of transport used by women, priests
Dotes+	Endowment, gifts
Escorbuto+	Scurvy
Escrivão+	Clerk
Fidalgo+	Nobleman
Firinghi rog	European disease
Fardo+	Bale
Feiticeiro+	Witch-doctor
Ghadi	Shaman
Girasal	Superior quality of rice
Hakim	Practitioner of Unani medicine
Hatar	Mat used to dry boiled paddy
Hatri	Small mat
Herbolario+	Herbalist
Hospital da Misericordia+	Hospital of House of Mercy
Hospital Militar+	Military Hospital
Hospital dos Pobres+	Hospital for the Poor
Hospital Real+	Royal Hospital
Kail	Frying pan
Kanso	Bowl used to eat soft boiled rice with water
Khandi	480 lbs. wt.
Kolso	Large vessel used to carry water from the well
Kompro	Vessel used to steam rice bread
Langoti	Loin cloth passing between the thighs and held by a cord or chain tied around the waist
Machila	A sedan chair carried by four to six men
Mainato+	Washerman
Merces+	Gifts, benefits
Modki	A vessel used to boil rice
Morambas+	Knee-length shorts
Moradias+	House rent

Glossary

Mordomo+	Superintendent
Mukdam	Leader of a professional group
Mundkar	Tennant attached to the land
Munz	Thread worn around the waist
Namasy	Rent-free land granted to village servants in lieu of service
Nachini	Eleusine caracona
Oitava+	An eighth part of an ounce
Ouvidor+	Judge
Ouvidor Geral+	Senior Crown Judge
Ordenado+	Salary
Pandito	Native physician
Prazos+	Private principalities
Patrão Mor de Ribeira+	Chief superintendent of shipyard
Patt	A low stool used by Hindus to sit
Pauta das mezinhas+	Price list of medicines
Pelo	Cup used to drink water
Pobre mendigo+	Beggar
Provedor+	Purveyor
Provedoria+	Institution of Public Assistance
Postura+	Municipal legislation
Pudvem	Garment worn by Hindu men
Quintal+	128 lbs. wt.
Recolhimento+	Home for the destitutes
Regedor+	Village magistrate
Regimento+	Standing order
Renda Verde+	Income from market fines on vegetables
Saguates+	Gifts
Sangrador+	Bleeder
Santa Casa Misericordia+	Holy House of Mercy
Senado+	Municipal Council
Shevgo	Machine used to prepare Goan rice noodles
Sigmo	Hindu festival corresponding to Holi
Soldo+	Basic pay
Sotel	Copper vessel used to prepare traditional Goan sweets
Sub-chefe+	Assistant chief
Sup	Winnowing fan
Tambio	Small vessel for water

Tanador	Chief revenue and judicial authority of a province
Taverna +	Liquor shop
Tirtha	Holy water
Tonga+	Horse-drawn carriage
Vaidya	Ayurvedic practitioner
Vatam	Copper plate used to eat food
Vatli	Metal plate for food
Vedor de Fazenda+	Chief revenue superintendent
Xeiçal+	Portuguese wine
Xetam	Devil

PREFACE

Health and Hygiene in Colonial Goa (1510–1961) contains an historical inquiry into the conditions and problems of health and hygiene during the period of Portuguese colonial rule in Goa.

The present work emerges out of the doctoral thesis entitled *Health and Hygiene in Goa – 1510–1961*, presented to the Goa University for the award of Ph.D degree in 1992. The work provides for the first time a comprehensive picture of the Goan society from the perspective of health and hygiene and related issues. In the process much documentary evidence is also made available for understanding the socio-economic conditions of life in Goa during the period covered by this study.

It is hoped that the contribution made by this work will enable those concerned about improving the quality of life in Goa to understand better the necessary background that has influenced and shaped many social attitudes and institutional strengths as well as handicaps.

I wish to express my gratitude to Rev. Dr. Teotonio de Souza, Director of the Xavier Centre of Historical Research, Goa, for his able guidance, constructive criticism and help in all stages of this research. I am also grateful to him for introducing me to the use of computers for word processing and for giving me some useful material collected by him at the Jesuit Archives in Rome and Brussels.

I am thankful to the authorities and the staff of various archives and libraries I have consulted in Goa and Lisbon (Portugal), specially to Ms. Lilia Colaço-Souza and Rev. Dr. Charles Borges of XCHR for their readiness to help and suggestions. I appreciate also the help given by Ms. Teresa Moraes-Almeida and Mr. Arvind Yalagi of Goa Archives, Rev. Benjamin Fernandes and Mr. Santana Diniz of *Paço Patriarcal*. Ms. Archana Kakodkar of Goa University, Ms. Pia Rodrigues and Ms. Lourdes Costa Rodrigues of Central Library, Panjim.

Inspiration to this work originally came from my father Dr. Francisco C. T. da Silva to whom I will be always grateful. My sincere thanks to Ms. Margaret Lopes and Ms. Isabel Santa Rita Vas for their encouragement and help. I am extremely grateful to Mr. Mark Pinto do Rosario for allowing me the use of his computer when my computer failed and for making time to help me with the graphs. I wish to thank also Dr. K.M. Mathew, Head of Department of History, Goa University for encouring me to go into research. Mr. Oswaldo Fernandes for giving me a collection of useful books; Mr. Ramachandra Naik for the map ; Dr. Zinia da Silva, Mr. Pedro Costa and Mr. Rajiv Pilgaonkar for the help they rendered.

Various persons have supplied me with interesting and significant information. They include: Dr. Adelia Costa, Dr. Carmo Azavedo, Dr. L. J. de Souza, Ms. Lia Alvares Colaço, Ms. Ivette Alvares Colaço, Mr. Aires de Sa, Ms. Mona Rebello, Dr. Celestino Afonso, Dr. Alvaro Pereira, Dr. Carmo Gracias, Dr. Ferdinando Falcão, Ms. Ivonne Costa Pereira, Brig. and Mrs. I. Monteiro , Dr. Manuel Dias and Mr. Adolfo Saldanha — to all of them I am very grateful.

I want to thank Prof. J. V. Naik, Head of the Department of History, University of Bombay and Rev. Dr. John Correia Afonso, Director Emeritus of Heras Institute, Bombay, for their appreciation and suggestions on my original work.

Finally, I thank my family - Tagore, Rohin and Nandita for their encouragement, support and understanding. But for their co-operation this work would have remained a dream !

Panjim-Goa 1994. FATIMA DA SILVA GRACIAS

INTRODUCTION

Problems of health and healing have always been a concern of, and a challenge to humanity. From the earliest attempts at witchcraft to the most recent resolution of the W. H.O. that aims to bring all the citizens of the world to a reasonable level of health by the year 2000 A.D. History records man's persistent efforts in improving the quality of life and the appreciation of the value of health as an essential component and indicator of it. Since the health and hygiene of a particular population at a given period of time can only be meaningfully studied within the context of a particular culture, an inquiry into the problems of health throws much revealing light on a variety of socio-economic, political and cultural conditions of the times, all of which are ultimately aimed at improving and sustaining a satisfactory quality of life. Given the fact that Eastern and Western cultures parleyed for a considerable length of time in what was a colony of Portugal in India, research into health in Goa also reveals a confluence of different systems of medicine, and arts of healing—parallel responses from within a composite culture to the question of life.

Health can be recognized by the absence of disease. It depends on basic material determinants of health such as nutrition, food, shelter, water, sanitation, clean environment, preventive and curative intervention. All these in turn depend on social opportunities or in other words on socio-economic conditions. Only a democratic society can offer such opportunities to all equally. Hence the situation under the Portuguese regime needs to be understood as part of its overall colonial rule.

Many have asked me what made me choose this topic for my thesis. Medicine has always appealed to me. Even as a child I was fascinated when my father, a medical doctor and his colleagues discussed medical issues. My mother too was extremely conscious of hygiene. She always sought to impress upon us the need for hygiene and good health. Years later, when I was considering a topic for research I felt that my work could be in the field of health. I felt the need to research, learn and contribute in some way to the medical history of Goa, as there was no comprehensive work done in this field. Most accounts available are limited to certain aspects of medical history.

Medical history has its value for the study of social, political and economic history. Besides in the recent times people have become conscious of good health and the necessity of maintaining the same in order to lead productive and satisfactory lives. Large sums are being spent on health. Health and Hygiene have become an important budget item of our public exchequer and as much as 13% is being spent on it. Hence it is important to know the state of health and hygiene in the past and how these conditions have affected the growth and prosperity or lack of it, of the inhabitants.

The material used in this work comes from a variety of sources. The Historical Archives of Goa yielded valuable material, much of it and hitherto unused. I have collected material from the manuscripts at Xavier Centre of Historical Research, (Porvorim) and Church records available at Patriarchal Palace (Paço Patriarcal), Panjim. I have also consulted published material at Xavier Centre of Historical Research, Goa University Library, Central Library, Panjim, Bibloteca National, Lisbon and material made available from private collections of various families. The more important archival, published primary and secondary sources have been described and assessed in the bibliographical essay. I interviewed some doctors who were directly involved in the health work carried out in Goa at the last few decades of the colonial rule.

Information concerning nursing homes in Goa is largely of oral nature obtained from the heirs of the nursing homes or persons closely related to the founders. This information has been crossed-checked for its reliability, as far as possible. My research has been restricted by the availability of sources. Nevertheless, I hope that my work will shed light on an area of much importance but not sufficiently studied.

The various chapters of this study seek to answer the following questions: What were the standards of living in Goa during the Portuguese regime? How did the living standards affect the growth of population? What were the health problems in Goa during colonial rule? Why were there frequent epidemics ? What was the role of Government and non-Government agencies in maintaining urban and rural health in Goa? How successful were the Portuguese attempts to provide medical care? What was the nature of various medicinal systems prevailing at the time? How did the Portuguese Government deal with the problems of health? These are some of the areas discussed.

This study consists of eight chapters besides a bibliographical essay: *Chapter I* discusses the *Standard of Living in Goa*. It does so with reference to the prevailing social stratification in the Goan society. It is observed that there were significant contrasts at all times, but these were sharper at certain times especially in the early period. The approximate cost of living, salaries of Government servants, wages of the labourers, role of domestic slaves, nutrition and mode transport have been studied with reference to our theme. The economic policies and practice were geared towards providing preferentially for the Portuguese colonial interests as it could be expected. Certain economic developments of more recent times helped to improve the quality of life more widely. The impact of these changes on the health and hygiene have been dealt with.

Chapter II deals with *Population Trends and Health Implications* in the pre-Census and Census period. It studies the density of population, sex ratio, standards of literacy and looks at the linkages of such demographic changes with the health and disease indicators like fertility, morbidity, mortality, epidemics and famines.

Chapter III covers *Personal Care and Environmental Sanitation* in rural and urban Goa. The inhabitants were very conscious of personal hygiene, but neglected their surroundings and general environmental sanitation. Poor water supply, and problems of housing, waste disposal, ignorance, poverty and poor enforcement of administrative policies are seen as responsible for the endemic and epidemic diseases during the period.

Chapter IV takes up the *Diseases and Epidemics* that were common in Goa throughout the Portuguese rule. The causes of most of these were poor nutrition, sanitation, poverty and lack of medical care. Many diseases were brought into Goa from outside the territory, particularly when the means of transport improved communications with British India. The Chapter studies also the preventive and curative measures introduced by the Portuguese administration to control diseases of epidemic nature.

Chapter V sketches the development of *Hospitals and Extension Services*. Although diseases were many, hospitals were few. New Conquests had no hospital facilities until the very end of the Portuguese rule. The chapter explains the role of the Government and its agencies in providing institutional care. The administration, policies of the hospitals and care provided to the inhabitants through extension services are also referred to.

Chapter VI delves on the *Indigenous Medicine and Traditions*. Since western medicine was not easily available to the masses, the inhabitants made use of indigenous medicine. The chapter discusses the indigenous systems and indigenous ways of coping illness. The majority of the population depended on them, but the colonial policies and practices restricted the scope of the indigenous systems of medicine and contributed to their decay. The chapter covers the role of the native rituals, beliefs, miracles, and the use of plants and minerals in the native forms of treatments.

Chapter VII is about the *Western Medicine: Training Facilities and Trained Doctors*. It narrates the history of medical training of Western type in Goa, starting with the informal training of doctors at the Royal Hospital and progressing with the establishment of the Goa Medical School. The chapter includes a sketchy listing of the contribution of some eminent doctors trained at the Goa Medical School, those who contributed significantly to health and hygiene of Goa as well as some Goan doctors who have made their contribution outside Goa.

Chapter VIII is an *Overview* which takes the place of a concluding chapter. It seeks to gather the insights and issues thrown up in the course of the various chapters of this study. Besides drawing some conclusions, the Overview also points out the limitations that could not be avoided in the process of attempting a first comprehensive study of the theme undertaken for this study.

A Bibliographical Essay has been included and it is meant to introduce the most important archival and published primary sources utilized in the study. It is hoped that such an introduction to the sources with some critical comments will assist the future researchers in this field of study. *Appendices and statistical documentation* to the various chapters provide a more detailed substantiation for many statements and conclusions in this study.

1

LIVING STANDARDS IN GOA

By living standards here is meant the amount of goods and services enjoyed by a community. They indicate the degree of material prosperity and the level of development of a people. The consumption pattern of the population is regulated by its income levels and manifested externally in measurable form by expenditure pattern, accommodation facilities, daily habits, life expectancy and other factors. The sources refer to extremes of income and wealth, especially from the sixteenth century onwards. We can form a picture of a small dominant class living a comfortable life-style and in sharp contrast with miserable living conditions of the masses, particularly in the city of Goa. Such contrast was not peculiar to Goa and such situation prevailed in the rest of the subcontinent and also in Europe. The upper social strata could enjoy high standards of living in " Golden Goa" which had become a world emporium where all necessities and many luxuries could be found.

The economy in the early period was geared to provide for defending Portuguese possessions and trade in the East as well as to cater for personal tastes and needs of the dominant upper class. The prosperity of the city of Goa lasted for about the first hundred years. The decline followed and the city inhabitants had to experience difficult times when other European powers challenged its earlier unrivalled control over profitable sea-trade. There were also the other native neighbouring rulers who challenged the Portuguese right to dominate in this part of the country. Expenses involved in resisting such challenges also told heavily on the Portuguese Goan economy and standards of living in the countryside.[1]

Goa had fertile soil, but produced little. Serious cultivation did not find encouragement from the Government. There were no industries of any importance. There were skillful local artisans, but there was no official promotion of their skills beyond production that ensured their subsistence. Such a decadent economy reflected on the living standards of all but for a few who could afford luxuries.² In the nineteenth century the annual income of the upper class did not exceed Rs.2000, while the poor had to do with just one meal.³ The economic situation improved somewhat at the turn of the nineteenth century, when the middle classes and the poor began to migrate to British India and to Africa. The remittances of these migrants to their families back home helped them to have better food, houses, clothes, education and other necessaries.⁴

The two World Wars and the great depression left their marks on the life conditions of the people in Goa. Inflation and lack of availability of commodities were felt in Goa. However, the development of mining at the fag end of the Portuguese rule helped to bring about some prosperity and provide employment to the poor.

The first two parts of this chapter may seem adequate to cover the matter under discussion. However, Part Three has been added to emphasize an important change in the urban-rural scenario of Goa from the late eighteenth century when the new capital Nova Goa (present Panjim) was only an administrative capital and no longer a trading-commercial centre. Hence, the urban-rural differences had been reduced to a minimum as the economic life was controlled by the upper classes in the countryside in close collaboration with the Portuguese administrative bureaucracy. Hence, Part Three refers briefly to the earlier period but concentrates largely on the latter part of the period under study.

I. Urban Goa

Social Stratification and Life Styles

During the early period the city of Goa was inhabited by people of all races. There were the native Christians and non Christians (including Goan Hindus, *Bananes* from Gujarat, and businessmen and artisans from elsewhere in India), and the Europeans (including the Portuguese and many of other nationalities) who could be classified into some broad groups, namely the high government officials (mostly *reinois,* the married settlers (*casados*) unmarried soldiers (*soldados*), missionaries and businessmen.

Urban Poor: It is difficult to describe the size of the urban poor at any time in the city of Goa. There is a record of urban poor in Goa from the times much before the arrival of the Portuguese. The development of Goa as an important centre in the network of coastal trade dates back at least to the period of the Kadambas, and a surviving inscription of

Jayakeshi I lists various countries in sea contact with Gopakapur. The same inscription refers to works of charity for the poor in the context of customs revenues set aside for looking after them. That was in the eleventh century.[5]

In this class we include the low class Government servants, artisans, domestic servants, soldiers, State and domestic slaves and vagrants in the category of the urban poor. The Jesuit reports from India, starting with the references to a hospital for the poor and the concern shown by St. Francis Xavier for the poor sick and lepers in the city of Goa, provide some indications about the plight of the urban poor from the first half of sixteenth century.[6] Pyrard de Laval, the Frenchman who was in Goa in the early seventeenth century, refers to many poor natives in the city of Goa living in dirt and as savages (*sem asseio e como selvagens*).[7] He also describes how the viceroy distributed alms to the native and Portuguese poor in the city as a bi-weekly routine.[8] We also come across an incident in the State shipyard in the late seventeenth century where a crowd of 500 poor employees are reported as protesting for not being paid their salary for seven consecutive weeks.[9] The *tombos and orçamentos* (land registers and budget records) of the State for different periods since the one of Simão Botelho in 1554[10] provide information about the salaries of different categories of State servants.[11] Information is also available regarding the wages paid to the artisans in the account books of the Religious Orders and they allow us to form a rough idea of the standards of living of the ordinary wage labourers.[12]

The soldiers were a visible component of the city population. They were never too many but were not paid well. The State paid them small salaries in summer when they worked in the fleets. During rest of the time when they were on the shore they had to fend for themselves. For this they sought patronage of *fidalgos* or female friends who could take care of them. Despite their hardships they sought to maintain appearances by dressing well and moving about with hired slaves.[13] Many of them depended on charities of various convents in the city of Goa and not rarely found their vocation for religious life.[14] Dissatisfied soldiers often crossed the borders to join the service of native rulers.

Slaves constituted an important base of the city economy. As many travellers have noted, hordes of slaves of different races were available and sold in Goa. It was a status symbol among the *fidalgos* to have as many of them as possible. These *fidalgos* derived a great part of their income from the manual labour of these slaves.[15] Majority of slaves were put to domestic work, particularly for distributing water, selling small wares and carrying palanquins and parasols for their masters. They were also used as personal guards and for settling scores. Female slaves were often engaged in prostitution. When slaves fell ill they were thrown away and even buried in the courtyards. There are reports of cruelties perpetrated against the slaves by male and female slave-owners.[16] The first Church Provincial Council in 1567 tried to check abuses and cruelties against the poor slaves and ordered the slave owners to care for their sick slaves.[17] The Council forbade export of slaves to other lands by non Christians traders. Any captain or master of a ship helping these traders was to be excommunicated and fined 50 *pardaos*. Natives also owned slaves, but there was a ban on non Christian natives to own slaves. It appears that the ban was not really observed in practice.[18] The fifth Provincial Council banned female slaves below the age of fifty years from selling goods on the streets.[19]

Sale of slaves was an organized market. *Rua Direita* in the capital city had a market where slaves were auctioned and bartered. One could obtain slaves from various nationalities and shades of colour, but the black female slaves (*Negras de Guine*) were much prized for their beauty.[20] Slaves who sought to run away were generally retrieved through the services provided on regular basis by the city Municipality.[21] According to Pyrard de Laval the best slave could be bought for a price ranging between 20-30 *pardaos*. Prices differed across the period. The Jesuits bought a boy slave in 1686 for 50 *xerafins*.[22] The Jesuits brought pressure on the Government to ban the importation of slaves, specially slaves from Japan and China as it was having negative effect on their missionary activity in those countries.[23] The Jesuits did not seem to have adopted a similar attitude towards the black slaves. Even the interest of the Jesuits in the Zambezi region was more in the gold and *prazos* than in humanitarian concern for the blacks.[24]

A small number of slaves were owned by the State. They were captured from vessels which failed to comply with requirement of *cartazes*. These slaves were sent to gunpowder factory or sold in the market. Slavery flourished till mid-nineteenth century, and even the French privateers were doing good business on it by taking black slaves via Goa to Mauritius.[25] Slavery was abolished in Goa officially in 1878.[26]

Besides soldiers and slaves there were vagrants and beggars in the city. They had no home and lived on the streets. Beggars were flocking from the surrounding countryside into the city. The viceroy Conde de Linhares had imposed a ban on such unwelcome city guests in 1630 while the situation in the city itself was critical.[27] The problem does not seem

Living Standards in Goa

to have been over in the following centuries. The records of the *Pastoral Visits* of the Archbishop has many indications of the problem during the eighteenth and nineteenth centuries. An order of the Administrator of Ilhas in August 1870 was forbidding able bodied men from begging and roaming on the streets. Only those who could not work for their living were permitted to beg. They had to carry a board with P.M. (= *pobre mendigo*, i.e. poor beggar) to identify themselves. They were allowed to beg from 6 a.m. to 6 p.m., but not near the temples and public offices.[28]

The urban poor also had their games and entertainments. The soldiers particularly idled away their time in the casinos of those days. Pyrard has left an account of the licensed gambling houses with police protection against rowdism.[29] The natives would play *tabola, circundio, follio* and similar games. *Sigmo* was an important festival which was celebrated with great enthusiasm, specially in the ward of Santa Lucia in the Old city of Goa. It was one of the major festival among carpenters and artisans.[30]

Urban Middle Clâss: From the accounts of travellers it is clear that there was considerable specialization of functions. Traders, wholesalers, shopkeepers, brokers, tax farmers, money changers belonged to this class. We may include in the middle strata the *fidalgos* who had lost their earlier wealth, some government functionaries and cleries who enjoyed institutional wealth despite their profession of personal poverty.

Goan Saraswat Brahmins and *banias* not only controlled the market by supplying goods and labour but were also revenue farmers for the State. They had a strong grip over the State economy.[31] Conde de Linhares remarks in his diary that worse than the Dutch of the sea are the Dutch of the land. The latter he defines as Sinays and the Brahmin Canarins of Goa.[32] Later in the same century D. Manuel Lobo de Silveira, a *fidalgo* who had been in Goa for nearly half a century; listed a number of wealthy Christian *canarins* and Hindus from Goa city and other outlying taluka. He believed that they were taking the cream off the Indo-Portuguese economy.[33]

The professional class also included physicians known as *vaidyas* or *panditos* lawyers, teachers and judges. Antonio Bocarro describes the quarrelsome nature of the Goans and their tendency to easily sue each other in courts of law. He refers to Goa as an academy of solicitors.[34] The religious were numerous and later during the period of this study the religious clerics were replaced in numbers by the native clergy. The Church officials were paid by the State and enjoyed other privileges in keeping with the understanding of the *Padroado* or the Crown Patronage of the Church. But while the Religious Orders were in control they had an immense say in the administrative circles, and the Jesuits in particular were suspected of accumulating large resources which attracted the attention of the Marquis of Pombal and brought about their suppression.[35] The *vaidyas* enjoyed prestige and certain privileges in the society. Their earning gave them a standard of living far above the common man.

Owing to decline of sea-borne trade and the epidemic attacks on the city of Goa the capital was shifted to Panjim after an unsuccessful attempt to shift it to Mormugão in 1759. The growth of Panjim as a capital city was also accompanied by the development of *vilas* or towns in the countryside provinces.[36]

The urban middle class had houses built of brick and stone covered with tiles. Some of these houses resembled the mansions of the rich but were not spacious or so well furnished. Such houses at the end of the nineteenth century could be built for 5000 *xerafins* to 7000 *xerafins*. The houses of the Hindus were built in different style. They had many rooms and could be built for Rs. 1000 to Rs. 2000 around 1880.[37] The houses were lit with lamps of kerosene or oil. Sometimes candles of wax and cloth were used. Merchants though prosperous lived at the back of their shops in badly ventilated rooms. Christian houses were furnished in European style. The Hindu houses were more scantily furnished.

There was a capitation tax on non Christians called *xenddy* tax. The tax affected mainly the middle class. A goldsmith and small shopkeeper paid 3 *xerafins* per annum. A broker paid 3 *xerafins* while others paid two *xerafins* each. The tax was abolished in 1840.[38]

During the second half of the nineteenth century the middle class could save very little due to high cost of living. The highest salary paid to a higher secondary teacher was 1880 *xerafins* and the lowest 900 *xerafins*.[39] Discrimination was made between the teachers of French and those teaching English and Marathi. A teacher of Philosophy earned 1060 *xerafins*. In the same period a *subchefe* (Assistant police chief) in the army received 300 *xerafins* as salary and an officer in the same department earned 240 *xerafins*. A *escrivão* (clerk) working for the captain of Ports earned 900 *xerafins*.[40]

Urban Rich : This category would include the high officials of the State, some wealthy merchants and landlords with palmgroves and rice fields in the countryside. Eventually, there arose in Goa during the last decades of the Portuguese rule other wealth owners such as mine owners, industrialists, importers, exporters and rich landlords. With rare exceptions the State officials reached their hands far beyond what they were legally entitled to. The *Soldado Pratico* of Diogo de Couto, the first archivist-historian of Portuguese India, has left a scathing account of corruption in the highest administrative circles of his time in Portuguese India. Describing a *vedor* or Director General of the Exchequer after his retirement, he writes: If you should walk into one of their houses you would find the whole veranda full of tailors, some making mantles of silk and satin, others, rich quilts. Inside, craftsmen hammered out silver carafes, Chinese-styled tankards, chains and bracelets for wives and daughters; other men trimmed caskets with tortoise shell, silver and coconut from the Islands. Below, in the courtyard, turners and carpenters were busy at orders for pleasure boats of all varieties, desks in marquetry work and wardrobes for commercial use. You might think yourself to be in a warehouse, rather than the home of a *vedor de fazenda*." Referring to the viceroys, he felt that they did better in the game of looting : "When they command an ambassador to be sent to Balghat or Mogador, he by custom must bring presents, and they enter on the ledger four, six or ten horses which the viceroy sells from his own stable at exorbitant prices: a horse worth two hundred cruzados goes for six hundred or more, and they enter the name of another on the receipt." The viceroys made most money on sale of offices and on renominations.[41] These high officials were not alone in their grafting activities. There were the members of their coteries who collectively managed to stagger off with as much or more booty than the viceroy.[42]

The other constituents of the rich upper class of the city besides the high officials and magistrates were generally the members of the municipal body and *fidalgos*. They controlled the city revenues, and more important was the opportunity they had of smuggling. As Disney has pointed out, smuggling up the Mandovi river and through the passes from Bardez into Bijapur was a thriving industry. He mentions two brothers, Nuno and Antonio da Costa, who were the owner and captain of Jua island in the vicinity of the city of Goa. From the obscurity and security of their island base the Costas conducted smuggling operations for various clients, including Gujarati *banias*. A number of the manchuas involved in smuggling up river were owned by important officials or prominent fidalgos including the archbishop.[43]

Housing: This class lived in stately mansions surrounded by beautiful gardens. Some houses were single storied and others double storied with one or two halls, and spacious dining room that could accommodate forty to sixty people at a time, several rooms, kitchen, store rooms, toilets and out houses. Houses were built of stone or mortar covered with tiles. The stone required was laterite of Goa but the black stone was ordered from Bassein. The view of the house was most important than observance of rules of hygiene.

Houses were painted in red and white. Hindu houses were built according to standard laid down in sacred scripts and this was followed upto early present century.[44] Their houses had small windows and doors to protect them from their enemies. Due to small windows houses lacked ventilation and were dark. Windows of the houses had polished oyster shells fitted in wooden frames as still seen in old houses in many Goan villages. The gentry had their summer houses too. The total cost of such houses in the nineteenth century was not more than 10,000 *xerafins*.[45]

Houses were furnished with tasteful and elegant furniture made of wood designed in European style – carved or covered with lacquer. It included bedsteads, mirrors, chairs, sofas, side tables, tables, stools, dressing tables etc., all richly decorated with inlay work. Plates, jars, mirrors, metal pots had functional as well as decorative use. Two dozen spoons of silver would cost Rs.120 between 1747-1885. Champagne glasses were sold for Rs.9 a dozen, 66 plates with gold rim were sold for about Rs.21, 5 *tangas* and 4 *reis*.[46]

Food: Next to the housing expenses; the upper class spent lavishly on their food. We can get an idea about their eating habits from various travellers. Among them Mandelslo who visited Goa in the seventeenth century describes the large spread by the Portuguese gentlemen consisting of variety of viands, pork, beef and poultry.[47] They ate vegetables, milk products, fruits and a variety of sweets prepared in the western and local styles. Fruits and vegetables were not easily available. Apples, oranges and other fruits were imported; a luxury which only the rich could afford.

Wine was imported from Portugal. On an average a gentleman would drink one or two glasses of wine for dinner. Wine imported from Portugal would cost forty *soldos* a measure. Some people drank wine made of raisins. It was cheaper than other wines available in Goa. In 1875 about 8 barrels of *tinto* wine (Portuguese wine) was bought for 880 *xerafins*. Coffee was a luxury imported from Arabia. It became popular for breakfast after the Commercial Treaty of 1878.[48] In the late nineteenth century a man of this class required 8 *tangas* a day for food, and a woman 6 *tangas*. The upper class made use of cutlery to eat their food. Many ate food with their fingers. They drank water in beautiful earthen containers. Water was stored in *Gorgoletas* of porous clay. Glass containers for water were not popular in the early period.

Mode of Transport: Regarding the mode of transport of this class

Living Standards in Goa

Mandelslo remarks that "persons of quality" never went on foot, they rode on horse palanquins and painted gondolas". They were attended by a slave who carried a fan or an umbrella.[49]

Horses taken out for a ride were beautifully decorated with gold and silver trappings. The saddle was covered with rich embroidered silk cloth brought from Bengal, China and Persia. The reins were studded with precious stones with jingling silver bells attached to them and the strings were of gold and silver. They were kept under care of trained persons who were well paid. Horses were imported from Persia and Arabia. According to the Englishman Ralph Fitch who was in India between 1583-1591 "All merchandise carried to Goa in a shippe wherein are horses pay no custome in Goa. The horses pay custome, the goods pay nothing".[50] The best horse could cost three hundred ducats to one thousand ducats each.[51] By an order issued by Governor Antonio Barreto Moniz, the Hindus were forbidden to move about on horses or palanquin.[52]

Palanquins were borne on the shoulders by *boyas* who demanded exorbitant rates there being no fixed hours of work. Conde de Linhares forbade the use of palanquins without prior permission to all people below the age of 60 years, because it was used by many women for illicit activities.[53] Despite repeated bans palanquins continued in vogue until the second half of the nineteenth century.

Palanquins were replaced in the late nineteenth century by *machila* a kind of sedan chain carried by four to six men. It was an expensive mode of transport because *boyas* had to be employed to carry the same. Ladies of upper strata also moved about in *dolim* a kind of hammock attached to a bamboo and carried by four men. This mode of transport was used during the second decade of the twentieth century. Priests also used *Dolim* for pastoral visits. Every Church had a *dolim* for such a purpose.

Cars were seen in Goa before World War I. It was the privilege of the few — the Governor, the Archbishop and some others, including the Conde de Mahem. Another mode of transport in early decades of the twentieth century was *Sarvotta Gaddi* or *Caixa de Fosforo*, as it resembled a match box. They were available on hire. In Bardez this kind of transport was mainly available at Saligão.

By 1925 *machilas* began to loose their popularity, its use was discouraged by the Government as it involved human labour. They were replaced by trams (horse carriages). *Machilas* and *Caixa de Fosforo* disappeared altogether in the fourth decade of this century. In their place cars, *carreiras* and *tongas* were used as means of transport. Inland water ways were common in Bardez, Ilhas and Salcete. Many gentlemen owned boats.

Dress: In the matter of clothes the rich made an ostentatious display of their wealth. When they moved out of their homes they wore rich clothes. Men of this class dressed in European fashion very often in outdated style. Elaborately tailored clothes for men are mentioned in some sources. Garments used by upper and middle strata in towns were similar, being distinguished by the quality of stuff used. Both these classes began to wear shoes at the end of the nineteenth century. A gentleman spent in this apparel about 20 *xerafins*. Bridegrooms of this class wore tailcoats designed in Louis XIV style with broad necktie shirt with stiff collar, long socks and shoes with silver buckles.[54]

Women seldom moved out. When they did during main festivals they wore costly apparel of velvet, damask, brocade and satin adorned with pearls and precious stones. Silk was cheap. It was used even by slaves for festive occasions. The apparel of native women for festive occasions cost no less then 1,000 *xerafins* at the end of the nineteenth century. This apparel was made of velvet embroidered with gold thread. The only concession to heat was that they wore no stockings. On their feet they wore slippers or *chappins* open in the upper side. The lower part was embroidered with gold and silver spangles studded with precious stones and pearls.

The rich wore ornaments profusely. They spent more on these ornaments than on clothes. They wore different ornaments such as bangles, pendants, rings, earrings, necklaces and flowers in the hair; all made of gold with precious stones.

Due to excessive heat during the greater part of the year both men and women wore bare minimum while at home. Men wore shorts and shirts. Women wore smocks of fine transparent material, which according to descriptions of some travellers, hardly covered anything. Smocks were replaced by western dresses in course of time. Before World War II women of this class wore hats and stockings when they moved out of their houses.

The upper strata in the city of Goa had plenty of leisure time helped by a number of slaves to take care of their needs. When slavery was abolished in Goa they began to engage servants. Each household had at least three servants who were paid at the end of the nineteenth century between one to four *xerafins* each. If the servant was a daughter of a *mundkar* (tenant) she was paid no salary. A cook was paid upto 10 *xerafins* and a *mukhadam* received 12 to 15 *xerafins*. Servants were provided with food and clothing in addition to their salary.[55]

Living Standards in Goa

The leisure was spent in entertainments. They played cards, dice, and chess. Slaves played music. Jugglers were hired to entertain them. The people spent their time visiting each other. They enjoyed equestrian exercises, boat cruises and games. At times of festivals folk plays were staged in their compounds.

II. Rural Goa

Social Stratification and Standards of Living

Majority of the rural population was engaged in agriculture. The village society consisted broadly of three sections: Firstly, the rich landlords who owned lands and cultivated them with the help of bonded (*mundkars*) or hired labour. This section got into the village administration in the course of the centuries following the arrival of the Portuguese. This process began as a result of the decline of the Portuguese trade fortunes by the end of the sixteenth century.[56] That is when many Portuguese settlers sought to invest money in land. Teotonio de Souza has studied this process of penetration of capital in the Goan villages in the seventeenth century. This process continued and many benefitted with the suppression of the Religious Orders and the auctioning of their large properties. Secondly, there were the conventional middle peasants or *ganvkars* of Goan villages who formed the bulk of the village tenants. Thirdly, there were the village servants and landless cultivators who received wages in cash or kind.

The middle class peasantry constituted the largest section of Goan rural society. For several reasons Goan villages had experienced an early monetisation of their economy. Possibly the need of paying revenue in cash to a sovereign always based across the Ghats, but also primarily due to the flourishing port economy of Goa and the urbanisation of the port city, the village crafts had grown earlier in independence from the agrarian control. The village artisans and craftsmen were able to produce for the market. Hence some crafts could develop to a very great perfection. Afonso de Albuquerque was writing to the king that guns manufactured by the blacksmiths of Goa were better than those made in Germany.[57] The emigration in the nineteenth century freed the artisans even further from the traditional village community control.

Villages were somewhat self-sufficient with most of the daily needs satisfied from the village resources. There were the seasonal inter-village fairs and the taluka town markets to provide what the village did not produce and in exchange for its surplus. Village artisans who served the village were maintained with *namasy* lands. These hereditary grants could be terminated only if the beneficiaries failed to provide the required services.[58]

The landed gentry, including the upper and middle peasantry had reasonably comfortable life. But the growing pressures of the Portuguese administration on the village communities by way of land tax and other taxes to meet the defence and administrative needs reduced greatly the profit margin of cultivation leading gradually to an agricultural stagnation in Goa.

Dress: Before the Portuguese conquest of Goa the dress of the inhabitants was to a great extent uniform but soon after the conquest, the natives who embraced Christianity were required to use European dress to distinguish them from the non Christians.

As regard clothing the landed gentry wore *cabayas*. This was also the outfit of the middle class in towns. *Pudvem* shirt and headgear were worn by the Hindus. In the nineteenth century men began to replace *cabayas* with *morambas* (kneelength shorts) and shirts. The women wore saris or *bajus*. These were worn along with tight fitting *cholis* or blouses. On an average a woman's clothes would cost about Rs.10, while the same clothes in silk could cost between Rs.15 and 100[59] in the nineteenth century. The Christian women, when they went to Church wore *hol*.[60] *Bajus* were placed by western-style clothes in the last decades of the Portuguese rule. The *kunbi* women worn *saris*[60] (*kapod*) in different style, with or without *choli*. In matter of dress it was the quality rather than variety that distinguished the upper classes from the poor. The rural poor wore fewer clothes than they do now. Adults of this class moved about in semi-naked conditions in rural and urban areas. Their males moved about with *langoti* worn around the loins and went about with their upper part uncovered. Legislation preventing such practice was issued from time to time. A legislative measure dated 4th November 1913 forbade adults from appearing without proper clothes in towns of Goa, in headquarters of New Conquests and ferry wharfs of Betim, Durbate, Rachol, Sanvordem, D. Paula and Piligão. Those disobeying the order in the capital city and towns were fined 2 *tangas*. In other places, they paid 1 *tanga* for the first time, 2 *tangas* for the second time, and the third time the person was arrested and jailed.[61] These orders were repeated in 1934.[62] Rural men had to wear a short skirt over their *langoti* when they visited the capital city. After 1934 they had to appear wearing a coat, a shirt or vest with pants or shorts. Non Christians were allowed to wear *pudvem*. Violation of this legislation incurred penalty of Re.1 as fine.[63] The women had to wear *choli* in public places.

The main ornament worn by men of the lower class was a *munz* of thread round their waist. Those little better-off had *munz* made of silver. They also wore a necklace of stringed green or red beads, sometimes bound in gold, costing 8 to 20 *xerafins* in the late nineteenth century.[64]

Housing: Upper class rural Goans lived in spacious houses, which combined solidity of structure with elegance. These houses were built on an elevated platform with broad steps. The Hindu houses were patterned around a central courtyard (*razangonn*). They had long narrow windows generally barred and with wooden shutters. The bigger mansions usually had ornate portals. The houses seldom had more than one storey.[65]

The bulk of the poor peasants lived in a single room huts, covered with straw or palm leaves, with a low door and no windows. The doors were so low that a person could not get through them in an upright position. The houses of the poor had no comforts. Their only furniture was mats, and during later period a stool, a table and a bench. Linschoten, the Dutch traveller who visited Goa in the late sixteenth century, says that "the household stuff of the people is mats of straw both to sit and lie upon".[66] The huts of the poor could be built for Rs. 10 to 20 in 1880.[67] The better sort had houses of mud with ceilings made of palm wood and bamboos covered with *ganvtti* tiles. The housing of the middle strata of villagers improved with the use of laterite and lime, and even cemented or tiled floors, as a result of income derived from emigration since the beginning of the last century.[68] The floors were covered with cow-dung. This practice was aimed at preventing flies and ants, and making the place ritually pure.[69]

The utensils used were mainly earthenware. Rice was served in *vatam* and curry in a circular dish called *gulam*. Christians in the nineteenth century made use of metal dishes to eat. Use of ceramic pottery is very recent in rural Goa, while it was a status symbol for the rich landlords to use China crockery that was more commonly found in the upper class urban households. The non Christians even those with better means, made use of banana leaves as disposable dishes. Banana leaves were extensively used to wrap food products. The other utensils used were *tambio, kolso, bindul, sotel, kopro, kail, shevgo, vatli, pelo, kanso*.[70]

Food: Rice was the chief item of the diet in Goa. Goa was considered as rice deficit area and the need for rice was satisfied by Basrur and Mangalore. The quality of rice suffered in transportation delays. Several kinds of rice were available. *Girasal* and *Chambasal* were good qualities of rice consumed by the upper classes. The poorer classes consumed low quality rice like black rice *(arroz preto)*. Pricewise the best quality would cost about 25 *xerafins* per *khandi* in 1629-30 (times of scarcity) while the cost of the inferior quality of rice stood at 15 *xerafins*. These prices varied proportionately at different times.[71]

Rice was eaten in different forms: Boiled in the form of *canjee* in a container called *modki*. It was popular for breakfast among the poorer classes with the accompaniment of condensed curry of the previous day (*kalchi koddi*). Rice for meals was boiled in water and salt among the Christians. The non Christians cooked it without salt. It was eaten with the accompaniments of curry and fish or pickles of mango and other vegetables. Rice flour was used in preparation of a variety of sweetmeats.

Kunbis and other lower classes consumed nachini (*eleusine caracona*) in large quantity in the form of *ambil, tizan* and *bakri*, until *nachini* was replaced in this century by wheat bread. Wheat was rarely consumed in Goa in the earlier centuries, except by the Portuguese.

Fish was available in plenty. Pyrard and other travellers of the seventeenth century mention fish being sold in the streets of the capital city of Goa.[72] Fish was consumed more than meat. From the eighteenth century onwards it became too expensive to obtain fish due to the taxes imposed by the Government. Cottineau de Kloguen who visited Goa in the nineteenth century remarks that the poor do not eat meat more than three or four times a year.[73] Milk and milk products were not a part of the diet due to their high cost. However, milk was cheaper in the villages than in the urban areas. In 1768 a can of milk was sold for 48 *reis* in towns, while it could be obtained for 26 *reis* in the villages.[74]

The inhabitants of Goa were fond of sweetmeats. The social habits of the period do not suggest that these delicacies were only for the affluent. The same appears to have been true of the popular intoxicant *feni*, which was consumed generously. Palm sugar was used to sweeten cakes and tea, until it was replaced by cane sugar during the second half of the nineteenth century.[75]

Bananas and seasonal fruits of the common kind, like mangoes, jackfruits, melons and few others were within easy reach of all. Cumin seeds, chillies and turmeric were also available to the poor. More expensive condiments like cloves, cinnamon were not easily available to them.

III. Cost of Living in the City and Countryside

Whatever details are available for the early centuries of the Portuguese

Living Standards in Goa

rule they have come to us through the accounts of travellers and missionary records. There is little information for the villages, but it can be presumed that daily necessities would be cheaper in the village, excepting perhaps in villages in the neighbourhood of the city and with possibilities of supplying to the city market for better prices. At the end of the sixteenth century a *khandi* of rice cost 10 *xerafins*. The same amount of wheat also cost 10 *xerafins*. About 62 *fardos* of *girasal* rice was sold for 75 *xerafins*.[76] Six *khandis* of cheaper quality rice was sold for 30 *xerafins* and 3 *tangas*. The following year 180 *fardos* of *girasal* was available for 270 *xerafins*.[77] Pyrard writes that Goa island had to import almost everything of daily necessity, but he also says that everything was very cheap.[78] In 1626 about 100 *fardos* of the same rice cost 160 *xerafins* and rice of cheaper quality 7 *xerafins* and 3 *tangas* a *khandi*.[79] The price of one *arroba* of onions was in 1787 about 7 *tangas* and beef was sold for 4 *xerafins* a *arroba,* salt for a *tanga* and half per *khandi* and garlic for 4 *xerafins* per *khandi*.[80] During this period an *arroba* of pork was sold for 5 *xerafins*. In 1794 one *arroba* of pork cost 24 *tangas*, 7 *arrobas* of beef were sold for 17 *xerafins*, 2 *tangas*, 30 *reis*. A chicken was available for half *xerafim*, about 1575 eggs for 24 *xerafins*.[81] Wheat was sold in 1850 for 47 *xerafins* a *khandi*, 9 measures of *asgo* rice was available for 1 *xerafim* and one measure of flour for 1 *xerafim* and 9 *reis*. Coconut was sold for 40 *xerafins* per thousand.[82] In 1860 5 measures of *asgo* rice was sold for 10 *xerafins*, 3 measures of *pancharil* rice for 10 *xerafins*, 1000 coconuts for 75 *xerafins*, one *khandi* of nachini cost 14 *xerafins*.[83]

To control excessive expenditure and probably to prevent people from following certain Hindu customs, the local Government issued orders to all Portuguese and native Christians not to observe Hindu customs regarding festivities to be performed after a birth of a child. It was custom among the Goans to celebrate the birth for eight days with entertainment and lots of food. However, Christian parents were allowed to celebrate the christening with close friends and relatives. Any one going against the order had to pay a fine of 100 *xerafins* for the first time. The second violation invited exile either to China or to Moçambique.[84]

The exact amount spent on marriages births deaths and festivals is difficult to determine. These celebrations provided a welcome relief to the poor from the monotony of their lives. Sums beyond their means were spent on such occasions on dowries, food, clothing, ornaments and entertainment, despite the *alvara* dated 1st February 1681 which banned excessive expenditure on marriages.[85] There are references to bans on marriage expenses from time to time. By another *alvara* of 1st October,

1729, it was decreed that the Portuguese and the native Christians could not invite relatives of third degree.[86] In 1876 the poor spent between 25-30 *xerafins* on marriage ceremonies in addition to dowry and gifts. The poor in Bardez taluka during this period spent 20 to 30 *xerafins* at the time of a birth, 100 *xerafins* for a marriage and 20 *xerafins* for a funeral.[87] In 1736 the custom of sending *saguates* (gifts) had been forbidden, but the same continued. Debts were often contracted to meet the expenses despite Government legislation to control it. Pilgrimages were popular, especially among the Hindus, who visited Pandarpur and other holy places.

The cost of living was high in the mid nineteenth century. A labourer earned a daily wage of 16 *reis*. About 30 wages were required to buy a *khandi* of rice. The whole year's wages could buy him only 10 *khandis* which were not sufficient to maintain the whole family. The estimated amount of rice required by an adult during a year was calculated as three *khandis* of unhusked rice.[88] The wages went up in the early twentieth century, but this rise did not correspond to the rise in prices. Hundred and eight wages were required to buy three *khandis* of rice. In 1914 the annual income of a labourer was Rs. 75. It could buy 8.33 *khandis* of rice, which was not enough to feed even three members of the family.[89] Rise in prices of the various commodities benefitted the landlords who sold their produce for profit. After the first World War the prices of coconut declined. On account of this situation the standards of living of the landed gentry suffered to some extent. A poor man spent about two *tangas* and a woman one *tanga* daily at the end of the nineteenth century.[90]

Economic conditions and the cost of living compelled many poor to migrate. Every year large numbers left for better prospects. Around 1871 a total of 16,795 Catholics were away from their homes in Ilhas, Bardez and Novas Conquistas.[91] In 1880 about 26,235 from Old Conquests and 2,981 from the New Conquests had left Goa.[92] By 1910 about 43,877 persons in Old Conquests and 3,557 persons in the New Conquests were away from their homes. In 1935 around 38,788 Catholics were absent from their homes in Ilhas, Salcete and New Conquests.[93] It appears that Goans first migrated after the British occupation of some parts of Goa during the Napoleonic Wars. During the war many Goans went to work in British ships anchored at Marmugoa. Later when the ships moved to British India the staff went along. Various events in the nineteenth and twentieth centuries provided additional impetus to the immigration of the Goans from Goa. Regular remittances to their families in Goa enabled them to have a better standard of living. Consequently the diet of these families improved. Many of them saved enough to build houses of their own separated from their ancestral home. Besides, emigration outside Goa there was intra-rural emigration all year around among skilled and unskilled labourers mainly pastoral nomads, quarry masons, carpenters and mine workers. People from outside Goa also came to work in mining areas of Goa during the later part of Portuguese rule.[94]

There was seasonal emigration as well from early twentieth century at the time of harvesting and early July. The harvesting of crops was given out to teams of seasonal workers on contract. Seasonal emigrants did not cross the boundaries of Goa. They travelled around the villages in small groups, returning again to their home base after a span of few weeks to a whole season.

Between 1919-1920 there was great scarcity of food-stuff all over India and Goa also suffered. The worst sufferers were the working class. The shortage of food affected the capacity to work. Due to shortage of rice the people fed themselves with *tero* and other wild leaves which caused diarrhoea.[95]

The standard of living of the poor cultivator appears to have improved after 1920, even though the cost of living had gone up. A man's wage had gone up to 8 *tangas,* and as a result he could have a better standard of living, if his income was supplemented by other working members of the family. A woman was paid 4 *tangas* and a boy 2 *tangas* per day. Skilled workers were generally paid weekly wages. The highest paid wages in the early twentieth century was in Bardez, Ilhas and Salcete. The best paid skilled workers were wood sawyers and carpenters. Probably because of demand and scarcity of such workers in Goa. A wood sawyer earned 10 *tangas.* By 1925 his daily wage had risen to Rs. 2 in Bardez.[96]

The great worldwide depression which started in 1929 was not without its impact on Goan economy, affecting specially those depending on meagre salaries. However, soon after the independence of British India, and the upsurge of freedom movement in Goa, the Portuguese Government tried to please the Government servants by raising their salaries. Before 1945 a school teacher was paid Rs. 60 and a medical officer Rs.90. These professionals could hardly meet their needs due to high prices in the war years. After 1947 a teacher began to earn Rs.400 a month. Also post masters were given a significant raise.

As regard transport, river navigation was the cheapest means for most. Some moved about in palanquins, *machilas* and later on horses and *tongas.* Physicians as late as 1930's used horses when they went around visiting the sick. Generally people walked with parasol as the upkeep of *machila* was expensive and *tongas* were not available in small towns and villages. *Carreiras* or brass chevrolets were popular after 1945.[97]

The upper class led a life of luxury and splendour during the first century years of the Portuguese rule in India but gradually their standard of living suffered badly due to lavish expenditure and declining economic fortunes. The trade of the Portuguese had been by then almost entirely taken away from them by their European rivals. Those who enjoyed earlier income of 2000 crowns were reduced by 1648 to the necessity of secretly begging for alms. They were reduced to such a degree of destitution that they had to part with furniture and jewelry in order to provide for the basic necessities of life.[98]

The annual income of the upper class in the early nineteenth century did not exceed two thousand rupees but then the standard of living was cheap. A quarter of a rupee or a half *pardao* was sufficient for a decent maintenance of a single individual for a day.

By the second half of the nineteenth century the standard of living of this class suffered due to inflation. During this period salaries of various government officials was raised. For instance, the Chief Surgeon earned 1800 *xerafins* and 3000 *xerafins* of allowances. In the accounts department the Controller was paid 3000 *xerafins* as salary and 250 *xerafins* as allowances yet they could not save much due to high cost of living.[99]

The prices of various commodities continued to rise in the early twentieth century but there was no increase in the salaries. The life of the upper class had a direct impact on the economic conditions of Goa. The traditional consumption pattern of the upper class created a demand for a wide range of goods, in the early period - household utensils, furniture, leather goods, tailored clothes, jewelry, perfumes and horses. Few of these items were manufactured in Goa. The rest were imported from various parts of Asia and Europe. Imports increased to cater to the demands of all kinds of luxuries. Luxuries from the rest of India were in keen demand but as the standard of the people went down due to rise in prices so also the demands for goods decreased during the two World Wars and the Great Depression between the two wars.

Introduction of railways and roads improved the quality of life. It helped for greater mobility within Goa and outside. Consequently there was greater uniformity of standards. The impact was more general on all sectors, though on different scale.

During the second half of the twentieth century shortage of rice and other foodstuff forced the landowners to convert their palm groves into paddy fields.[100] This change contributed to decrease in the production of coconuts and consequent decrease in exports. The impact of World War II was felt by all classes. The landlords suffered due to the fall in coconut prices. Salt and arecanut had no demand.

Portugal was greatly disturbed with independence of British India in 1947. The Portuguese Government decided to improve the economic and social conditions of the Goans. They promoted rapid expansion of the mining industry. This gave rise to a new class -the mine owners. Some mine owners lived in *Novas Conquistas*[101] and others in *Old Conquests*.[102] Since mineral ore was the chief item of export. The mine owners came to play an important role in this field. They also formed the importing class. They imported goods from abroad and distributed the same to local salesmen and small traders. The later opened their shops in developing vilas and towns with administrative and other offices around them. There were also schools, cinemas, hotels, restaurants and markets. Weekly bazaars were held to which village artisans and farmers brought their goods for sale and purchased factory made goods from Europe.

In July 1954 Goans involved in Goa's freedom together with local population liberated two Portuguese possessions in India, namely Dadra and Nagar Haveli. The Portuguese fearing military action by the Indians on Goa sealed the border and cut-off rail links with Goa and India. India replied by imposing an economic blockade. All trade between Goa and the rest of India stopped officially in 1954.[103] Portugal dumped consumer goods from different parts of the world into Goa creating an impression of self-reliance and trying to keep the upper classes happy with luxuries.

REFERENCES

1. Teotonio R. de Souza, ed., *Goa Through the Ages*, New Delhi, 1990, pp. 111, 263 ff.
2. *Loc. Cit.*,
3. Dennis L. Cottineau de Kloguen, *An Historical Sketch of Goa*, Bombay, 1910, p. 117. (Henceforth Kloguen).
4. Stella Mascarenhas-Keys, "International Migration : Its Development, Reproduction and Economic Impact on Goa upto 1961", *Goa Through the Ages*, 11, op. cit., p. 243.
5. P.S.S. Pissurlencar, "Inscrições Pre-Portuguesas de Goa", *O Oriente Portugues*, n. 22, 1938, pp. 381-460.
6. Georg Schurhammer, *Francis Xavier : His life, his times*, II, Rome, 1977, pp. 170-1, 227. More will be said about the hospital and also the activities of the Holy House of Mercy *(Casa de Misericordia)*, later.
7. *Viagem de Francisco Pyrard de Laval*, II, ed. Magalhães Basto, Porto, 1944, p. 32. (Henceforth Pyrard). Pyrard was a French traveller who arrived in Goa in 1608 and left in 1610.

8. *Ibid.*, p. 65.
9. Teotonio R. de Souza, *Medieval Goa*. New Delhi, 1979, p. 153.
10. Rodrigo Jose de Lima Felner, ed., *Subsidios para a Historia da India Portugueza*, Lisboa, 1868.
11. Artur Teodoro de Matos, "Financial Situation of the State of India during the Philippine period", Indo-Portuguese History : Old Issues, New Questions, ed. Teotonio R. de Souza. New Delhi, 1985, pp. 90-101.
12. Teotonio de Souza, *op. cit.*, pp. 168-173. A barber, for instance, received 5 *xerafins*, a cobbler 4 xerafins, a cook 3 *xerafins*, and a palanquin bearer 6 *xerafins* as quarterly pay in the seventeenth century.
13. Pyrard, *op. cit.*, pp. 92-100
14. Conde de Ficalho, *Garcia da Orta e o seu tempo*, Lisboa, 1886, pp. 151-152.
15. *The Travels of Pietro Della Valle*. vol. 1, ed. Edward Grey. London, 1892, p. 157.
16. Jeanete Pinto, *Slavery in Portuguese India 1510-1842*. unpublished thesis submitted to the University of Bombay, pp. 88-98.
17. *Bullarium Patronatus Portugalliae Regum*, Tomo I, ed. V. de Paiva Manso, Olisipone, 1872, p. 24, (Henceforth Bullarium).
18. HAG: *Ms. 9529 – Leis a favor de Cristandade, fl., 187*. C.R. Boxer, *The Portuguese Seaborne Empire* 1415-1815. London, 1973, p. 308 : states that in the seventeenth century a Mulatto blacksmith at Goa was alleged to own 26 slave women. Rich ladies sometimes owned 300 slaves. Many fidalgos besides being fascinated by slaves were fascinated by Indian nautch girls; PP:*Visita Pastoral*, X, fl. 18: During pastoral visits non-Christians were told not keep Christian slaves in their houses.
19. *Bullarium*, op. cit., pp. 131-140.
20. Pyrard, *op. cit.*, p. 51.
21. Teotonio R. de Souza, *Medieval Goa*. Appendix B-3, p. 267.
22. HAG: *Ms. 2088 – Receita e despeza de Jesuitas*, fl. not numbered.
23. J. Wicki, ed. *O Livro do Pai dos Cristãos*. Lisboa, 1969, pp. 90-3, 329-31. In the case of China the reference is to female slaves.
24. William F. Rea, *The Economics of the Zambezi Missions. 1580-1759*. Roma, 1976; Teotonio R. de Souza, "The Afro-Asian Church in the Portuguese Estado da India", *African Church Historiography : An Ecumenical Perspective*, ed. O. Kalu, Bern, 1988, pp. 36-72. Antonio Gomes was a rare Jesuit who was sympathetic to the cause of the blacks and could write: "quem diz que os Cafres são brutos paras as couzas de Deos he grande engano, faltão-the vizinhos a quem imitar" (*Ibid.*, p. 72)
25. Teotonio R. de Souza, "French Slave-Trading in Portuguese Goa, 1773-1791", *Essays in Goan History*, ed., Teotonio R. de Souza, New Delhi, 1989, pp. 119-131.
26. B.S. Shastry, "Slavery in Portuguese Goa (A note on the nineteenth century scene)," paper presented at the Workshop on *Slave Trading in the Indian Ocean*. SOAS, London, December 17-19, 1987. There are several works on this subject among these: Teotonio R. de Souza, "French Slave-Trade in Portuguese Goa (1773-1791)" in *Essays in Goan History*, ed. T.R. de Souza, New Delhi, 1989; P.P. Shirodkar, "Slavery in Coastal India", *Purbhilekh-Puratatu*, vol. III, n. 1, January-June 1985; Jeanete Pinto, *Slavery in Portuguese India 1510-1842* (unpublished thesis submitted to the University of Bombay, 1985).
27. Wicki, *O Livro do Pai dos Cristãos*, pp. 155-7. This must have been the occasion of nation-wide famine in India. Since the city was better provided with imported foodgrain, the poor from the countryside must have been moving into the city. Cf. Teotonio R. de Souza, *Medieval Goa*. p. 145, n. 76. The State tried to control the prices but the farmer in charge of *Renda de Mantimentos and Renda Verde* tried to

inflate the prices. These measures failed to control the prices and improve the conditions of the people. Many shopkeepers left for the mainland because of the measures taken against them. Rice was now procured directly by the Government from Mangalore. The shortage of food was acute. Adulterated food was sold at higher prices then fixed on the door. Many *boticarios* were punished for this reason – three were burnt and some sent to the galley (HAG: MR 14, fl.48; Ms. 1498 – *Ordens Regias*, n. 2, fls. 8v-9v).

28. *Relatario Annuario do Governo Geral do Estado da India Administração do Concelho das Ilhas da Goa,* 1904, Nova Goa, 1904, p. 269; Maria de Jesus dos Martires Lopes, "Mendicidade e Maus Costumes em Macau e Goa na segunda metae do seculo XVIII". Unpublished paper presented at the 6th International Seminar on Indo-Portuguese History, Macau, Oct. 1991.
29. Pyrard, *op. cit.*, pp. 84-85.
30. Antonio, Bāio, A Inquisição da Goa, vol. I, Lisboa, 1949, p. 118.
31. M.N. Pearson, "Indigenous dominance in a colonial economy: The Goa Rendas, 1600-1670", *Mare Luso-Indicum,* 1973, II, 61-73; Teotonio R. de Souza, "Glimpses of Hindu Dominance of Goan Economy in the 17th Century", *Indica,* XII, n. 1 (March 1975), pp. 27-35.
32. Diario do 3° *Conde de Linhares,* II, Lisboa, 1943, p. 150.
33. C.R. Boxer, *Portuguese India in the Mid-Seventeenth Century,* New Delhi, Oxford University Press, 1980, p. 43.
34. Teotonio R. de Souza, *Medieval Goa,* p. 99.
35. Teotonio R. de Souza, "The Portuguese in Asia and their Church Patronage", *Western Colonialism in Asia and Christianity,* ed. M.D. David, Bombay, Himalaya Publ. House, 1988, pp. 11-29.
36. Teotonio R. de Souza, *Goa through the Ages,* op. cit., p. 102.
37. XCHR: J.N. da Fonseca's Collection: *Customs and Manners.* (Henceforth Fonseca's *Customs and Manners.*)
38. Teotonio R. de Souza, "Xendi Tax – a phase in the history of Luso Hindu Relations in Goa," *Studies in Foreign Relations of India,* ed. P.M. Joshi, 1975, p. 467.
39. HAG: *Ms.* 1828 – *Informação Annuais,* fl. 120.
40. *Ibid.,* fl. 126.
41. G.D. Winius, *The Black Legend of Portuguese India,* Delhi, 1985, p. 18.
42. *Ibid.,* p. 19.
43. A. Disney, "Smugglers and Smuggling in the western half of the Estado da India in the late sixteenth and early seventeenth centuries", *Indica,* XXVI, nn. 1 & 2, March-September 1989, pp. 57-75.
44. Caroline Ifeka, " The image of Goa" *Indo-Portuguese History Old issues New Questions,* New Delhi, 1985, p. 189.
45. XCHR: Fonseca's *Customs and Manners.*
46. HAG: Ms. 2799 – *Papeis dos Conventos Extintos,* fls. 3-9.
47. *Mandelslo's Travels in Western India,* ed., M.S. Commissariat, London, 1931, p. 81. (Henceforth Mandelslo).
48. Constancio Roque da Costa, *O Tratado Anglo-Portuguez de 26 de Decembro de 1878 – o Sr. João de Andrade Corvo e Os povos da India Portugueza,* Margão, 1879. The treaty was signed to bring uniformity in currency, weights and measures, etc. By this treaty the British Government in India was given monopoly in the distribution of salt in Portuguese India. Both the countries agreed also to build a railways connecting Goa with British India.
49. Mandelslo, *op. cit.,* p. 77.

50. *Early Travels in India of Ralph Fitch,* ed. William Foster, Oxford University Press, London, 1921, p. 12.
51. James Forbes, *Oriental Memoirs,* I, New Delhi (reprint 1988) p. 300.
52. HAG: *MR* 93B, fl. 363. Palanquin consisted of chair hanging from a bamboo having an overhead silk cloth or leather cover.
53. Antonio Baião, *A Inquisição de Goa,* Vol. I, Lisboa, 1949, p. 97; Bullariun, op. cit., fl. 142.
54. Fonseca's *Customs and Manners.*
55. XCHR: Fonseca's *Customs and Manners.*
56. Teotonio R. de Souza, *Medieval Goa,* New Delhi, 1979; Teotonio R. de Souza, "Rural Economy and Life: *Goa through the Ages,* II, 1990, pp. 78 ff.
57. *Cartas de Afonso de Albuquerque,* ed., Bulhão Pato, Lisboa, 1884, 1, p. 203; Teotonio R. de Souza, *Goa through the Ages,* op. cit., pp. 85-7.
58. Teotonio R. de Souza, *Medieval Goa,* pp. 82-3.
59. XCHR: *Mss.* J.N. da Fonseca's Collection: *Administração Fiscal da 4ª Divisão de Novas Conquistas,* fl. 12.
60. A. Lopes Mendes, *A India Portuguesa,* vol. 1, Lisboa, 1886, p. 48, (Henceforth Lopes Mendes) Hol was a white sheet worn over saree by Christian women to the Church.
61. *Boletim Official,* no. 89, 7th November 1913. (Henceforth B.O.).
62. B.O. no. 27, 3rd April 1934.
63. *Legislação relativa ao Estado da India* 1934, Nova Goa, 1936, pp. 136-37. (Henceforth LREI).
64. XCHR: Fonseca's *Customs and Manners.*
65. Mario Cabral e Sa, "Thresholds of Leisure", *Goa: Cultural Patterns, ed. S.V. Doshi,* Bombay, Marg Publications, 1983, pp. 103-114.
66. The voyage of John Huyghen van Linschoten to the *East Indies,* ed., A.C. Burnell and P.A. Tiele, Vol. 2, London, 1885, p. 225.
67. XCHR: Fonseca's *Customs and Manners.*
68. Mascarenhas-Keyes, *op. cit.,* p. 251.
69. A. Lopes Mendes, *A India Portuguesa* vol. 1, New Delhi, (reprint), p. 256 says that the inquisition issued a decree on 14th April 1736 forbidding the people from covering the floors of their houses with cowdung at the time of a delivery or after a dead body was moved out of a house.
70. A.B. de Bragança Pereira, *Etnografia da India Portuguesa,* Vol. 2, Bastora, 1940, p. 380. (Henceforth *Etnografia).*
71. Teotoni R. de Souza, *Medieval Goa,* Delhi, 1979, p. 172.
72. Pyrard, op. cit. p. 82.
73. Kloguen, op. cit., p. 118.
74. *Ibid.,* p. 22.
75. Fatima Gracias, "Quality of Life in Colonial Goa: its Hygienic Expression (19th-20th Centuries) in *Essays in Goan History,* ed., Teotonio R. de Souza, New Delhi, 1989, p. 192.
76. HAG: Ms.2785 – *Despezas do Convento da Graça,* fls. 80-81.
77. *Ibid.,* fl. 191v.
78. Pyrard, op. cit., p. 28.
79. HAG: Ms. 4396 – *Papeis dos Conventos Extintos,* fls. 2 and 9.
80. HAG: Ms. 7513 – *Livro da despeza do Convento de N. Sra. Graça,* fl. 8.
81. *Boletim do Governo,* no. 33, 16th August 1850, p. 253. (henceforth B.G.).
82. Francisco Maria Bordalo, *Ensaio sobre a Estatisca do Estado da India in Jose*

Joaquim Lopes de Lima, *Ensaios sobre a estatisca das possesões Portuguesas no Africa, Asia e na Oceania,* Lisboa, Impren sa National, 1844-1862, pp. 88-90.
83. Eduardo A. de Sa Nogueira Balsemão, *Os Portugueses no Oriente,* Part II, Nova Goa, (year of publication not mentioned) p. 121.
84. Lopes Mendes, op. cit., p. 243.
85. *Ibid.,* p. 42.
86. XCHR: Mss. J.N. da Fonseca's Collection *Questions and Responses – Regedor de Assolna.*
87. *Appendice I-A gives an idea of the expenses of this class as well as the middle and rich classes* around 1870. Some items such as bread was consumed by the upper classes only. Extra-ordinary expenses at the time of births, marriages, feasts and funerals have not been included.
88. Pedro Correia Afonso, "O Problema da Mão d'Obra *agricola na India Portuguesa,* 70. Congresso Provincial, *Secção* II, Nova Goa, 1927, p. 53.
89. XCHR: Mss.J.N. da Fonseca's Collection, *Questions and Responses,* no. 67, fl. 21.
90. PP: *Rois das Ilhas, 1870-1889; Rois de Bardez, 1870-1889; Rois de Novas Conquistas, 1870-1889.*
91. PP: Rois das Ilhas, 1870-1889; Rois de Bardez, 1870-1889; Rois de Novas Conquistas, *1870-1889.*
92. *PP:* Rois de Ilhas, 1934-1941; Rois de Salcete, 1934-1941; Rois de Novas Conquistas, 1934-1941. Many literate men also migrated during this period to British India, Africa and Burma.
93. *Alguns aspectos demograficos de Goa, Damão and Diu, Goa,* Government Printing Press, 1965, p. 188.
94. Daily expenses of two families of cultivators, one Hindu and the other one Christian, are provided in the Appendix I-B. Certain commodities such as bread consumed by the middle and rich classes have not been included.
95. Pedro Correia Afonso, op. cit., pp. 20-21.
96. Teotonio R. de Souza, *Goa through the Ages,* II, pp. 229-30.
97. Klogen, op. cit., p. 14.
98. HAG: Ms. 1828 – *Informações Anuais,* fls. 3-70.
99. J.B. Amancio Gracias, *Historia Economica Financeira da India,* Parte II, Lisboa, MCML, p. 606.
100. Zairam Neugi, Babi Patkar, are some of those mine-owners who lived in New Conquests.
101. V. Salgaocar, V.S. Dempo and V. Chowgule, Marzuk Kadar, Damadar Mangalji, Nazaziano da Costa, Cosme da Costa, Lidia Simões lived in Old Conquests. Biographies on first three have been published.
102. Sarto Esteves, *Goa and its Future,* Bombay, 1966, p. 87.

2

POPULATION TRENDS AND HEALTH IMPLICATIONS

Population trends always have a direct relation with the prosperity and progress of a place. The study of population trends is relevant to health and hygiene. Health conditions are obviously a determinant of mortality and fertility and consequently of quantitative population trends.

The size of the population and its growth in Goa were influenced by economic conditions of life that were based predominantly on agriculture and its impact on the health conditions. Majority of the people could be called poor. The prevailing living standards were responsible for the level of nutrition, lack of hygiene and diseases. Since most people lived in chronic economic stress they could not afford to spend much on food and basic amenities. The diet of the majority of people was faulty due to poverty and certain irrational food habits sanctioned by tradition. Faulty diet was responsible for many diseases prevailing in Goa. It also affected the ability of the people to work. Poor diet together with lack of hygiene, polluted water and scarcity of food led to morbidity and mortality. The vulnerable age group were pregnant women, infants and children. This chapter has two sections. Section one will deal with population changes in pre-census period. Section two deals with population trends in census period that is from 1881 to 1961.

I. Pre-Census Period

The population figures for the pre-census period for the district of Goa are not complete nor very accurate. The information available is restricted to areas where the Jesuits and other missionaries exercised their missions. It is based on Church records. They are the prime sources of population figures since the early centuries of Portuguese regime. Parish registers were started as a result of the Council of Trent (1545-1563). Parish registers provide some information about socio-economic problems and specially the health conditions of the time. Figures for births and deaths for the first centuries are not available.

The Jesuit records reveal that in 1603 the population of Salcete consisted of 34,238 inhabitants.[1] This number went up in 1606 to 35,500.[2] In 1608 Salcete had 82,200 Catholic inhabitants. The increase in Catholic population was due to large scale conversion and natural growth.

The total population of Ilhas, Bardez and Salcete between 1631-1643 was 1,22,840 inhabitants. Out of these 60,000 were Catholics and 40,000 non Catholics. Among these were 22,840 soldiers. In the late seventeenth century the total population of Ilhas consisted of 30,000 inhabitants. Salcete had 80,000 inhabitants and the population of Bardez was about 70,000.[3]

Between 1719-1721, the total population of Ilhas taluka consisted of 70,186 inhabitants including 62,328 Christians. Among the Catholics there were 1,038 Portuguese. The non-Christian population of this taluka consisted of 7,719 Hindus and 39 Muslims.[4] At the same time Salcete had 66,965 inhabitants: 64,916 Catholics, including 76 Portuguese, 2,280 Hindus and 153 Muslims. The population of Bardez in the north of Goa was 1,19,490 with 1,05,260 Christians, 13,330 Hindus and 900 Muslims.[5]

In 1723 the total Catholic population (including slaves) of the city of Goa, adjoining islands, Anjediva, Salcete and Bardez consisted of 1,81,565. In 1749 the population of Ilhas taluka amounted to 52,781 including 1,156 Portuguese, 5,573 Hindus, 11 Muslims and 2,218 slaves. The city of Goa had 368 Timoris, Chinese and Bengalis. In the meantime the total population of Salcete was 65,182 including 1,539 Hindus, 45 Muslims, 294 Europeans and 803 slaves. In the case of Bardez the population was 61,171 with 351 Portuguese, 5,567 Hindus, 147 Muslims and 433 slaves. The island of Anjediva had only 817 inhabitants — 36 whites, 32 Hindus, 1 Muslim and 11 slaves.[6]

The total Catholic population of Goa (Bardez, Salcete and Ilhas) was 1,79,175 in 1773.[7] In 1775 this number decreased to 1,68,079. This could be due to epidemics and famines.[8] In 1790 Bardez, Ilhas, Salcete and Ponda had 1,36,844 Catholic inhabitants.[9] This number rose to 1,69,019 around 1795.[10]

In the year 1810 the population of Ilhas amounted to 31,586. During the same year the population of Bardez, Salcete, Ponda, Canacona, Bicholim, Pernem and Tiracol were 22,071, 69,287, 32,620, 32,583, 14,583, 8,723, 23,293 and 456 respectively. The figure must have been higher as most of the births, deaths and marriages were not registered. Salcete had a total population of 69,287. About 2,077 births took place in this taluka. The Catholic population of Goa was around 87,039 in 1810.[11] In 1820 the Catholic population of Goa was 1,24,097.[12]

In 1825 the population of Goa amounted to 2,60,000 including 1,000 Europeans (Portuguese) and their descendants.[13] As per the census carried out in Goa in the year 1848 the total population of Goa was 3,55,402 including 1,79,466 males and 1,75,936 females. There were 2,30,983 Christians, 1,31,527 Hindus and 1,461 Muslims.

The census of 1851 shows that the population of Goa was about 3,63,474 including 1,80,240 males and 1,83,234 females. A report issued by the Health Services around 1860 stated that the Old Conquests had about 2,48,217 inhabitants and the New Conquests (including Anjediva and Tiracol) had 18,006 inhabitants.[14] The population of Goa in 1877 was 3,92,234. including 1,94,590 males and 1,97,644 females. The population of *Velhas Conquistas* (Old Conquests) consisted of 2,64,740 inhabitants. At the same time *Novas Conquistas* (New Conquests) had a population of 1,27,494.

In the year 1878, there were a total 7,641 births, 5,816 deaths and 3,039 marriages. Between 1600 to 1700 the population of Goa declined. This decline can be attributed to many epidemics that broke out during the period including the ones that took place in 1618, 1635, 1648 and the wars with Shivaji. During this conflict many people migrated to the neighbouring kingdoms. Famines too must have contributed to the decline in population. For instance during the famine of 1630 about 4-6 persons died daily due to scarcity of food. Jesuit missionaries daily fed about 900 persons with boiled rice and canjee. In Salcete there was acute shortage of food resulting in many deaths mainly among children.[15] However, between 1700-1800 there appears to be a rise in population even though epidemics continued to take a toll of life.[16] This could be as a result of the acquisition of New Conquests during this period.

II. Census Period

The Anglo-Portuguese treaty of December 26th, 1878 paved the way for the uninterrupted decennial series of substantial censuses starting from 1881. The British Government had agreed to supply salt to *Estado da India* and wished to know the exact population of the territory. The British Government asked the Portuguese Government to carry out a census. In August 1899 Portuguese Government ordered that decennial census

Population Trends and Health Implications

should be carried out in all Portuguese colonies from 1900 onwards. The censuses have been a major sources of information on trends of population and its character. The other official demographic data such as registration of births was started much later. The censuses specially in the early period are not fully reliable. Sometimes door to door enumeration was not carried out. The *regedor* (village magistrate) was asked many times to fill up the forms.

The first census was carried out on 17th February 1881. The census took into account all population present and those temporarily absent. The census of 1881 gives 4,45,263 as the total population of Goa. In 1900 Goa had 4,75,513 inhabitants. This population steadily increased upto the third census of 1910 which registered 4,85,752 inhabitants. Between 1881-1900 there was increase of 30,250 persons - a rise of 6.75%, whereas during the decade 1900-1910 the population showed a marginal increase of 10,239 persons which was an increase of 2.36%. During this period large number of Goans living in Bombay returned to Goa panic-stricken due to plague that ravaged Bombay between 1896-1914.[17]

The mortality rate was high in Goa. The Government appeared to be concerned with the problem. It appointed a committee to investigate the causes. The high mortality could be associated with poor standards of living, lack of medical facilities and epidemics of cholera, plague, smallpox as well as endemic diseases such as malaria, typhoid, and tuberculosis. The mortality caused by malaria was high in Sanguem taluka where the disease existed in endemic form. Between 1900-1910 about 6,000 inhabitants died in Sanguem due to malaria and more than 15 villages disappeared from the map. Malaria was also responsible for the disappearance of four villages in Canacona (South Goa).[18]

During 1910-1921 a decrease was noted in the population of Goa. The decrease of 3.55% was attributed to emigration and epidemics, particularly to the pandemic of influenza and to certain economic conditions.[19] Ilhas taluka was densely populated until the nineteenth century. After this period Bardez emerged as the most densely inhabited region. This density decreased after 1931 because of emigration flow.

An increase of 35,787 inhabitants was registered in the decade 1921-1931, presumably because of expansion of port activities at Marmagoa and absence of severe epidemics as well as famines. Between 1931-1940 the population of Goa rose from 5,05,281 to 5,40,925 – a percentage growth of 7.05%.

In the decade 1940-1950 the increase in population was low. Only 6,523 persons were added. Between 1950-1960 there was a mere 1.21%

increase. In the early 1950s many Goans on account of economic blockade left Goa because their family earners in the rest of India could not remit money to Goa freely. At the same time, the blockade gave impetus to the development of ore extraction. The emergence of mining brought about a shift of population to the mining areas of Sanguem, Bicholim, Quepem and Satari. The population of these talukas noticed an increase of 44.6%, 26.95%, 27.41% and 17.05% respectively.

A corresponding increase of population was also experienced in Marmagoa port region. Around 1961 there were 5,89,997 inhabitants in Goa, including 3,30,219 in the Old Conquests and the remaining in the New Conquests.[20]

The increase in population in the mining areas were not only due to working facilities but also due to control of diseases such as malaria. In 1950s malaria campaign was carried out at Canacona, Sanguem and Quepem talukas. As a result malaria that was endemic in these areas almost disappeared. During this period Government agencies made strenuous attempts to improve the conditions of health by controlling diseases. Although financial reasons did not permit large scale policy measures, still it was responsible for marked decline in mortality in the last decade of colonial era. Improvement of nutrition, immunization and mass public health measures helped in deep reduction of infectious and parasitic diseases from the beginning to the end of a life span.

Before 1914 all births were not registered in Goa. Catholics registered births at their respective parishes at the time of baptism. The compulsory birth registration in the territory of Goa, Daman and Diu was started in 1914, with the publication of the Civil Registry Code. Every new born had to be registered within 30 days, failing which the parents were to be fined.

Despite the law making birth registration compulsory, many births remained unregistered particularly in rural areas either through neglect of the parents or their ignorance. Births many times were registered only at the time of a child going to school or at the time of a marriage.

Birth rates were high among the Muslims. In the year 1900 the birth rate in Goa was 17.65%. The following year a decrease was noticed with 16.83%. In 1910 the crude birth rate was 59.87% and in 1920 it was 52.82%. A total of 15,805 births took place in 1921 out of these 7,974 were Catholics and 7,831 were non-Catholics.

Still births were common in Goa throughout the period due to lack of medical aid and other factors. Most of these still births were not registered.

Sex Ratio

Sex ratio was favourable to males during the years 1848 and 1881 with 980 and 990 females per thousand males. This could be because males were better looked after in the early days of birth and very often survived diseases. Pronounced preference for sons led to poorer feeding and neglect of daughters. Women spent a considerable part of adult life pregnant or nursing. They suffered from higher level of infectious diseases. Along with poorer nutrition, lack of knowledge of asepsis in delivery contributed to the adult female excess of deaths over males through child bearing ages largely from maternal mortality, tuberculosis and malaria.

The following table show excess of females over males between 1900 to 1931.[21]

Year	Male	Female	Female
1900	2,25,825	2,75,973	50,148
1910	2,61,596	2,86,646	25,050
1921	2,52,096	2,79,856	27,760
1931	2,79,398	3,00,572	21,174

The highest number of females per 1,000 males was in 1950. In this year there were 1,128 females for 1,000 males. However, in 1960 there was a slight decline with 1,066 females for 1,000 males.

The ratio in favour of the females was due to variety of factors. Among these emigration was an important one. Large number of Goans migrated to British India and East Africa right from the nineteenth century. Bardez, Salcete, Ilhas, Sanquelim and Pernem had excess female rate between 1900-1931. Excess of the females could be attributed to the fact that the above mentioned talukas had large paddy fields where women labour was required. Until 1950s Satari, Bicholim, Sanguem and Quepem talukas had more women then men. This trend changed due to development of mining industries as more men worked in the mines.

Marital Status

In 1848 there were around 56.64% married persons, 4.53% widowers, 5.12% widows and 30.50% unmarried persons in Goa. The highest number of married people were found in New Conquests among non

Christian inhabitants probably because among the non Christians marriage was a necessity and girls did not remain unmarried after certain age. In 1948, Bicholim had the highest percentage of married people (79.51%), followed by Pernem (75.75%) and Canacona (72.98%). Salcete had the highest number of unmarried persons (50.23%), apparently because it had large number of minor population or many people in the taluka married late or never. [22]

The census of 1851 gives 45% married persons, 41% unmarried and 14% widows and widowers. The marital distribution of population based on 1881 census suggests that there were 48% unmarried persons, 39% married persons and nearly 13% widows and widowers. The highest number of married people according to census of 1881 was found in Pernem (46.93%).[23]

The census of 1900 reveals that there were 47.47% unmarried,[24] 39.71% married and rest widows and widowers. Salcete still continued with the highest number of unmarried population.

Single persons maintained excess over married persons throughout the census of 1900, 1931, 1940, 1950 and 1960. Again Old Conquests had relatively lower proportion of married persons compared to New Conquests. People from Old Conquests usually migrated to other countries, thus delaying marriages. The economic conditions of the time also might have compelled some people to postpone their marriages. On the other side in New Conquests girls were married early as an assurance to the husband of purity and chastity. There were more married women then men particularly among Hindus. Hindu men often had two or more wives who lived in the same house.

Divorces were few in Goa specially among Christians as it was not encouraged by the society. The census of 1931, 1940, 1950 and 1960 show negligible percentages for divorced persons namely 0.02, 0.02, 0.02 and 0.04 respectively.[25]

In 1950 only 17% of women of 15 and above remained unmarried. Among the men the percentage of unmarried was 33%. Unmarried men were more then unmarried women particularly in the age group of 20-34 years. Men usually married after completing their studies and when they were settled in life.[26]

According to census of 1950, there were in that year 1,923 married women and 355 married men with less than 15 years of age.[27] Among those was one man and one woman below one year.[28] Married state must have had its effect on mortality, both physical and psychological. This was particularly so for women who were liable to extra risks to health arising from child bearing. Bereaved women and more particularly men, must have suffered poorer health than those still married and their mortality was higher too specially in the years immediately following the loss of the partner.

Fertility Behaviour

The fertility of a population depends on the first place, on the fecundity of its members, that is, on their ability to achieve conception. A wide variety of cultural practices influenced fertility. Fertility was evidently related to age at marriage, marriage practices, post-partum sexual activities, religious norms, birth control practices and by health and mortality status of the population.

Among the above mentioned factors probably the most important factor that reduced fertility in Goa and rest of India was the wide spread practice of extending breast feeding till the infant was 36 months old. This practice was reinforced by Hindu custom that required abstinence from or at least limitation of sexual intercourse during the period of lactation. Similar regulations existed at time of religious festivals. Hindus were prohibited to have sexual relations on the anniversary day of the dead parents, nights previous to the anniversary, in the day time, at sunset, midnight and during an eclipse.

The poor health and nutritional conditions responsible as they are for spontaneous abortions, still births and excessive mortality in reproductive age groups must have had a pronounced effect on fertility. The level of fertility was associated with the incidence of malaria. Birth rates were low in areas were malaria was endemic. Women in these areas frequently experienced miscarriages and abortions. Other important causes of still births included anemia, pelvic deformity and venereal diseases. Epidemics and famines also affected fecundity.

In Goa marriage age varied among different communities. Christians had the highest mean age at marriage while the Hindus had the lowest. Although there were laws forbidding early marriages, child marriages prevailed in Goa. In the Gauda class girls married between ages of 5 to 9 years. Hindus also married early sometimes before reaching puberty. Early marriages contributed to high fertility rate as well as high maternal and infant mortality. Christian girls married between 18-30 or even in older age. Hindu males married at any age.

Married couples had large families, specially among the poor class. In the healthy villages the average number of births to each marriage was

6 to 8 children and in unhealthy areas 2 to 4 children. Barren people were few. Infant mortality was one of the many factors that contributed to large families. Women who lost their infants had shorter lactation and non-ovulatory periods before becoming fecund again and in part because they needed more children to replace those they lost. They continued to bear children even at later ages. Men and women wanted to have as many children as they could or "as many as God wills".

The census of 1940 for the first time revealed the number of children born and those that survived. The records available show that there were 3 Hindu women with 20 or more children each. About 64 women gave birth to 15 to 18 children each, out of these women 37 were Catholics, 24 Hindus and 2 Muslims.[29]

In 1940, there were 3,541 children for every 1,000 Catholic mothers, 3,531 children per 1,000 Hindu mothers and 3,903 children for every 1,000 Muslim mothers. It was noticed that fertility rate was high among Muslims women compared to Hindu and Catholic women.[30]

The high Muslim fertility followed general pattern of fertility among Muslims around the World. In Muslim tradition the permanent state of celibacy is considered abnormal for men and unthinkable for able bodied women.[31] The Catholic Church also fostered the doctrine of large families. Majority of the Catholics believe that children are a gift of God. Hindu scriptures emphasize numerous children as blessings of God, but there was lack of central authority to enforce these tenets.

The highest number of unwed mothers were among the Hindus. In 1940 there were 942 unwed mothers with 2,898 children. This high number of unwed mothers among the Hindus was due to the fact that many women from this community were *bailadeiras* (temple dancers) who often engaged in prostitution.[32] According to the census of 1940 there were 64 Catholic unwed mothers with 117 children in Goa. The rate might have been higher. Many did not register the births of their illegitimate children.

The period from 1950-1954 show a higher birth rate among the Catholics (36.98%) even though many of these women had their husbands abroad. The birth rate among the Hindus for the same period was 24.7%.[33]

Population density

Population density is a demographic index which helps to evaluate density of population in a given area. There are various reasons for this density in certain areas. The density of population has its impact on health and hygiene.

We know that the city of Goa was over-populated in the sixteenth and seventeenth centuries. This overcrowding had its impact on health and hygiene of the place. The inhabitants suffered from all kinds of diseases some of which erupted many times in epidemic form. Potable water was not sufficient to meet the needs of the population. Facilities for disposal of waste were primitive. These conditions contributed to infections and diseases which finally led to the decay of the city.

In 1848 Salcete taluka had the highest concentration of population namely 358 persons per sq.km. followed by Ilhas, Pernem, Ponda and Bardez. *Velhas Conquistas* were highly populated because of better socio-economic conditions. They were the first to profit from various health improvements introduced by the Government. These areas had many waterways and roads. Many inhabitants from this region migrated to British India and British Africa. They sent regular remittances home thus helping to create better standard of living.

The census of 1931 showed that the density of population was 153 inhabitants per sq. km. Ilhas, Salcete, Bardez, Marmagoa and Ponda had density above average, while Pernem and Sanquelim had medium density and Sanguem, Satari, Canacona and Quepem had low density. These last four talukas had large areas but small population. Poverty, poor hygiene and malaria were responsible for the low density of population. However, the density of Bardez taluka began to decline after 1931. One of the causes for the decline was emigration.[34]

During the years 1940, 1950 and 1960 the density of population in Ilhas was 423, 440 and 478, in Salcete it was 417, 428, and 426 whereas Bardez registered 402, 391, and 369. Marmagoa showed an increase of population of 100 persons per sq.km. probably due to port activities. In the early 1950s many people left their land on account of economic blockade. At the same time the blockade gave an impetus to the development of ore extraction. The emergence of mining brought about a shift of population to the mining areas of Sanguem, Bicholim, Quepem and Satari. These talukas saw an increase in population by 44.6%, 26.95%, 27.41% and 17.05% respectively.[35] A graph in the appendix shows percentage distribution of population religion-wise in Goa from 1881 to 1960.[36]

Standards of literacy

Literacy index is one of the factors that helps to evaluate the development of a place. The early census in Goa defined as "literate" those who were able to read and write. The literacy rate increased in Goa from 10.91% in 1881 to 17.5% in 1931 and 31.23% in 1960.

The Old Conquests had the highest number of literate and educated persons. Among the Old Conquests talukas Bardez had a high literacy rate, even though it had less number of schools per 100 sq.km. This could be because of greater contacts with the outside world and better economic conditions. In its turn literacy helped to maintain better living conditions.

Among the New Conquests talukas Ponda had higher literacy rate of 7.85% in 1881. It rose steadily to 14.2% in 1921 and 22.46% in 1960.[37] Minimum literacy rate was in Satari. The literacy rate was higher among the Catholics and Muslims. Many Hindus knew to read and write in more than one language.

Mortality and Morbidity

Mortality is one of the three components of population change. The other two are fertility and emigration. Mortality has played a dominant role in determining the growth of population, the size of which fluctuated in the past mainly in response to variations in mortality. Mortality is an important indicator of health conditions of a population. In fact it is total absence of health.

The W.H.O. defined death as follows: Death is the permanent disappearance of all evidence of life at any time after birth has taken place.[38] Unlike births, events of deaths had to be registered in Goa. No corpse could be buried or cremated unless the death was registered in the parish or with civil authority.[39]

The causes of high mortality rate were primarily epidemics, famines and wars. Poverty, malnutrition, insanitation, diseases, lack of medical care were the long term underlying cause of morbidity and mortality. Insanitation and lack of potable water promoted cholera, typhoid, fever malaria, dysentery or diarrhoea as well as hookworm diseases and other helminthic infections. Malaria led to morbidity and death. Tuberculosis also killed people. About 1,513 persons died of tuberculosis in Bardez between 1915-1924. Majority of them suffered from pulmonary tuberculosis. The highest number of death due to the disease occurred in Mapuça followed by Aldona and Siolim.[40]

Mortality rate was high in the sixteenth and seventeenth centuries. One estimate claims that between 1604-1634 about 25,000 soldiers died in the Royal Hospital in the city of Goa. Among these 500 died every year

Population Trends and Health Implications

of syphilis and other sexually transmitted diseases. A report dated 1655-1656 says that out of 3,000 soldiers who arrived from Portugal in 1655 about 1010 died in the Royal Hospital. Again in September 1699 a total of 100 soldiers died in the same hospital. Another document of the early seventeenth century states that 15-25 patients died daily in the Royal Hospital of various diseases.[41] Manucci, the Italian traveller mentions that between mid seventeenth century and early eighteenth century around 25 patients died everyday in the hospital. Upto mid seventeenth century about 22 governors died of dysentery and fevers. In 1876 a total of 573 patients died of fevers in the Military Hospital of Goa.[42]

Recurrent epidemics and diseases killed many people in the late nineteenth and twentieth centuries. Tuberculosis killed large numbers in the Old Conquests. It was considered the worst killer after malaria in the post World War I era. Tuberculosis was associated with substandard living.

Most of the records available about mortality do not indicate the cause of death. In Goa most deaths occurred outside the hospitals and when they took place in homes they were largely unattended by doctors. The cause of death was occasionally stated by the informant. There was a tendency to record the cause of death as "natural death" even in case of a new born infant. A study of Parish registers of Anjuna (Bardez) between 1930-1961 reveal that majority of deaths occurred due to senility, cardiac and brain problems, bronchitis and cirrhosis of liver.[43]

Infant and child mortality

Infant mortality was by far the largest source of deaths. Even now, about 40,000 children under the age of five die in the world of preventable causes every year.[44] Around 150 million children under five are malnourished despite the fact that the medicine has made tremendous progress and there are better sanitation and standards of living. Infant mortality is a sensitive index of general health status of a place.

Infant mortality (0-1 year) was high in Goa during the colonial period. The situation improved only during the last few decades of the Portuguese rule in Goa due to immunization against infectious diseases such as cholera, tetanus, typhoid, smallpox, tuberculosis as well as better nutrition.

Figures concerning infant mortality are difficult to obtain particularly concerning early period. Many infant deaths and still births were not registered due to neglect and ignorance. However, among the Catholics most infant deaths were registered in the Church at the time of burial.

In the early twentieth century in Sanguem taluka around one third of the new born children died. The percentage of still births was 8% in the same taluka. In 1927 about 1,614 infants died in Goa. During the same period there were 501 still births.[45] The following year infant mortality in Goa amounted to 1,700 and still births to 670. About 2,000 infants died in Goa in the year 1941. The highest number of infant mortality was in Salcete. A total of 652 still births took place during the same period. Between 1931-1941 about 158 Catholic infants died in the village of Anjuna (Bardez).[46] During the same period in Carmona there were 147 infant deaths.[47] About 42 Catholic children died at Anjuna between 1942-1945 and again from 1952-1961 around 16 infants died in the same parish, victims of various diseases.[48] Infants who survived death in the early period suffered from various physiological and morbidity problems.

Infant mortality can be divided into two major groups — neonatal (within the first month of life) and post-neonatal mortality (after the first month but within the first year). Most neonatal mortality resulted from genetic defects or from infections or injury received at the time of delivery. Neonatal deaths were due to mother's poor nutrition during pregnancy, poor midwifery services and largely as a result of tetanus because the cord was not cut or was not tied in a sterile way. This infected the umbilical stump.

Tetanus was one of the most common cause of infant mortality throughout the period. In 1914 about 22% of the deaths among infants were caused by tetanus in the villages of Aldona and Moira of Bardez taluka.[49] That explains why *sotvi* was considered a curse of Durga Devi. The disease was known as *sotvi* as it usually appeared on the 7th day of the birth. Goddess Devi was worshiped in a special way to avoid the disease. Houses of the lower strata lacked basic amenities. It is not surprising therefore, that death due to tetanus occurred. Second cause of neonatal mortality was nutritional status of the mother. Complication during pregnancy, delivery and low weight babies were closely related to maternal weight and height.

Infant mortality was high among economically backward class. These infants suffered from malnutrition and were vulnerable to all kinds of infections. Infants of the low income group were breast fed upto 36 months, but the milk was inadequate because no supplementary food was there excepting water mixed with jaggery that was administered to clear the intestines. The water used was often not boiled and it was fed with the help of a piece of cloth dipped in water and then squeezed into the mouth of the child. Children under five were most susceptible to the ill effects of malnutrition. Statistics show that more than 28% of the deaths, during the early decades of this century were registered among children below five years of age. During the years 1938-40 and 1948-50 the mortality rate upto one year compared to general death was equal to 21% and 22% respectively. Poor diet had its effects on the height and weight of the poorer children as compared to the children of the upper classes.

In an inquiry carried out in 1943 among 36 families of school going children from Panjim primary school, it was found that 11% of the children in the family died before school going age. This percentage rose to 12% in 1951. Out of 673 students more than half suffered from lack of vitamins and tongue fissures which were signs of malnutrition.[50]

Malnutrition was mainly due to poverty and lack of knowledge of dietics. Even in conditions of poverty the education of women might have helped in improving the nutritional status and health.

Another fatal infection among the infants was pneumonia and bronchopneumonia. The infection that in combination with nutritional status was often fatal in children was diarrhoea. A child suffered from diarrheoa at least 8 to 10 times in a year. Diarrheoa often led to dehydration and many times to rapid death. In Goa it was responsible for large number of deaths under the age of five. Diarrheoa could have been prevented by proper nutrition, clean food, water and general hygiene.

Dysentery, measles and malaria also took heavy toll of life. Many still births were results of malaria. These were the children whose mothers had suffered from malaria. Superstitious beliefs played an important part in taking a toll on the infant life bound by traditions of customs and castes to the observance of habits which were conducive to infections and diseases. Linschoten, the Dutch traveller says that once he went to the house of a Canarin to ask for water to drink, and he saw the woman washing her newly born with cold water. After the wash the infant was placed on a fig leaf as it was believed this would bring the child good health.[51]

Few inoculations were available in Goa to prevent infections such as measles, whooping cough, diphtheria, typhoid and tetanus. Even when they were introduced people influenced by superstitious beliefs were reluctant to subject their infants for such inoculation. Alcoholism and syphilis among the parents also led to infant mortality. Many undiagnosed causes of the time might have contributed to still births and infant mortality among them Rh negative incompatibility of the parents.

As a result of improved antenatal and intra-natal care plus increasing availability of medicine, establishment of maternity homes in rural areas, expansion of education and means of transport, mortality incidence among infants declined in the last few decades.

Maternity deaths

Child bearing is a term that can be used to refer to human procreation from conception throughout birth, puerperium and early parenthood with all its physical, psychological and social ramifications. Childbearing was a difficult process in Goa as still is in many developing countries. Around 2,30,000 women still die in South Asia during pregnancy and childbirths.

Such high mortality rate was the result of the conditions surrounding the pregnant mothers before, during and after the delivery. Antenatal care did not exist in Goa during those days. No prenatal tests were carried or urine examined. The swelling of the feet was paid little attention. This often led to eclampsy.

Deliveries during major part of the colonial period was conducted at home. A wide spread custom required that the young woman returned to her mother's house for the birth at least of her first child. The birth was attended by a *dai* a woman of low caste or a servant in the house. The *dai* had no formal training. It was a hereditary skill or lack of skill that was greatly responsible for high infant mortality. According to certain cultural norms prevailing mainly among Hindus, the actual event of birth was considered ritually impure. That is the one of the reasons for lack of hygiene in the delivery room. The *dai* had little knowledge of hygiene and even less of obstetric science.

In New Conquests lack of medical facilities, poverty and poor transport facilities prevented the people in need to seek help of trained doctors. No wonder they had to be contented with *dais* and quacks. At the same time people resorted to their Gods, Goddesses, saints and healers at the time of the delivery.

During the First Sanitary Conference 1914, it was suggested that *dais* should be prevented from practising their trade due to high infant and maternity deaths. Further, it was suggested that trained nurses from Bombay should be sent to rural areas to educate the women in matters of hygiene.[52] A proposal was made that village Communidades should contribute towards the upkeep of nurses in the village. These suggestions were not accepted by concerned authorities.[53]

Childbirth among the people mainly Hindus was looked down upon as unclean process. Therefore, a woman at the time of delivery was kept in most unhygienic conditions under strict diet.

Dais rarely made preliminary examinations of the patients. They were usually called once the labour set in. She examined the patient with unwashed hands to find out if the head was straight in the middle. In case the head was not in the middle she would do so by external manipulation. Many *dais* did not take the trouble to do this examination as they did not understand the position of the head. The *dai* not only conducted mature deliveries but also abortions. The result was high mortality rate due to the methods used. They were at loss in complicated cases such as when the child's legs appeared first or when the umbilical cord got entangled around the child's neck. There was no cleanliness in the delivery room.

There were five major, though common reasons for the deaths of the mothers in Goa during colonial time. At the top of the list was haemorrhage which required immediate treatment. This was not possible as in rural areas medical facilities were not available and lack of transport made it impossible for her to seek help in urban areas. *Dais* had often no idea how to control such problem and many times a mother bled to death.

Obstructed labour was another cause which required immediate surgery. Such things were unheard especially in rural areas for a long time. In urban area where hospital facilities were available women often times refused to avail of such facilities. Often mothers contracted infection and fevers soon after delivery due to unhygienic conditions around. In those days there were no antibiotics to control such infections. High blood pressure also led to death. The largest number of maternal deaths occurred during abortions. Abortions performed by quacks in filthy conditions led to death due to haemorrhage or sepsis.

Furthermore, as mentioned earlier in Goa most girls especially of the lower strata married early, even before they completed their growth. Poor body built and stature were major causes of obstetric risks. Women had large number of children due to religious influence. High mortality led to economic necessity of bearing many children so that some may survive to provide much needed manual labour in agriculture. More births were needed to ensure surviving adults when the parents became old. All these factors contributed to maternity deaths.

Mortality rate decreased to a large extent in the last decade of the Portuguese rule in Goa. Increasing availability of medicine, absence of major epidemics, better standards of living, expansion of education, improvement in medical facilities helped the decline of mortality specially among the vulnerable groups of mothers and children.

Despite all that has been said Goans enjoyed greater longevity. There are references to several old people in the sixteenth century. The age is sometime mentioned as 90 and 117 years and once even as 120 years. In 1931 there were 4 (1 male and 3 females) in Salcete, 2 males in Bardez, 1 in Pernem, 1 in Satari of about 105 years of age.[54] There were eleven individuals over 94 years, 34 with 95 years.[55]

The census of 1950 states that there were about 6,638 persons between the ages of 80-89. There were 283 persons of 100 years and above and about 1,000 of 90 years and above.

REFERENCES

1. ARSJ: *Goa 33*, I, fl. 116.
2. ARSJ: *Goa 33*, I, fl. 185.
3. ARSJ: *Goa 35*, Annual letter, fl. 324.
4. HAG: *Monções do Reino*. 86 A, fls. 10-21. (Hence-forth *MR*).
5. *Ibid.*, fls. 35-50.
6. Balsemão, E.A.S.N., *Os Portugueses no Oriente*, Part 3, Nova Goa, 1882, p. 161; HAG: *MR*. 122, fl. 270.
7. PP: *Rois de Christandade de Goa*, 1773-1775, fls. 1-30. (Henceforth *RC*).
8. PP: *RC*. 1775-1783, fls. 1-130.
9. PP: *RC*. 1784-1797, fls. 126-144. In the cholera attack of 1786 in Marmugao alone about 911 died of the disease. Around 500 persons died in the cholera attack of 1897.
10. *Ibid.*, fls. 217-236.
11. PP: *RC.*, 1810-1829, fls. 1-10.
12. *Ibid.*, fls. 121v-130.
13. HAG: *MR*. 203 B, fl. 579.
14. *Jornal de Pharmacia e Sciencias Medicas*, ed., Antonio Gomes Roberto, Nova Goa, 15th November 1862, p. 57.
15. ARSJ: Goa 34, II, Goana Historia 1648-1649, fl. 290.
16. Appendix 2-A.
17. João Bareto, *A peste na India Portuguesa*, Proceedings of Ia. *Conferencia Sanitaria*, Nova Goa, 1917, p. 821.
18. Francisco C.T. da Silva, "Luta anti- sezonatica em Canacona 1950-1951" offprint of *Anais do Instituto de Medicina Tropical*, vol. IX, no. 2, June 1952, Lisboa, p. 671.
19. J.C. Almedia, *Alguns aspectos demograficos de Goa Damão e Dio, Panjim*, 1967, p. 92 says: The epidemic of influenza killed thousands of people in Goa. There were 48 deaths for every thousand persons in 1918 and 25 deaths for every thousand person in 1920.
20. Appendix 2-B.
21. Census of 1931.
22. Census Report 1950.
23. Census Report 1881.
24. Census Report 1900.
25. Harish C. Shrivastava, "Demographic History and Human Resources", *Goa Through the Ages*, ed., Teotonio R. de Souza, New Delhi, 1989, p. 65. The data used by him from the Historical Archives Goa and Census volumes have been given by me.
26. Census Report 1950.

27. Census Report 1950.
28. Census Report 1950.
29. Census Report 1940.
30. *Loc. Cit.*
31. Kirk, Dudley, "Factors Affecting Moslem Natality" in *Moslem Attitudes Towards Family Planning.* ed., Olivia Schifellin, New York, 1967, p. 570.
32. Census Report 1940.
33. Census Report 1950.
34. Census Report 1940.
35. *Appendix 2-C.*
36. *Appendix 2-D.*
37. *Census Reports,* 1921-1960.
38. Peter Cox, *Demography,* Bombay, 1976 (reprint), p. 163.
39. J.C. Almeida, *Alguns aspectos demograficos de Goa, Daman e Dio,* Panjim, 1967, p. 240.
40. Filipe F. de A. Mascarenhas, *A Luta Antituberculosa em Bardes,* Nova Goa, 1923, p. 27.
41. Nicolau Manucci, *Storia do Mogor,* vol. 111, ed., W. Irwine, Calcutta, 1966, p. 265.
42. *Estatistica Medica dos Hospitais das Provincias Ultramarinas referida ao ano 1876,* Lisboa, 1883, p. 201.
43. PP: Parish Registers of Anjuna, 1930-1961.
44. *Time Newsmagazine,* n. 40, October 1, 1990, pp. 2 and 37-43.
45. *Arquivos da Escola Medico Cirurgica de Nova Goa,* 1930, Bastora, 1930, p. 636.
46. PP: Parish Registers of Anjuna, 1931-1941.
47. PP: Parish Registers of Carmona, 1931-1941.
48. PP: Parish Registers Anjuna, 1942-1961.
49. Honorato Elvino de Souza, "*A mortalidade infantil e o tetano*", in proceedings Ia. Conferencia Sanitaria 1914, vol. II, Nova Goa, 1917, p. 692.
50. Pacheco Figueiredo, J.M. de., "A alimentação na India Portuguesa" offprint of *Anais do Instituto de Medicina Tropical,* 6th September 1953, Lisboa, p. 1211.
51. *The voyages of the Jonh Huyghen van Linschoten to the East Indies,* ed., A.C. Burnell and P.A. Tiele, II, London, 1885, p. 262.
52. Alfredo Antão, "Algumas notas sobre mortalidade infantil no concelho de Sanguem", *Proceedings Ia. Conferencia Sanitaria de Goa, 1914,* Nova Goa, 1917, p. 872.
53. Proceedings of *Ia. Conferencia Sanitaria 1914,* Nova Goa, 1917.
54. Census Report 1931.
55. Census Report 1931.

3

PERSONAL CARE AND ENVIRONMENTAL SANITATION

Hygiene both personal and environmental is important in the maintenance of health. Environmental sanitation is a major concern today. People are deeply worried about the way our world is rapidly being destroyed. Our environment is threatened by a host of man-made ills from toxic landfills to ozone depletion. In recent years, scientists have warned of the destructive effects of acid rain, deforestation, toxic waste, pollution of our oceans and rivers, extensive desertification and climatic warming. Major disasters like Chernobyl nuclear disaster, Bhopal gas tragedy, Texas oil spill and the more recent Arab Gulf oil slicks have set off alarm bells in public consciousness. The disasters have created dire health problems and ecological devastation. Today much attention is paid to green life, protected water and garbage disposal by scientific methods.

Few decades ago people were hardly aware of environmental problems. Chimneys belched out black smoke, refuse was seen scattered everywhere, poisonous effluents were discharged freely into the rivers and oceans, destructive gases rose up into the atmosphere. And no one cared ! In the past there were no problems of greenhouse effects and oil spills, but there were other important problems due to lack of certain facilities essential for the maintenance of health and hygiene.

During the Portuguese regime Goa was an unhealthy place due to lack of sanitation caused by scarcity of protected water, drainage system, proper toilets as well as means to dispose garbage and night soil. Hygiene was generally given a low priority. Lack of sanitation was a major cause of different diseases. Though much attention was paid to personal cleanliness probably on account of climatic conditions, habits and religious outlook, the inhabitants neglected their surroundings and general environment.

Majority of people lived in small, overcrowded and insanitary houses. Houses lacked basic amenities such as running water, drainage system or proper toilets. Protected water was scarce in Goa. The inhabitants depended on natural sources of water supply. These natural sources were often highly contaminated and unfit for human consumption.

River banks, open fields, hills and streets were used to defecate. In some cases, even courtyards were used for such purpose. The rivers were endangered with germs. There were no facilities for disposal of garbage. Garbage was dumped on the streets, open fields or rivers, making the whole area a dangerous place to live. In the absence of proper drainage system, water accumulated around the houses and lanes. Rural areas had many ponds, culverts and marshes with stagnant water. Very little was done to clean them and other water sources or to use disinfectants.

Since early days some legislative measures were issued to improve the sanitary conditions of the city of Goa and later of Panjim. But these measures were not strictly enforced, probably because of lack of finance, poor administration and community participation. The participation of the people was important for effectiveness of the legislation. Many defended insanitary practices, because they were economically advantageous. Dumping of cowdung near the houses to be used later as manure in the fields is one example.

Insanitary conditions led to diseases and pestilence. Diseases such as typhoid, gastro-enteritis, skin diseases, eye infection, malaria, encephalitis and intestinal infections took heavy toll of life. Repeated attacks of epidemics in the century made the Government concerned about the hygienic conditions in the territory.

Personal Hygiene

The inhabitants were clean in appearance. Travellers such as Linschoten who visited Goa in the sixteenth century, were greatly impressed by the level of personal cleanliness in Goa, specially of women folk.[1]

Women used to bathe sometimes twice a day. They used sweet herbs, perfumes, frankincense and rubbed their bodies with sweet sanders. Pyrard de Laval remarks that unlike people of Africa, in India, people were free of body odour.[2] This was probably due to daily bathing.

The Hindus bathed everyday before lunch as religious rite. However, many times people of lower strata did not change to clean clothes after a bath. People made use of water when they eased themselves. They washed their hands before and after meals as well. People cleaned their teeth with leaves of a caju or a mango tree. Toothpaste or tooth powder was not known among the masses during a major part of the Portuguese rule. Betle was chewed presumably to keep the teeth strong and to prevent bad breath. In rural areas and coastal areas, people were fond of swimming in the rivers and the sea. The inhabitants took good care of their hair, using oil and washing it with herbs. Women maintained their hair long but men cut off their hair as often as every week.

Some of the personal needs were taken care of by barbers. The inhabitants availed of their services to clean their ears, nails, cut hair, shave off their beards and rub their legs. Barbers acted also as bleeders and surgeons. They followed their trade in the streets. The native inhabitants felt no embarrassment to use the services of the barbers on the streets. However, the fidalgos called them to their homes.

To protect themselves against excessive heat, the people often wore light clothes or dressed scantily. They changed their clothes everyday. The poor had limited number of clothes. Underwear was generally used only by members of the higher strata. Children moved about naked upto the age of seven as it was considered a healthy habit.[3]

The upper classes among the Christians in the present century wore western style clothes for formal occasions. This was unsuitable to the climate and harmful for health. In early 1930s several doctors including Baronio Monteiro, Peregrino Costa, Sales de Veiga Coutinho, Jose Filipe Meneses, Constancio Roque Monteiro and others established *Liga Economico-Social da India Portuguesa* to combat certain aspects of the western culture, including the trend to wear heavy western clothes which did not suit our climate. The Liga condemned also the custom of wearing black for funerals and for mourning. It advised the people to wear sandals instead of socks and shoes. Many of its members wore cabayas which was considered a practical outfit specially for the doctors.

The clothes were washed regularly at a well, spring or river by the women folk. They would beat the clothes on a stone to clean them. The affluent people gave their clothes to mainatos (washermen). The lower strata of population did not have special night wear. The poor went around barefooted. The unhygienic consequences were easy to imagine as bare feet were exposed to hook-worms and other infections.

Housing and waste disposal

As already discussed in Chapter I, housing standards varied from class to class. Although the upper strata in the society lived in spacious houses of stone and mud, some of the rooms of these houses were permanently closed. These made the room dark and airless. Store rooms were breeding grounds for rodents, which many times caused diseases, and even plague. Kitchens were usually situated at the back of the houses beyond sleeping area and close to the well and toilets. The houses of the middle class were often dirtier than of the despised poor, because of the middle class attitude to menial work. They were reluctant to handle dirt.

Despite abundance of space in rural areas, majority of its inhabitants, lived in poorly built and insanitary houses. Village housing promoted disease in several ways. Most houses were leaky, damp, ill-ventilated and overcrowded. These houses were scantily furnished and lacked basic amenities. Fifteen to twenty people lived in a single squalid hut. Most villagers kept farm animals but few could afford sheds for them, so at least during rainy season people shared their living quarter with them. Very often, these animals were domiciled in the house all year around to prevent theft. Samuel Purchas writes that " they account the oxe, cow or buffle to be holy which they have commonly in the house with them and they besmeere, stroke and handle them with all friendship in the world and when the beasts ease themselves, they hold under their hands and throw the dung away.[4] Fr. Eduardus Leitão, a Jesuit missionary mentions in the late sixteenth century that the houses of the poor resemble pigsties. The poor slept on the ground often without any mat to lie on or a cloth to cover. Due to lack of basic necessities many died of disease.[5]

A typical house of the poor was made of mud and palm leaves with a thatched roof. Majority of these houses consisted of a single room, rarely of two or three rooms. The single room served as a living room, dining room, bed room and kitchen. Fresh air could not circulate freely as there were no windows. The Government appears to have been concerned over the lack of ventilation in the houses. In 1847 the Government issued orders to the Municipality to fix the number of windows for each new house.[6] Lack of ventilation was responsible for many diseases. The floors smeared with cowdung, helped breeding of flies, ants and other insects. Till the second half of the nineteenth century, some church floors too were covered with cowdung. The soft mud floors encouraged rats to burrow in them. These houses had no chimneys and consequently the inhabitants often suffered from eye, throat and lung problems caused by smoke. The insanitary atmosphere was mitigated only by strong sun. Walls of the houses were rarely cleaned or white washed. They were dark with kitchen smoke and soot.

During the influenza epidemic of 1918, it was found out that in a single hovel at Taleigão about 70 people lived together.[7] The habit of keeping cows, fowls and goats in the houses is still followed in rural areas. Animal urine and dung created health problems. The houses were infested with rodents and insects. Overcrowding together with inadequate sleeping arrangements helped the spread of transmittable diseases, especially since a sick member of a family could be rarely hospitalized.

Bakers and artisans such as potters, blacksmiths, goldsmiths and others carried on their trade in or around their homes. These conditions were not conducive to the good health of the children and adults. Most houses had no bathrooms and toilets.

The greatest problem perhaps was the disposal of human waste. Night soil has been a major source of insanitary conditions and diseases both in villages and towns. It was a common practice to defecate in fields, river banks, bushes, hills and streets near human habitation. When it rained the parasites that thrived in human waste were washed into rivers, streams, wells and tanks. Indiscriminate defecation was greatly responsible for general ill health, promoting cholera, typhoid, fevers, hookworms and other helminthic infections.

Dr. Fryer, an English traveller, who visited Goa in the seventeenth century, refers to a curious habit of throwing excreta on the roof tops for the birds to do the cleaning.[8] In some houses the courtyards were used for washing and these became breeding ground for mosquitoes, causing malaria as there was no water drainage. This water never evaporated entirely leaving unhealthy and foul-smelling cesspool, injurious to the inhabitants.

Houses had no proper toilets. The upper class people in the capital town made use of pots, which were emptied by a class of scavengers known as bongis. These bongis brought from British India were employed to empty the waste pans in the rivers. This practice still continues in some areas of the capital city. Bongis performed their job indifferently and their carelessness increased the health hazards. They carried pots on their heads. They were exposed to virulent germs and many of them acted as carriers.

Efforts to improve the disposal of night soil were not successful, despite a postura (Municipal order) which directed that all excreta were to be emptied only between 5 a.m. and early evening in the sea, that is, during low tide.[9] Otherwise the high tide deposited everything back on the shore. Those who failed to follow the order were to be fined. As in the case of most regulations, the above regulation was not always enforced

Personal Care and Environmental Sanitation

strictly. Dumping of excreta into the rivers and sea without proper treatment endangered the health of the people. Many times, the bongis emptied their pots on the streets and drains meant for rain water, making living dangerous for the inhabitants.

Besides movable toilets, houses in Panjim and other areas had fixed dry toilets. These toilets were cleaned by pigs. The system of cleaning toilets by pigs was considered harmful to health, as these pigs were later consumed by the people.

In 1863 some individuals from Panjim put forward suggestions to improve the sanitary conditions in the city. Very often people tended to keep the night soil in the house the whole day, as they had no one to carry it to the river. It was suggested that one hundred blacks be brought from Angola to do the job. No action followed on the part of the Government due to alleged lack of finance. In the absence of better alternative the Medical Board (*Junta de Saude*) suggested that all excreta should be disinfected. Separate pots for solid and liquid excreta were to be distributed among the poor. Night soil carriers were to be employed to carry the excreta within twenty four hours. However, no improvement followed and epidemics continued to take a heavy toll of life year after year.

In 1950 less than three hundred and fifty houses had septic tanks. The highest number was in Panjim with one hundred and eighty-six septic tanks, followed by Mormugåo.[10]

Water Supply

Protected water which is essential for the diet and maintenance of health and hygiene was not readily available in Goa, during major part of the Portuguese regime. No efforts were made to supply water to the people by means of pipes. Throughout this period majority of the people had to be content with natural resources of water-supply, namely rains, rivers, springs and wells. Even the famous "Golden Goa" had no facility of running water during its heydays. The water supply was remarkably deficient. The inhabitants had to avail themselves of fresh water from two suburban springs one at S. Domingos and the other one at Banguenim.

Water from Banguenim spring was preferred for drinking. It was supposed to possess ingredients conducive to health. Pyrard remarks: "With regard to the water which is ordinarily drunk in the city and its suburbs, the best and the most wholesome as well as the lightest in my opinion is the one which is sought for a quarter of League's distance from the city where lies a great fountain of pure and humid water called Banguenim which issues from the rocks".[11]

The spring of Banguenim served the entire city. The water was carried by slaves in earthen vessels at five bazarucos a pot and sold in the main junction of the city. It would have been far better if the authorities had supplied water to the city by means of pipes or aqueducts. It appears that the Government and slave owners were not in favour of such a step, as they would lose income, which they collected by sending slaves to sell the water in the city.[12] Around Banguenim, there were many reservoirs where mainatos (washermen) and others washed their clothes.

The first attempt, to provide piped water to Goa city was made in 1535. For this purpose Nuno da Cunha issued an alvará to the Municipality of Goa in order to collect thousand pardaos from the inhabitants of the city. It was planned to bring the water from the Spring of Our Lady of the Mount.[13] Colonial politics also killed another proposal in 1601. It was proposed to start a limited project to direct the waters from Timmaya's tank above Trindade to the city below. The plan was aimed to provide water to the city during the hot summer months. The city during this period faced scarcity of water.[14] Since the budget of the city could not fund the project, it decided to impose 1% additional tax. The plan was approved by the King, but could not be implemented as the King disapproved the use of funds from 1% revenue, which was reserved for works of charity (obras pias).[15]

In 1618 the Municipality of Goa issued a Postura which forbade under penalty of five xerafins from washing at the *bicas* (water flow) of the two springs at Banguenim and S. Domingos. This measure was introduced to stop pollution of the water.[16]

Two more attempts were made to provide the city of Goa with running water. Once in 1630 when Conde de Linhares granted a sum of six thousand xerafins for this purpose.[17] A second time at the end of the eighteenth century.[18] The religious of S. Domingos de Graça, S. Filipe Neri and Santo Agostinho offered 30,000 *xerafins* for the purpose and remaining was to be spent by the Municipality.[19] But the plan failed as many workers fell sick due to prevailing diseases.

Majority of native population all over Goa depended on wells for their water supply. In the Old Conquests upper classes had wells attached to their houses. These wells were built in the courtyards of the houses and sometimes close to the toilets. Wells were always kept open. Water from the wells was often unfit for human consumption as it contained chlorides, nitrites and decomposed organic matter.

Personal Care and Environmental Sanitation

These peculiar habits of the natives gave rise to sources of contamination. When a native went to the well, he did so to wash as well as to drink. Water was drawn with copper or mud vessels with the help of dirty ropes. Some wells also served to wash cattle. The lower class people had bath around the wells. The filthy water then seeped back into the well. These wells were not cleaned inside and outside.

Drinking water was seldom boiled, though drawn from the same wells and tanks that were used for watering animals and for washing clothes. Water was stored in mud pots and copper pots which had not been tinned for years. One of the causes of cholera in Goa was tirtha (holy water) brought by pilgrims from Pandarpur and other places where cholera existed in endemic form. This holy water was frequently mixed with larger quantities of water in Goa and distributed to friends and relatives to drink.

In areas situated along the river banks, particularly in the New Conquests, people consumed contaminated water from the rivers. Even today in remote areas people drink water from rivers in the absence of better alternatives. The same rivers were used to transport or to dump waste. Most villages and towns had no sewage. Refuse was thrown into the lanes and backyards. This waste was washed away into water sources by rain. As a result, these sources were polluted.

Panjim, the new capital of Goa, depended on water of two springs till the end of the nineteenth century. Even the Military Hospital had no running water. Lack of water in the hospital greatly affected the maintenance of hygiene. Majority of inhabitants continued to use contaminated water from the wells.[20] There is reference to attempts made in 1896 to provide Panjim with running water. This water was to be brought from Banguenim spring by means of pipes to Panjim.[21]

Orders were issued by the Health Authorities at the end of the nineteenth century, to prevent people from bathing around the wells. These orders were repeated again in 1922, but they were hardly observed.[22] No efforts were made to cover and flag the wells or to build saucer drains to carry the water. The only factor that saved the people in the midst of such situation was their natural immunization. The Portuguese made no effort to provide potable water and thereby to improve the health and hygiene.

In 1907, the Government earmarked 6,20,000$000 to start a scheme of water supply in Panjim, when it was realized that lack of water affected food, hygiene and growth of population. Mortality rate exceeded birth rate in Panjim during this period.[23] In 1914 Panjim had one hundred wells with potable and others with contaminated water.

The improvement of environmental hygiene not only depended on financial, material and human resources, but also on the attitude of the masses. They were unco-operative and suspicious of any change that was introduced. When, for instance, wells were opened, springs were cleaned and reservoirs built to tap water in the Sanguem Taluka, the people still preferred to use water from the rivers, rather than draw it from the wells. In order to attract them to the wells, pumps were set in many wells, but these stopped working due to carelessness.[24]

Water supply was a serious problem in Goa during the months of April and May. Lack of pure water was responsible for many diseases. As late as 1950s, only a small section of the population had access to protected water supply with pipes in Ilhas, Marmugoa and Margão talukas. In Panjim, two hundred and six houses and in Marmagoa fifty-one houses received tap water.[25] In 1956 the Government approved a plan to provide tap water to several villages in Goa.[26]

Environmental sanitation in urban Goa

The inhabitants of Goa throughout the Portuguese period displayed a remarkable indifference to environmental problems.

Goa and especially the city of Goa, was a dangerous place to live in during its "golden" days. The city of Goa was overpopulated, had no facilities of running water and drainage system. Garbage was found scattered all over the place. These conditions were responsible for various epidemics that broke out at regular intervals throughout the early period. The geographical conditions of the city played an important role in the health and hygiene. The city was surrounded by chains of small hills which blocked the free movement of the breeze.[27] Besides, the tropical climate favoured the spread of micro-organisms, which alone or in combination acted as agents of infectious diseases.

In 1542 two officials were appointed to maintain cleanliness of the city. They were given the powers to arrest the people polluting the place. However, it appears that they neglected their duties.[28]

After 1570 the sanitary conditions of the city deteriorated.[29] Besides being over populated the city was surrounded by marshes and stagnant pools of water. No attention was paid to hygiene, which was essential for the preservation of health.

Throwing out refuse from the house to the streets below was a common practice. The common people with the permission of the

Personal Care and Environmental Sanitation

authorities, made use of the river banks to defecate. Although labour was cheap, the Government did not seem eager to take effective steps to remedy the situation. More than thirty years later, in the early seventeenth century, the Viceroy Ayres de Saldanha was forced to issue an alvara forbidding the people from throwing filth on the streets. The Viceroy directed the Senado (Municipality) to appoint a gentleman of good conscience and habits as an Inspector to prevent people from throwing dirt in the city of Goa.[30]

Inspite of the measures introduced by the Municipality the situation had worsened in the course of the years. To remedy the situation, the Municipality of Goa issued a postura on 3rd November 1618. This postura was valid up to mid-nineteenth century. It imposed several restrictions on the inhabitants of the City of Goa, so as to improve the hygiene of the city.[31]

The postura forbade the inhabitants to dump filth in places other than those fixed by the Municipality for the purpose. A penalty of 100 reis was imposed on the defaulters. Half of this penalty would go to the Municipality and the other half to the denouncer. People throwing filth around Se Cathedral and other churches were fined 5 pardaos. Anyone messing up the place had to pay 1 tostão. Furthermore, the inhabitants of the city were prevented from throwing dirty water between Rua Direita and Fortaleza in the drains meant for rain water. The city of Goa had a number of drains to carry rain water to the river.

During this period, it was common to see people frying fish and other foodstuff in the streets of the city of Goa. The postura of 1618 put an end to such practice because the smoke and the smell polluted the area. Anyone found frying fish was fined 2 pardaos.[32] The inhabitants of the city were also forbidden to have cooking fire outside their houses.

No beef and pork could be sold in places other than those fixed by the Municipality. Those who failed to follow these orders were fined 20 pardaos. Lamb and mutton could not be sold to convents, hospitals and private individuals without prior license. It was forbidden under penalty to kill female pigs. The city regulations did not permit anyone to rear pigs or let them move within the city limits. All cattle to be slaughtered had to be registered at Paço.[33]

The postura of 1618 directed that dead animals should be buried away from the city. However, dead cats could be disposed off in the sea. It appears that many *tavernas* (liquor shops) and *boticas* (general stores) sold meat of dead horses which died of old age or disease. The postura put an end to such practice, as it was bad for health. Bread meant for public consumption had to be prepared under hygienic conditions.[34]

The city of Goa faced difficult times at the end of the seventeenth century on account of economic problems and diseases.[35] Eventually, by mid-eighteenth century, officials and other inhabitants left the city. Buildings were demolished and stones were carried to Panjim. Some buildings decayed due to lack of maintenance. Others were allowed to fall to ruin so that the owners could sell the material and obtain means of subsistence. The whole city was deserted. The city was an unhealthy place to live in due to prevailing endemic diseases. These diseases were caused by lack of environmental hygiene. There were dense trees. The soil was humid and full of dry leaves. Lack of water facilities and acute scarcity during the hot season had forced the inhabitants to build hundreds of wells almost as many as the people living in the city.[36] When the city started to decay, many of these wells remained unused and uncleaned. They were covered with dry leaves and were responsible for diseases.

The above mentioned conditions forced the Government to introduce a few measures to improve the hygiene of the city. By an alvara dated 17th May 1777 the Governor of Estado da India ordered felling of trees in the city. Trees that could not be used for timber had to be burnt to purify the air.[37] The alvara also ordered opening of more drains to carry rain water. The work was carried out despite high expenses. Sewers and cesspools were cleaned. The cistern of St. Rock College was opened and cleaned.

By another order the Government directed the Municipality of Goa to close over 300 wells in the city of Goa.[38] The lake of Carambolim was also a source of disease. The lake and the springs around were cleaned during this period.[39]

In 1779 the Municipality of Goa appointed a committee comprising of the Chief Physician, other physicians, army officials and judges to study the unhygienic conditions of the city of Goa and find out the probable causes. It was important to investigate these causes as they appeared to be responsible for several diseases specially the one that struck the people who spent the night in the city. Separate reports were submitted by various members of the committee. The Chief Physician offered the following suggestions to improve environmental hygiene:

All wells which did not receive direct sunlight were to be closed. Drains attached to the convent of Santa Monica were to be cleaned every year. Toilets in unused houses were to be closed. No buildings should have small windows. These windows were to be opened in the direction of the breeze. Trees were to be felled because they did not allow penetration of sunlight and responsible for dry leaves scattered on the ground.[40]

Apparently, the Government was concerned and interested in improving the conditions of the city of Goa. In 1779 it asked the Municipality of Goa to find out ways to improve the situation.[41] It directed that high walls should be build around the cemeteries not only to prevent pollution but also to prevent foul smell. Further, the Municipality was asked to light fires in the city to burn all the filth and to purify the air. It was expected that these measures would eradicate diseases prevailing in the city and make it possible for the people to live in the city at night.[42] James Forbes, a traveller who visited the city in 1784 remarked that the conditions of the city were really bad.

In mid-eighteenth century, the headquarters of the Government were finally shifted to Panjim, a small village on the banks of Mandovi. Just like the city of Goa, the new capital was an unhealthy place. Some areas in the new capital such as Fontainhas and Santa Inez were filthy and full of stagnant ponds of water. In 1853 the government was debating whether to fill up ponds belonging to Francisco Paula Fonseca at Fontainhas. During this period Panjim had only two narrow roads and was full of huts.

These areas resembled more a village than a town. The inhabitants lived together with their animals. There were pigsties and cowsheds in the compounds of the houses. Cattle and pigs moved freely on the streets.

The inhabitants of Panjim emptied garbage on the streets, as they had no alternative arrangements. Many small lanes were inaccessible in the morning on account of the excrement found there. This poisoned the atmosphere. Houses were overcrowded and small.

In 1861 under pressure from various quarters, including the press, the Government was forced to adopt measures to improve the conditions of Panjim. Culverts and fields which were breeding grounds of mosquitoes at Santa Inez were filled up. Ponds close to the Phoenix spring and the one belonging to Francisco Paula Fonseca at Fontainhas were also covered. The latter emitted foul smell. Trees and shrubs near the river banks and springs were cleaned. Still the sanitary conditions of Panjim left much to be desired. The use of fish manure in the paddy field had been banned earlier in 1795 by the Communidades de Ilhas. This practice was considered a health hazard.[43] A committee was appointed in 1885 to frame rules to keep clean Nova Goa, Margão and Mapuça.[44]

In the early twentieth century posturas were issued by Municipalities of various talukas in Goa to improve hygiene.[45] One of the first urban posturas in this century was passed by the Municipal Council of Salcete in 1902.[46] It prescribed rules to be observed in building houses. No construction work could be carried out without the license of the Municipality. Houses had to be white washed or painted before 30th November of every year in any colour other than white. The white colour was considered dazzling to the eye. Those disobeying the orders would be fined Re. 1.

Dogs, fowls and other animals were forbidden from straying on roads. Any animal found straying was to be captured by Municipal inspector or any other person. A penalty of Re. 1/2 was to be imposed. Dead animals could not be left on the roads. Dumping of manure near the houses was banned by the postura. Material emitting foul smell had to be destroyed away from dwellings.

Wells had to be maintained clean and were to be flagged 75 cms high. The inhabitants were forbidden from washing clothes and animals near the wells. Milk of sick animals could not be sold to the public. Begging was punishable by law.

Toilets had to be built thirty metres away from the roads, railways and public places. A fine of Rs. 25 was to be imposed on those not obeying the order. In case of complaint toilets could be demolished and moved elsewhere at the expense of the one who complained. A notice of eight days was to be issued to the owner.

Cowsheds and horse stables could not be built near the roads and public places. Those who failed to comply with these instructions were fined Rs. 8.

The Municipal Council of Ilhas issued a Codigo das Posturas on 15th September 1906 with 375 clauses.[47] It sought to take some measures as noted below:

The inhabitants of Panjim were banned from throwing filth and dead animals in public places but the alternate arrangements made by the Government did not meet the needs of the city. There were only ten bullockcarts to carry garbage of the whole city. The garbage was collected in wooden containers often in bad shape. The system of collection had many drawbacks and lacked hygiene. The carts were always overflowing with garbage. The garbage was usually collected from areas occupied by the upper strata of the society. Places such as Alto de Guimaraes and Bairro de Pilotos were completely neglected.

People using mobile toilets were required to use jars of porcelain, zinc, iron or wood covered with tar. Night soil had to be removed by bongis between 4 a.m. to 7 a.m. and 7 p.m. to 10 p.m. failing which the owner was fined Rs. 5. Bongis still carried pots on their heads. Pots were to be emptied at Gaspar Dias river. All pots carried were required to be covered before they were moved out of the house.[48]

Several restrictions were imposed on sale of foodstuff, bakery, meat shops and restaurants. Foodstuff could not be sold in paper other than white. A fine of Re. 1 was imposed on those selling foodstuff wrapped in newspapers. The sale of contaminated food in eating houses and pastry shops was banned. The owners were instructed to maintain their places specially the kitchen clean. Brass and copper vessels had to be tinned. The transgressor had to pay Re. 1 for the first time, Rs. 3 for the second time and Rs. 4 for the third time. Owners of eating houses that failed to maintain cleanliness or prevented sanitary inspections were imposed a fine of Rs. 8.[49]

Bakers were directed to maintain their bakeries clean. Baked bread was to be placed on white sheets of cloth or clean baskets. No milk could be sold before it was checked by an inspector appointed by the Municipality. The Codigo das Posturas initiated the process of collecting data about health, diseases and the number of people vaccinated in Ilhas taluka.

It appears that cows, ducks, turkeys and hens moved freely in the streets of the city. To put an end to this habit owners of cattle found straying had to pay 4 *tangas* and one *tanga* for the birds.

Cattle was not allowed to graze from Rua de Malaca onwards. Rearing of pigs was strictly forbidden in the capital. Although the Municipality banned such practice it made no provisions to provide the inhabitants with public toilets or funds to the owners of houses to build proper toilets. Cattle for consumption was to be slaughtered in a slaughter house. Meat had to be inspected before sale.

In Panjim death rate exceeded birth rate around 1907. This cause was attributed to lack of general sanitation and specially to scarcity of water. Lack of water affected nutrition, hygiene and growth of population. Therefore, the Government earmarked 62,0000$000 to start a scheme of water supply to Panjim.[50]

The plague of 1907 in Panjim led the Government to appoint a committee consisting of Directors of Public Works Departments, Health Services and the President of the Municipality of Ilhas to suggest new measures to improve the sanitation of the capital.

In 1917 the Municipality of Ilhas decided to engage the services of Jal Jahangir Chichgar from Bombay and residing in Panjim to remove the excreta and urine from the city. A contract was signed between him and the Municipality for the purpose.[51] The excreta was to be collected twice a day in metallic jars. The expenses were to be met from the taxes collected for the purpose by the Municipality. Residents paying a rent of Rs. 5 had to contribute with 6 tangas, paying rent upto Rs. 10 were taxed 10 tangas, above Rs. 20 paid one rupee and those whose rent was upto Rs. 40 had to pay Rs. 2. Houses that remained closed for a period of a month were exempted from the tax for that period.

The contractor was responsible for cleaning the jars at his own cost. In case the contractor failed in his duties the same had to be reported in writing to the Municipality for necessary action. The contractor was also responsible to maintain clean the public toilets as well as the ones in Government offices, hostels and boarding schools. He had to sign a contract with these institutions through the department of Accounts.

The collection was to be carried out in carts between 5 a.m. to 8 a.m. and between 8 p.m. and 11.30 p.m. The arrival of the cart was to be announced by hooting of a horn. Jars had to painted and covered with a lid. Fines were to be imposed on contractor whenever he failed in his duties. There were different fines for houses, Government offices and other places. The contract was for nine years.

A report from Health Services states that the sanitary conditions of Panjim improved after the plague of 1919. Soon after the plague broke out certain measures were implemented. Wells were cleaned and disinfected. This reduced the incidence of typhoid and paratyphoid.[52]

During the third decade of this century, the capital town still had no protected water supply and drainage system connecting the houses. It also had no proper toilets. Drains along the streets were permanently clogged. The town had no sanitary police to maintain hygiene. Drains from the streets were connected with the river, and at high tide the water and filth returned to the drains. Radical changes were necessary.

The ground floors of many houses belonging to the merchants in Panjim were used to store grains. These places were breeding grounds for rats that caused plague. Besides rats, store rooms were infected with cockroaches. In 1920 the Director of Health Services suggested to the Government to ban storage of foodgrains in private houses and proposed that the Government should build a granary. This granary could be used by merchants to store grain.[53]

In 1935 a Sanitary Police was organized because of constant epidemics in Goa. The immediate aim was to improve the sanitation of the capital town.[54] This was the first concrete step taken by the Government to see that an effective machinery was provided to look into the sanitary problems and to introduce measures to prevent spread of diseases. The Sanitary Police was effective in furthering the cause of vaccination. It initiated the process of collecting data about diseases.

The Sanitary Police had wide powers. It was under the charge of a Health Officer who was helped by a nurse and two other workers. Additional staff could be recruited in times of emergency. The Sanitary Police was empowered to inspect only during day time houses, restaurants, bakeries, biscuit industries and other manufacturing foodstuff. In case of a residential house prior notice had to be issued to the inhabitants. Stagnant water around the house had to be cleared. No person could throw urine near the house. House had to be cleaned, white washed and open for ventilation. Markets were cleaned and washed daily. Shops selling cold drinks were asked to use protected water. Sale of milk of sick cattle was banned. Persons suffering from tuberculosis, leprosy and other contagious diseases could not be employed in bakeries and restaurants.

The Sanitary Police was responsible for implementing various sanitary posturas issued by the Municipality. The regulation of 1935 applied also to Bardez taluka. Expenditure involved in implementing the above mentioned measures were to be met by the taluka Municipalities. Many of these measures could not be implemented due to lack of necessary finance, material and human resources. Besides it was difficult to educate the masses concerning hygiene.[55]

Environmental Sanitation in Rural Goa

Environmental hygiene in rural Goa was equally bad. Heaps of refuse was always seen scattered around threatening the lives of the people. In rural areas no attempt was made for the collection and disposal of household refuse. In some areas cowshed refuse was collected along with household refuse and piled in the backyard to be used as manure. This refuse attracted vermin and rodents.

Cattle, pigs and goats moved freely messing up the place. During rainy season roads were inaccessible. Most roads were in bad shape. In rainy season these roads were full of stagnant water. Dead bodies of animals were often found on the roads.

One of the causes of insanitary conditions in rural areas were permanent ponds of stagnant water and lakes. The inhabitants of Taleigão were concerned about a lake in their locality. It was responsible for diseases in the area. The stagnant water was covered by dry leaves and dead plants. The lake was surrounded by dense trees.

Cemeteries in Goa were built in close proximity to human habitation.

This constituted a health problem. To prevent such situation the Church issued a decree in 1779 providing guidelines to be followed when building cemeteries.[56] In 1894 the Government issued orders to concerned authorities that in future all cemeteries should be built away from human habitation. Health officers were asked in 1896 to accompany taluka administrators during their visits to check the sanitary conditions of their talukas.

People of all communities were reluctant to adopt preventive measures which were introduced by the end of the nineteenth century to control diseases. They were reluctant to accept inoculation against cholera and smallpox.

In the beginning of the twentieth century several villages such as Chincegal, Motto Patim, Caranzal, Oxel, Sirxarem, Sonaulim and Talauli in Sanguem taluka disappeared from the map due to malaria, cholera and smallpox. Sanguem had dense forests and stagnant waters which led to malaria. The people lived in most unhygienic conditions.

On festive occasions food was cooked in large quantity in copper vessels. This food was kept exposed to flies and other insects. During the fairs sweets were exposed to flies and dust. These sweets were sold in coloured paper which was harmful for health. It was not unusual to notice food exposed in open utensils close to the toilets.

The conditions in which food was cooked in restaurants and other eating places was unsatisfactory. Bread was baked in most unhygienic conditions and in ill-ventilated places. The dough for the bread was kneaded with feet because of large quantity and more pressure. This method contaminated the dough. The quality of meat available was poor. Generally meat of undernourished and diseased animals was sold.

One of the first Municipalities to issue a Codigo das posturas was the Municipality of Sanquelim. It issued postura to improve the sanitation of the town. In 1908 few more clauses were added to this postura. The cleaning of the houses, shops, cowsheds, wells and springs was made compulsory. This work was to be supervised by the Health Officer, Municipal doctor or regedor twice a month. It was the duty of the regedor to inform the Municipality the name of those who failed to comply with the orders. A penalty of 8 tangas was to be imposed on such individuals with the obligation of cleaning the place in the presence of the concerned authority.

The Municipality of Sanquelim issued guidelines to the working class who wished to build houses. All houses of this class had to face northeast. Every house was required to have a veranda in front and two rooms. One of these rooms had to face the veranda. It required to have two side windows and three doors. One of the doors had to open towards the veranda. These guidelines were applicable only to those who could afford to build such houses.

No cowsheds could be built in the vicinity of the house. Cowsheds had to be maintained clean. Dumping of cowdung near the houses was banned. The postura directed that palm leaves of all huts had to be changed with new ones every May before monsoons.

The Municipality of Ponda issued a postura on 25th April 1903 with 162 clauses and 4 tables.[57] The Codigo forbade the inhabitants of Ponda to dump garbage and dead animals on the roadside. Any person found throwing garbage in public were to be fined Rs. 2. No dead animal could be thrown in well or in river. The guilty person was to be fined Re. 1 per animal. However, if the animal was small only Re. 1/2 was to be collected from him. Washing around the well was prohibited under penalty. House owners were asked to clean stagnant water around the house and to white wash the exterior of their houses as well as the compound walls. Those who failed to comply had to pay a fine of Rs. 2.

The Municipality of Canacona issued a detailed postura on 12th May 1908, covering all aspects of environmental hygiene. It had 136 clauses. By this postura the inhabitants were banned among other things from defecating in public places. Any person found answering the call of nature in public was to be fined Re. 1. Dumping of stones, garbage, wood and other material near the houses was strictly prohibited. The inhabitants of Canacona had to appear before the taluka headquarters properly dressed.[58] Similar postura, was issued by the Municipality of Quepem in 1908.[59]

Generally the Government appeared to be indifferent to the possible dangers facing the environment until recurrent epidemics broke out in the early twentieth century. These epidemics of cholera, plague and smallpox forced the local Government to issue a regulation on 14th March 1913 concerning environmental hygiene. The regulation required all unused wells, tanks, culverts to be covered. Tanks, cisterns and wells were to be covered with a metallic net and pumps set in. The inhabitants were advised not to keep containers with water and food stuff exposed to nature. Vessels were to be emptied every two days to prevent breeding of mosquitoes.

Roofs of the houses, compounds and land around were to be cleaned twice a year. All empty boxes, coconut shells, husk and similar material had to be destroyed by setting fire to them. No houses could be built or repaired without the approval of the Municipality and Health authorities.

Administrative and Health authorities were given permission to inspect shops and residences during day time. Any one disobeying the regulation could be penalized.

The regulation made provision for the appointment of a committee in each taluka to implement the measures. The committee would consist of taluka administrator, health officer and another member either from agricultural class or landed gentry. In addition certain number of workers were to be appointed to help the committee to execute the measures.

In 1950s the mining activities in New Conquests were responsible for deforestation and dust pollution in the mining areas. This pollution gave rise to various chest diseases including tuberculosis. There was no legislation to control health problems caused by mining activities. However, regular check of the workers by health officers was carried out.

In July 1956 the local Government approved and implemented a legislative measure providing inspection of animals to be slaughtered, their meat and sub products. The regulation forbade slaughtering of animals without being checked by veterinary doctor or health officer. Animals such as cows, buffaloes and pigs had to be slaughtered in the slaughter house. Pigs could be killed privately provided it was done under hygienic conditions. No meat or fish could be sold without approval of competent authority.[60]

No significant environmental improvement took place during the Portuguese period. Major reasons for the lack of improvement were probably lack of finance, apathy on the part of the Government, poverty and lack of responsiveness among the people.

Personal hygiene was difficult to achieve when public sanitation was inadequate. The value of bathing, washing hands, hair and mouth was negative when water was polluted. In 1961 only few towns had protected water supply. The remaining population had to still depend on highly polluted water from rivers and wells which were responsible for typhoid, paratyphoid and cholera. Even where there was protected water supply, sewage and drainage facilities were not provided simultaneously. Inadequate maintenance of water system created health problems. Sewage facilities were introduced in Goa much after the Portuguese left the territory.

Sanitary conditions were closely associated with housing conditions. These conditions were responsible for many transmissible diseases. Improvement in housing was not possible due to high cost.

Proper toilets were few hundreds in towns and some villages. Even now soil disposal in many areas of the capital town and other parts of Goa is primitive and conducive to the spread of diseases and such hazards as presence of worms in the intestine. Public toilets are also few and badly maintained. People are exposed to uric acid and urine vapors discharged by the people in public places.

Garbage disposal continues to be a major problem. Overflowing waste bins, garbage dumped around street corners and footpaths, all unattended to for days, is a common sight and serious threat to our health. There are no incinerators to destroy garbage. Scavengers very often salvage papers and other materials and sell to vegetable vendors for use. Garbage is collected from the towns and dumped carelessly in certain areas. This litter attracts pests. Birds many times carry the waste from dumps and spread it around. Sun, rains, pigs and birds destroy a part of the filth. But, for these natural friends it would be difficult to live in Goa.

REFERENCES

1. *The voyage of John van Linschoten to the East Indies Linschoten*, vol. II, ed., A.C. Burnell and P.A. Tiele, London, 1885, p. 223.
2. *Viagem de Francisco Pyrard de Laval*, vol. II, ed., Magalhães Basto, Porto, 1944, p. 51. (Henceforth Pyrard). He states that the Portuguese and mestiço women also followed the Indian custom of bathing daily.
3. John Fryer, *A new account of East India and Persia*, II, London, 1698, p. 54.
4. *Early Travels in India*, ed., J. Talboys Wheeler, Calcutta, 1956, p. 106.
5. *Documenta Indica*, ed. Josef Wicki, vol. III, Rome, p. 316 (Henceforth DI).
6. BNL: S.A. 19946v — Providencias para urbanizaçãoeo saneamento de Goa. The Government also advised the people to have a chimney in their kitchens.
7. Relatorio dos Serviços de Saude 1919.
8. Fryer, *op.cit.*, p. 152.
9. HAG: Ms. 7795 — Livro de Posturas, fl. 108.
10. Census of 1950, pp. 139-175. Many houses even in the capital city of Goa still do not have proper toilets. Appendix 3-A.
11. Pyrad, *op. cit.*, p. 111.
12. *Ibid.*, p. 54.
13. V.A.C.B. de Albuquerue, *Senado de Goa: Memoria Historica Archaeologica*, Nova Goa, 1909, p. 444.
14. HAG: Ms. 7765 – Assentos da Camara, fls. 124-126v; T.R. de Souza, *Medieval Goa*, New Delhi, 1979, pp. 268-269. Appendix 3-B.
15. HAG: Monçoes do Reino, 7, fl. 120. (Henceforth M.R.). Appendix 3-C.
16. HAG: Ms. 7795 — Livro de Posturas, fl. 74.
17. HAG: M.R. 14, fl. 168.
18. HAG: M.R. 159 C, fls. 718-718v.
19. *Ibid.*, fl. 723.
20. Relatorio de Serviços de Saude, 1879, p. 28.
21. HAG: Ms. 11670 — Correspondencia diversa, fl. 67. (Henceforth CD).
22. HAG: CD 10552, fl. 19.

23. B.O., no. 39, 17th May 1907.
24. Arquivos da Escola Medico Cirurgica de Goa, 1937, Bastora, 1937, p. 1687.
25. Census 1950, pp. 139 and 175.
26. Legislação Relativa ao Estado da India, 1956, Nova Goa, 1957, pp. 369-393. The water was to be supplied to houses situated along the roads, railways and airports.
27. HAG M.R. 190, fl. 744.
28. A.P.O., Fasc. II, Nova Goa, 1857, p. 77 Appendix 3-B.
29. A.P.O., Fasc. III, p. 33.
30. A.P.O., Fasc. II, p. 228, Oriente Conquistado, I, p. 22; HAG: Ms. 7765 – Assen tos da Camara, fls. 144-144v. Appendix 3-C.
31. HAG: Ms. 7785 – Livro de Posturas, fl. 72.
32. HAG: *Ibid.*, fl. 72.
33. *Ibid.*, fl. 72v-73.
34. *Ibid.*, fl. 69.
35. Porous soil allowed drainage to seep into the wells from where the people drew drinking water. This aided the transmission of fecal-borne diseases and increase in malaria cases due to stagnant water. (C.R. Boxer, The Portuguese Seaborne Empire 1415-1825, Middlesex, 1973, p. 131).
36. HAG: MR., 190 C, fl. 743.
37. HAG: Ms. 1214 – Ordens aos Senadores, fl. 21.
38. *Ibid.*, fl. 23., HAG: M.R. 159 C, fls. 718-718v.
39. HAG: Ms. 1214, fl. 13.
40. *Ibid.*, fl. 75.
41. HAG: M.R. 159 C, fl. 721. Orders were issued by the local Government to Brig. Henrique Carlos Henriques to open drains for running water and to clean the city of Goa. (HAG: Ms. 1214, Ordens aos Senadores, fl. 81).
42. *Ibid.*, fl. 721.
43. Filipe N. Xavier, Collectão das Leis Peculiares, p. 220. In 1865 a committee under Eduardo Freitas Almeida, the Chief Physician of Estado da India, was appointed to frame rules in order to keep clean Nova Goa, Margeo, Maputa. (HAG: Ms. 4472 – *Pessoal de Saude e Empregados do Hospital Militar*, 1886, fl. 2.
44. HAG: Ms. 4472 – *Pessoal de Saude e Empregados do Hospital Militar*, 1886, fl. 2.
45. HAG: Ms. 11674 – Correspondencia Diversa, fls. 3 and 15.
46. Legislação Relativa ao Estado da India 1902, Nova Goa, 1903, pp. 106-138. (Henceforth LREI).
47. Codigo de Posturas do Concelho das Ilhas de Goa, 5th September 1906, Nova Goa, 1928, pp. 20-66.
48. The owners of the toilets were asked to white wash and keep the toilets clean. Those who failed to follow these orders were to be fined Rs. 5.
49. *Ibid.*, pp. 20-66.
50. B.O. no. 39, 17th May 1907.
51. LREI 1917, Nova Goa, 1918, pp. 183-84. The same Codigo approved the plan to build tanks at Borbota (Taleigão) to dispose excreta.
52. Relatorio anual desde Junho de 1919 a Junho de 1920 de Secretaria dos Servitos de Saude do Estado da India, Nova Goa, 1926, p. 10.
53. *Ibid.*, p. 21.
54. LREI, 1935, Nova Goa, 1938, pp. 40-49.
55. B.O., no. 8, 25th January 1935.
56. Sumario Chronologico dos Decretos Diocesanos do Arcebispado de Goa Desde 1775-1900, ed., Manuel Jação Socrates d'Albuquerque, Bastora, 1900, p. 7.

Personal Care and Environmental Sanitation

57. Codigo de Posturas de Concelho de Ponda, 25th April 1903, pp. 2-4; HAG: CD, 11674, fl. 15 refers to a project to improve the sanitation of Margão; HAG : CD, 10471, fl. 43 indicates that Rs. 100 were advanced to the Satary administration in order to improve the conditions of the place.
58. LREI 1909, Nova Goa, 1910, p. 98.
59. LREI, 1909, Nova Goa, 1910, p. 82. It prescribed the rules concerning building of houses. No house could be built of less than five metres of height.
60. LREI, 1956, Nova Goa, 1958, p. 59. The regulation banned slaughtering of sick animals, female cows or pigs in advance stage of gestation and animals less than 21 days old. The authorities were empowered to destroy animals and birds (fowls) suffering from T.B. and other infectious diseases.

4

DISEASES AND EPIDEMICS

Several diseases prevailed in Goa throughout the Portuguese regime. The city of Goa in particular was a very unhealthy place. Poor hygienic conditions, malnutrition, impure water supply, bad drainage and absence of preventive measures favoured diseases. During later period emigration contributed to diseases such as tuberculosis, hepatitis and meningitis. Cholera, smallpox, dysentery and fevers were the main killers throughout the period.

Linschoten writes that common diseases in Goa made their appearance according to seasons.[1] Another traveller, the Italian Manucci was of the opinion that the climate of Goa was not suitable to man below forty years.[2]

Diseases erupted many times in epidemic form. They occurred at regular intervals, even after inoculation was introduced. Probably, the improved means of communication with British India and emigration were responsible for the frequency. Epidemics often followed famines and this is particularly true of epidemics which appeared after 1870 in Goa and rest of India. Majority of epidemics that broke out in Goa originated in British India, where many diseases existed in epidemic form.

Until the mid-nineteenth century no preventive measures were implemented to avoid epidemics. During colonial period health services were dominated mainly by curative measures, and preventive aspects were confined to providing environmental sanitation, water supply and immunization coverage to particular areas, usually urban, inhabited by the ruling class. For the rest of the population, anti-epidemic measures were adopted only when there were epidemic outbreaks of serious proportions.

Preventive measures when finally introduced, were not easy to enforce. The natives refused inoculation on various grounds. There were

Diseases and Epidemics

other problems besides the attitude of the people, such as scarcity of personnel, funds, equipments, clinics, poor remuneration to the workers and low level of environmental sanitation.

The chapter has four sections. Section I is largely concerned with diseases and epidemics in the sixteenth and seventeenth centuries. Section II of the chapter deals with the same in the eighteenth and nineteenth centuries. The third section considers major epidemics in the twentieth century including new diseases and epidemics that made their appearance as a result of greater contact with the outside world. Finally, the fourth section of this chapter, deals with the preventive and curative measures introduced to control diseases and epidemics.

I. DISEASES AND EPIDEMICS IN THE 16TH AND 17TH CENTURIES

Cholera

Cholera was widely prevalent during the period. It was known by several names, *Mort-de-chien*, *xirxirem*, *xirxiry*, *modxi*, *nermuly* or *xirly*. This infectious disease was characterized by profuse stools, griping, vomiting and muscular cramps. The disease sometimes killed the victim within few hours. The incidence of cholera increased from the third quarter of the nineteenth century due to greater contacts with British India.

It was believed that cholera was transmitted through air and was caused by consumption of certain vegetables that grew wild in the rainy season such as *allum (Arum)*, *terem (Colocasia)*, and *taiquillo (Cassia)*. In addition new rice, over-ripe jackfruit, pineapple and melon were believed to cause cholera. However, in the nineteenth century, it was discovered that cholera virus was the cause of cholera. This virus was found in the stools of cholera victims. The disease was transmitted by flies, contaminated foodstuff, water and articles belonging to cholera patients.

Some people considered cholera a curse of goddess Durga when she was not given due recognition and reverence. To pacify this goddess they offered a red flag, iron, fire sacrifices, flowers, coconuts and performed rituals. After these rituals they believed the victim was free from the curse. When the health of the victim deteriorated, the victim was carried in a beautifully decorated boat with flowers and flags to the accompaniment of music and was left in the middle of the sea to die.[3]

Merchants, fishermen, labourers and pilgrims were responsible for carrying cholera from rest of India to Goa. Fishermen who visited the Malabar coast brought the disease to Salcete and Canacona in the south and Tiracol in the north. Hindu pilgrims often visited sacred places in Pandarpur, Gokarna, Kasi, Tirupati, Kanpur and elsewhere outside Goa. These places of pilgrimages were always overcrowded and lacked proper hygiene. Furthermore, many of these places were situated on the banks of important but highly polluted rivers of India. The pilgrims had their bath, consumed water and carried *tirtha* (holy water) from these rivers. The *tirtha* was distributed to their relatives and friends in Goa. This way they, also carried cholera to Goa.

Cholera was endemic in British India. The disease originated in Bengal, and particularly in Calcutta. Dry season seems to have prevented the spread of cholera and the wet season promoted the outbreak of the disease. In Goa, the disease usually appeared in places situated along the railway line and rivers originating in the *Ghats* (British India). Cholera was eradicated from Goa in the last 30 years of colonial regime.

Native practitioners prescribed canjee with pepper and cummin seeds. During the attack of cholera, it was a custom to burn the middle of the heel with hot iron until vomiting stopped. Yet another treatment prescribed by native practitioners was to tie the body with ligaments, probably to prevent cramps.

The first well-known outbreak of cholera was in 1543. Garcia d'Orta the famous Portuguese physician living in Goa at that time gives a vivid description of this epidemic in the city of Goa.[4] People of all ages fell victim to the disease. The death toll was high, even animals and birds were not spared. The disease caused panic among the inhabitants, leading the Governor Martim Afonso to ban tolling of bells at the time of burial. Everyday bells tolled for fourteen to sixteen Christians. Bells were not tolled for non-Christians, who were in a majority.[5] The Christian population being one fifth of the total population an average of eighty persons died daily. It caused considerable havoc, reducing the population to some degree. The exact number of the dead is not known. Patients treated by the Portuguese physicians lived for a day or two, whereas those treated by the natives practitioners seem to have done better.

In 1570 several epidemics broke out simultaneously, possibly due to a famine. This was the result of a siege imposed by Ali Adil Shah to expel the Portuguese from Goa.[6] Cholera of virulent nature appeared in the ward of the potters in the city of Goa. People in this ward lived under dreadful conditions. The disease affected nine hundred persons, killing one third.[7] It was alleged that the disease was caused by a dead elephant in the lake of Carambolim. There is no evidence of any measures adopted by the Government to control the epidemic. However, the Jesuit missionaries were prompt to provide care to the victims. The area was divided into three zones and a list of the sick was prepared. Food and medicine were distributed to the victims. The ward was fumigated with smelling herbs. Inspite of these measures, many died within a short time. In one instance a missionary during his routine visit to the area found a mother and her child without sufficient clothes. The missionary went around to collect some clothes. By the time he returned both the mother and the child had died.[8]

Between 1618 - 1619 two epidemics broke out in the city of Goa. The first was cholera epidemic of 1618. The Hindu inhabitants of the city of Goa were considerably reduced due to this cholera attack.[9]

Cholera did not disappear from the city of Goa but there seems to be a respite from great epidemics between the end of the seventeenth century and the one that raged all over Goa at the end of the eighteenth century. Probably, cholera cases in small scale appeared during this period. Manucci writes that cholera was one of the diseases prevailing in Goa during the period. The epidemic of 1630 killed many Portuguese in Goa. In Gujarat and Cambay three thousand people were reported dead.[10]

Smallpox

Next to cholera, smallpox was most feared in Goa. It was the greatest killer, causing misery and suffering by way of mortality, disfigurement and blindness. Children below ten years of age were the worst sufferers of smallpox. Goddess Devi was said to produce pustular diseases, including smallpox. She was worshiped with cloves, betelnuts, coconuts and fire sacrifices to prevent smallpox.

In 1545 smallpox erupted in epidemic form. In just three months more than eight thousand children died of the disease including children of the King of Ceylon.[11]

Fevers

In the sixteenth century, when the Portuguese arrived in Goa, they found wide prevalence and different kinds of fevers much more than they occurred in Portugal and far more fatal. Fevers were endemic in Goa even before the Portuguese occupation of the place. Therefore, the Muslim rulers left their residence in the city of Goa during the hot months of the years. The disease attacked large number of Portuguese including several viceroys, noblemen and inquisitors. Linschoten recorded that the Portuguese were victims of fever because of scarcity of meat, nourishing drinks and much company of women.[12]

The Portuguese had no idea of the exact cause of the disease. They classified fevers as remittent and intermittent. These fevers were often ascribed to *mal-air*. Fevers took epidemic form in 1570 and again in 1619. During this latter epidemic many Portuguese left the city for more healthy places. Jesuit accounts refer to many Jesuits affected by these fevers.[13]

The famine of 1631, the locust invasion in Bardez[14] and other socio-economic vicissitudes seem to have contributed to many epidemics in 1635. Epidemic fever started with unprecedented violence and contributed to complete the ruin of "Golden Goa". The struggle between the Dutch and the Portuguese had drained the public exchequer, and as a result the state was unable to introduce measures to control the disease.

In April 1648 Goa suffered from an earthquake. Soon after there was a cyclonic storm that brought down palm trees, took away roofs and destroyed fields. The following year during the monsoon there was a terrible famine in which at least four people died daily in the city of Goa.[15] It is probable that, as usual, epidemics followed.

Bubonic plague

Apart from cholera, fevers and smallpox, other epidemics such as dysentery and plague were widespread. Bubonic plague was a great fear in those days. The disease was two-fold, pulmonary plague and older Bubonic plague known as black death. In Goa plague killed several people around 1570. However, Linschoten who lived in Goa between 1583-1588 says that "the plague has never been in India neither it is known unto Indians."[16] There was a respite from plague for sixty five years until it reappeared in 1635.

Dysentery

Dysentery another water borne disease, was common in early days. It was known as *Doenças das Camaras* or Bloody Flux. The disease afflicted the people in Goa during the rise and fall of the Portuguese influence. Several viceroys suffered from the disease. Dysentery was many times confused with colitis and enteritis. Dysentery is a painful diarrhoea, with

Diseases and Epidemics

blood and slime in the stool. There is inflammation of the inner lining of the large bowel accompanied by fever.

There were constant epidemics of dysentery. Dysentery, particularly amoebic dysentery, was endemic in the city of Goa. The *Vaidyas* had a remedy for dysentery. It consisted of roasted *Rhuibarb* and cumminseeds. These two ingredients were mixed either with lime or rose water. A strict diet was followed consisting of canjee mixed with sour milk. Western medicine was ineffective in early days. In fact the Italian doctor Careri says that the Portuguese physicians learnt to cure dysentery from their native counterparts.[17]

Deficiency Diseases

Nutritional disorder and deficiency disease due to malnutrition were estimated to be common. Scurvy was first known as caused by malnutrition. Scurvy was known in Goa as *Escorbuto* or *Mal de Luanda*. The disease prevailed among the newly arrived Portuguese soldiers and native children. About 1,000 men died annually of scurvy during their journey to Goa. Much mortality during the journey was caused by contaminated beef, pork diet, absence of fresh vegetables and citric fruits. The Portuguese unlike other European rulers did not acquire meat, sour lime and vegetables on the way.[18] Unlike the ships of other colonial powers, the Portuguese ships did not carry necessary medicine to tackle scurvy. Therefore, it was considered a miracle to reach India safely.[19]

Another disease provoked by malnutrition was beriberi. First reference to beriberi appears in 1571. Three hundred passengers died on the fleet of D. Antonio Barretto Moniz. Majority of these passengers were victims of beriberi.[20]

Venereal Diseases

Venereal diseases such as syphilis and gonorrhoea are said to have entered Goa with the Portuguese. In Goa venereal diseases were known as *firinghi rog* (European disease) and *baili pidda* (foreign disease).[21] The disease affected people of all classes, including high Government officials and physicians. The morals of the society was lax. Young men of upper strata spent time with women of low moral character, which included slaves as well as ladies of high society.[22]

Information available refers to amorous activities of the Portuguese men and native women. Afonso de Albuquerque disapproved of casual alliances which he termed "living in sin". He preferred men to marry their women. Albuquerque encouraged unions between Portuguese men and native women by giving them incentives. Each couple was granted 18,000 *reis* and a piece of land to settle.[23] There is a rather odd incident, where Albuquerque got several couples married in a private home. The place was poorly lit and overcrowded. In the confusion Portuguese men took the wrong wives home and tried to exchange them for the right ones next morning.[24] In one of his letters, Albuquerque complains that Portuguese men carried native women along with them out of Goa without his approval.[25] Many times, Portuguese men took women to the ships for casual sex, termed by Albuquerque as "infernal play". Apparently, all hell broke loose in such occasions. However, there is an order dated 3rd December 1513, from Albuquerque to the Factor of Goa, stating that he was sending eight women for the use of Portuguese men and that they should be looked after well and paid. He further mentioned that in four months time, these women would be replaced by new ones from Cananor.[26] There appears to be some double standards in these matters.

Albuquerque was not above caste and colour prejudices. He did not encourage his men to marry Malabari women, because they were "dark in complexion and corrupt". The Portuguese appeared to show a special preference for Muslim women as they were "white and chaste". These women in turn preferred the Portuguese, because of better treatment given to them and the general belief among these women that conversion to Christianity would absolve them of their sins. There is evidence that Canarin women readily accepted alliances with Portuguese men, unlike high class Nair women.[27]

Prostitutes were found all over the city of Goa, and specially in area known as *Ilha de Fogo*. Prostitution helped the spread of veneral diseases. Above 5% of total deaths among the soldiers occurred due to the disease. In those days it was not a disease to be ashamed of.

Several legislative measures were taken to curb or control prostitution and prevent the spread of venereal diseases. The Church Provincial Council in 1567 asked the Municipality to fix certain areas for prostitutes beyond the Hospital of St. Lazarus.[28] Those disobeying the order were to be exiled for 5 years to Ceylon and fined 50 *pardaos*. But just like other regulations this one was not strictly followed. The nautch girls from the main land were found in the island of Kumbarjua.[29] The Jesuits who collected a tax from the prostitutes in this area, were accused of encouraging the trade.[30]

King Phillip, the ruler of Portugal issued a decree in 1593 forbidding

Diseases and Epidemics

women from soliciting all over the city. As a result of the above regulation prostitutes began to move about in palanquins from house to house. To end such practice another legislation was issued in 1597. By this legislation individuals under 60 years of age were forbidden to move in palanquins. Anyone disobeying the order was to be fined 200 *crusados*.[31]

Smallpox

Apart from cholera the other major killer specially of the young ones was smallpox. The first outbreak of smallpox in the eighteenth century was in 1705. The disease struck many villages of Bardez. In Anjuna (Bardez) several people died due to lack of medical assistance. During this epidemic the ecclesiastical authorities sent to Anjuna four native priests belonging to St. Phillip Nery (Oratorians) to render medical assistance to the victims.[32]

In the second half of the nineteenth century several epidemics of smallpox broke out in different parts of Goa in 1870, 1872, 1882, 1884, 1889, 1891, 1892 and 1897.

Deficiency Diseases

Scurvy was still responsible for high mortality rate during the journey from Portugal to Goa. In 1716 a small ship *S. Francisco Xavier* arrived with only 4 passengers. The remaining 46 had died of scurvy.[33] In a letter dated 14th January 1749 Viceroy Marques de Alorna states that majority of the passengers suffered from scurvy during the journey and many succumbed to it in the Royal Hospital.[34] Out of 513 passengers on board the ship *St°. Antonio e Justiça* only 21 passengers were free from scurvy.[35] Again in 1769 about 27 persons died of scurvy during their journey.[36]

Cholera

In 1777 there was an epidemic of cholera. Soon after this epidemic the Portuguese Government made a feeble attempt to investigate the causes of cholera and the means to control the same. Suggestions made by Dr. Costa Portugal were not implemented on the grounds that they were not practical.[37]

Two important epidemics of cholera raged in Goa at the end of the eighteenth century. The disease was carried by pilgrims and traders from British India. It appeared first at Loutolim (Salcete) and subsequently it spread to the neighbouring villages and Mormugão. During 10 months at least 911 people suffered from the disease in Mormugão.[38]

The second epidemic of virulent nature was *Epidemia de Rachol* which raged from 1789 to 1792. Rachol (Salcete) was an important military station. Six hundred soldiers suffered from cholera. Nearly 470 succumbed to the disease. One third of the soldiers were Portuguese. The Government adopted an unusual method to control the disease. Large number of cattle were brought to the village to clean the place.[39] Gun shots were fired to kill the germs and purify the air. This measure was very popular in Daman and Diu in times of epidemics. A ward was set up at Rachol to treat the victims. The Portuguese soldiers were moved from Rachol to Ponda.

The State for the first time distributed medicine to the cholera victims in 1818. It was supplied through Parish Priests and military officials. The most common medicine was *calomel* (a mercury compound) and *laudanum* (opium compound) A total of 1,371 *xerafins*, 3 *tangas* and 25 *reis* were spent on these medicines.[40] These medicines failed to cure the victims, who finally resorted to indigenous medicine. In Ilhas taluka, Francisco de Paula Fernandes, a diploma holder from the Military Hospital, was appointed to render help to the victims.[41]

From the meager information available, we know of cholera epidemics in Goa during two consecutive years, 1831 and 1832.[42] The mortality rate fluctuated, depending on the season. It was high during the monsoons. These epidemics gave rise to clear beginning of public health policies. A proper regulation to control epidemics was under preparation. In the meantime the local Government issued a *Regulamento Provisório de Saúde Publica* (Provisional Regulation of Public Health).[43]

The regulation was introduced soon after the cholera attack of 1845. During this period, a virulent epidemic raged in India. In Goa the disease started in January 1845 at Sanquelim and Calapur and later in S. Braz including Kumbarjua. Cholera appeared in Panjim at the end of the month. By June the disease had spread to Mapuça, Penha da França, Reis Magos, Taleigão, Goa Velha, Mandur, Quepem, Ponda and Salcete. Cholera was widespread in areas situated along the rivers.

In 1845 the Government published a list of medicines for the treatment of cholera victims.[44] The medicine consisted of a mixture prepared with or without opium.[45] They were also prescribed some kind of tablets. Physicians were advised to bleed the patient, only if the pulse was normal and there were strong cramps. Hot bricks and hot sand was prescribed for fomentation of the spine and legs followed by the friction of the arms and legs. Patients were advised to drink water sparingly, to prevent vomiting. A total of 77 cholera patients were admitted at the Military Hospital and 25 died of the disease. Cholera in 1845 spread from India to other parts of Asia, Europe and America.

In spite of control efforts cholera appeared again in Goa during 1854. When cholera made its appearance in Panjim, the Health Board appointed a doctor to handle the situation. The sale of fruits, shell fish and vegetables were banned. The affected areas were cleaned. The following table indicates cholera spread taluka-wise from 13th May to 31st July 1854.[46]

Talukas	Cases	Cured	Dead
Ilhas	421	351	70
Bardez	27	19	8
Pernem	36	21	15
Total	484	391	93

In 1857, 553 cases of cholera occurred with 151 deaths.[47] This information was published at the end of December 1857 and it is presumed to cover whole year. It is reported that in Loliem 20 persons died daily.[48] The attack was mild in Pernem and Canacona but virulent in Bardez and Salcete. The rains were normal during the year. No more details are available.

The poor inhabitants of Ilhas were struck by cholera in 1865. The table in the Appendix 4-B gives cholera cases in a single month of September 1865.[49] The death toll was high in the epidemic of 1870. Many inhabitants fled Panjim for their ancestral village homes in Bardez and Salcete. At times there was no one to carry the sick or bury the dead as even grave diggers had disappeared. A report from the Health Services mentions that in a single house seven died of cholera. The healthy members of the family moved away leaving behind the sick and the dead.[50] Yet in another house a mother and a child were left helpless. At least 18 persons died daily in Santa Barbara (Ilhas). Cleaning of streets, markets and compounds, fumigation with gunpowder and tar was carried out to control cholera in Panjim. Out of 289 reported cases, 46 died of the disease in Salcete.[51] In this taluka cholera repeatedly appeared in S. Jose Areal. This village was far away from a river or sea. The only possible explanations for the repeated attacks in the area could be the poor hygiene and food habits of the inhabitants. A remarkable feature of this epidemic was the immunity enjoyed by the Portuguese from the disease, probably because of better hygiene and food habits.

The first victim of cholera epidemic (1869) in Panjim was a *boia* machila bearer. In Panjim 50 persons died out of 122 cases. The total reported cases in Goa were 823 with 306 deaths due to the disease. [52] Besides Ilhas cholera raged in Ponda, Salcete, Mapuça and Assonora.

Cholera in epidemic form appeared every year in Goa during the last 20 years of the nineteenth century. The introduction of railway at this time ensured easy and fast travelling, between Goa and rest of India, and at the same time making it difficult to checkmate the spread of contagious diseases.

On account of repeated cholera epidemics in Jua, Velim, Curtorim, S. Lourenço de Agaçaim, Kumbarjua, S. Bras and S. Pedro, the local Government sanctioned a sum of Rs. 4,000. These funds were used to improve hygiene of the above mentioned areas.

A family from Ponda was responsible for cholera epidemic at Sanvordem in 1896. This family had gone on a pilgrimage to Kanpur where one of its members died of cholera. Two other members fell ill during their journey back home. They stayed approximately 10 hours in Sanvordem before returning to Ponda. In Ponda three members of the family died due to the disease.[53]

The following year labourers working in the Ghats carried cholera to their homes in Salcete and New Conquests. The disease appeared at Loutolim and Raia in the wards of fishermen and sailors. From Loutolim the disease spread to Velção, Cansaulim, Cortalim, Nagoa, Verna and Margão. This epidemic of 1897 was accompanied by a famine caused by excessive rains and floods. Quarantine was introduced at Colem to prevent the spread of cholera from British India.[54]

Fevers

Fevers continued to prevail in the eighteenth century. Several viceroys were victims of the disease including Conde de Ega, Marques de Alorna, Jose Pedro de Camara and his family.[55]

In 1778 all village *communidades* were required to send certain number of people to work on the reconstruction of the city of Goa. Workers who were reluctant to go on account of prevailing diseases, were dragged by soldiers. Out of one thousand six hundred workers from Salcete, nearly six hundred and sixty five fell sick. The city had only 35 permanent inhabitants and majority of these inhabitants were taverna owners and their families. Most of the workers and their families retired at night to their villages.[56] It was noticed that those who spent even a single night in the city were victims of fevers. Dense trees, rotting leaves, polluted wells, decaying buildings and stagnant drains contributed to the disease.

From June to December 1849 a total of 300 patients were treated for fevers at the *Hospital Regimental*. Five hundred and twenty-six patients suffered from recurring fevers between June to December 1850 in the same Hospital. The following year another 400 patients were treated at *Hospital Regimental* for recurring fevers.[57] In 1869 around 1,199 patients were treated for recurring fevers at the Military Hospital.[58] A total of 573 patients died in the same hospital of fevers in 1876.[59]

The Portuguese resorted to bleeding even for slight fever. They bled several times and took away 18 to 20 ounces of blood. Conde de Linhares, the Viceroy of India has recorded in his diary that he was bled many times as a cure for fevers.[60]

The most common fevers were caused by malaria. Malaria is believed to be one of the factors responsible for the decay of Golden Goa. Besides the City of Goa, the disease was widespread in Quepem, Sanguem and Canacona. Dense and humid forests in the area, combined with poor hygiene were the cause of malaria. Malaria was spread by mosquitoes. Nearly 14,261 persons suffered from malaria in 1878.[61]

Epidemics occurred at regular intervals throughout the nineteenth century, even after inoculations against some of them were introduced. This was probably due to greater contacts with rest of India, where many diseases existed in endemic and epidemic form. The Governor of Goa in a report sent to Home Government states that in 1820 intermittent fevers were common in Goa.[62]

Venereal Diseases

Venereal diseases were widespread in the nineteenth century. Large numbers of soldiers were treated in the Military Hospital for venereal diseases. It appears that the Government was concerned about the problem. In 1858, the Government repeated its order to Health Board making it compulsory for all prostitutes to undergo weekly medical examination. The following year the same Board was asked by the Government to advise soldiers and others to refrain from frequenting prostitutes[63] and to calculate funds necessary for the treatment of V.D. patients.[64] A total of 127 patients with V.D. were provided treatment in

1868 at Military Hospital. The number of patients treated for venereal diseases between 1869-1880 in the Military Hospital is given in the appendix.[65] There are references too to homosexuality.

Water Borne Diseases

The incidence of water borne diseases, such as typhoid, dysentery, diarrhoea and diseases caused by intestinal parasites was high in Goa. Typhoid and paratyphoid fevers were frequent in Old Conquests among the Hindus. Typhoid was fatal in hot months of April and May, when there was scarcity of water. The disease was mainly caused by polluted water. For instance in 1862 the high incidence of typhoid in Taleigão was due to a polluted lake in the area. Orders were issued by the Government during the same year forbidding the people from using the polluted lake.

Bubonic plague

A terrible bubonic plague raged Bombay between 1896- 1897. There are references of plague in Goa as well but it did not take epidemic form.[66] Large number of persons affected with plague entered Goa in their incubation period from 1896-1914.[67]

III. DISEASES AND EPIDEMICS IN THE 20TH CENTURY

There were recurrent epidemics of cholera, smallpox, plague, fevers and dysentery in the first thirty years of this century.

Cholera

A virulent epidemic of cholera raged in 1900 throughout *India Portuguesa* killing 400 persons in Salcete. Altogether 5000 persons suffered from cholera in *India Portuguesa* (including Daman and Diu) and 2000 died of disease.[68]

In 1907 the death toll on account of cholera in Salcete and Quepem were 135 out of 285 cases. The following year in the month of January alone another 95 persons died of cholera in Salcete, Quepem and Sanguem.[69] During cholera epidemic of 1909 which started in Benaulim about 193 persons fell victim to the disease and 121 died. Deaths due to cholera were high. In a single month of July 1913 around 82 cases of cholera occurred at Margão and Curtorim killing 40 persons. In 1914 in

Diseases and Epidemics

Bardez and Salcete 64% of the victims succumbed to the disease.[70] Between November and December 1917 a total of 163 persons were struck with cholera and nearly 129 died.

Cholera which broke out in epidemic form in 1906, 1907, 1908, 1909 and 1912 originated in British India. Fishermen who returned from South of India carried cholera to Cavelossim, Varca, Benaulim, Colva, Majorda, Velção and Mormugão. The disease was also brought by labourers from Ghats to their homes at Paroda, Molem, Guirdolim, Macazana and Curtorim. During these epidemics Ilhas, Salcete, Sanguem and Canacona were most affected, perhaps due to closer proximity to the sea or railways. Between 1900 to 1927 at least 500 persons were affected by cholera. Cholera that broke out in epidemic form in 1922 was carried by fishermen and pilgrims from Pandarpur. The death rate from cholera began to show a remarkable decline after 1941. This was due to the fact that more stress was laid on sanitation and there were less famines in India. Besides cholera inoculation was proving its efficacy.

Bubonic plague

The first detailed account of the bubonic plague in Goa is available from a report submitted in 1901 by Dr. Wolfango da Silva to the Health Services. The plague started in 1901 at Ribandar and struck the poor who slept on humid floors.[71]

Rats propagated the disease to other parts of Ilhas. A tobacco merchant who visited Belgaum in connection with his trade carried the disease to Ribandar and from there the sick person was transported to his ancestral home in Piligão (Bicholim). In Bicholim he infected those around him. Initially the doctors failed to diagnose the disease. Vigorous measures were adopted at Ribandar by Health Services. Patients were isolated in a special ward. Their belongings and houses were disinfected.[72]

Twelve plagues occurred in Goa from 1901-1920.[73] The bubonic plague in Margão appeared in 1916. Margão a small town with 8,000 inhabitants, lacked proper hygiene. It was the commercial centre of Salcete and neighbouring talukas. This town had 250 shops, ill ventilated and full of dust. The market area was filthy, so also several wards including Comba, where shopkeepers lived in small ill ventilated houses. Their store rooms with imported food stuff remained closed almost permanently. These rooms were breeding grounds of rats.[74]

How did the plague start in Margão? The disease appeared in the first week of February 1916. Two members of Alvo family died of fevers. This family lived close to the godown of one Vasu Borodo, a merchant who imported contaminated foodstuff from Dharwar.[75] Doctors failed to diagnose the cause of deaths. It was only few days later, when there was another death nearby, that they realised they were cases of bubonic plague.

Immediately after the plague was confirmed, several measures were implemented to contain the disease. Nevertheless, plague spread to Raia, Varca, Chinchinim, Loutolim, Benaulim, Colva and Navelim. The attitude and behaviour of the people was responsible for the spread. Many times they denied the occurrence of the disease and were very secretive. For instance at Varca only after the death of five members of a family, the head of the family informed the authorities about the disease.[76] The plague of 1916 ended in the year 1919. It was noticed that bubonic plague broke out usually in Goa during the cold season from November to March. Just like cholera the death rate from plague declined in the third and fourth decade of the twentieth century.

Smallpox

Smallpox appeared in Goa in epidemic form in 1900, 1904, 1906, 1909, 1911, 1915 and 1924-1926. The epidemic of 1900 was severe in Goa. Hundred and forty people died of smallpox in 1922. The disease affected mainly the *Deuli* community, which refused vaccination on religious grounds. Smallpox continued to rage over Goa during the third and fourth decade of the twentieth century. At least 23 people died in 1941.[77] A total of 257 cases of smallpox occurred in Goa in the year 1945. The incidence must have been higher as many cases were not registered. The attitude of the people played important role in the delayed smallpox eradication.

Deficiency Diseases

Many cases of beriberi occurred in 1908 among soldiers of a Portuguese ship "Rio Sado" anchored at Panjim. Beriberi appeared again in epidemic form in the year 1913 among the African soldiers stationed at Valpoi.[78]

Fevers

Between 1910 - 1914 about 35% of total deaths in Sanguem were caused

Diseases and Epidemics

by malaria.[79] Since persons stricken with malaria were prone to other diseases the full toll must have been higher. Malaria fevers were widespread during and after the rains.

In the second decade of the twentieth century in a population of over 4,00,000 inhabitants on average there were 2,000 deaths due to remittent fevers. These fevers were popularly known as *febres nervosas* (fevers caused by mental problems) because they were accompanied by convulsions. These fevers prevailed among age group of 20-30 years. They were contagious and appeared in July-August and September-October. Dr. Froilano de Mello discovered that these fevers were para-typhoid and they were endemic in Goa.[80] There were also cases of "Malta fever" in Goa during the second decade of the twentieth century.

Epidemic fever prevailed in Goa. Malaria was epidemic in the city of Goa, Canacona, Sanguem and Quepem. The disease was widespread because of dense forest and poor hygiene.

Tuberculosis

Tuberculosis was rare in Goa until the end of the nineteenth century. The rapid spread of the disease, after the beginning of the present century was due to emigration of Goans to British India, and the introduction of railways. Pulmonary tuberculosis was common among the adults. In children the disease was found in the glands and intestine. It accounted around 1914 for 18.4% of deaths.[81] These were registered cases. The rate must have been higher. In rural areas very few resorted to western medicine and tried to conceal the disease because of stigma attached to the same.

T.B. incidence was low in the New Conquests, probably because majority of its inhabitants were non Christians who did not migrate from Goa. Furthermore, the New Conquests were thinly populated. Among the non-Christians the disease attacked soldiers and artisans who lived in poor unhygienic conditions.

Tuberculosis prevailed in Bardez and Salcete talukas with large emigrant population. About 75% of deaths among the emigrants and their families were caused by tuberculosis. This figure may be an exaggerated one. Probably it was not so high. For instance, at Tembim, a ward of Raia (Salcete) out of 24 houses, about 20 houses had at least 1 person suffering from T. B. in 1914.[82]

The emigrants in large cities of Bombay and Calcutta lived in congested places, very often in one single room known as "Kud" shared by several persons in most unhygienic conditions. Their nutrition was also poor. These conditions contributed to diseases such as T.B. Emigrants suffering from T.B. contaminated their families when they came down to Goa on holidays.

From 1916 - 1927 deaths due to T.B. amounted to 6,120 in Goa. The incidence was high among the poor, *mestiços* and newly married women. Four hundred and fifty one patients died of T.B. between 1929 to 1933. In 1934 nearly 39 deaths occurred in Ilhas on account of T.B.[83]

In 1942 a total of 40 cases were treated at *Enfermaria Anibal Mendes* attached to *Hospital da Misericordia*.[84] The admission of T.B. patients in *Sanatorio S. Jose* amounted to 145 during the year.[85]

Tuberculosis was feared because of high mortality rate. As the disease was communicable, persons suffering from T.B. were isolated in a room, away from the family quarters or in an outhouse. Members of the family disinfected themselves with vinegar on slight contact with a T.B. patient. When the patient died all his belongings were destroyed. Tiles from the roof of the house were removed to allow sunlight. Walls of the house were white-washed. In case the room occupied by the sick was in an outhouse, this room was demolished. Tuberculosis was considered a hereditary disease. Therefore, people refused to marry in families with history of T.B. cases.

Venereal Diseases

The incidence of venereal disease continued to be high in the beginning of the present century. Participants of the first Sanitary Conference (1914) made several suggestions to control the disease. Mass education about venereal diseases, establishment of special wards for V.D. patients and a compulsory medical check up for those desiring to get married.

In the early years of this century a number of children died of hereditary transmitted syphilis. In some families with 10 to 12 children, about half died on account of the disease and the remaining suffered from some kind of physical or mental deformities.

There are references to open flesh trade in the capital town around 1925. In 1934 there were about 1,000 known prostitutes in Goa.[86] High incidence of venereal diseases among the soldiers and prostitutes forced the Government to start a clinic in the *Hospital Central (Old Hospital Regimental)* in Panjim. In 1927 14 military men, 3 prostitutes and eight others were admitted in the clinic. In addition 200 persons received treatment at the outpatient department of the hospital. During the same

Diseases and Epidemics

years 125 servicemen, 23 prostitutes and five children suffered from the disease at Valpoi (Satari). Two clinics, one in Panjim and other in Valpoi, provided treatment for V.D. patients. Because of lack of medical facilities in other parts of Goa, poor transport and stigma attached to the disease the majority of V.D. patient resorted to quacks. This played havoc with health and life of the patients. A table in the appendix provides information regarding the deaths due to syphilis between 1916-1935.[87]

Water borne Diseases

Typhoid alone accounted for some 3 % of all deaths in Goa around 1914. Between 1916-1927 at least 3,701 were reported dead due to typhoid.[88] In 1928 there were 212 cases of typhoid. This rate must have been higher, as many cases were not reported. Typhoid was endemic throughout 1930s in Ponda taluka. In 1933 out of 89 reported cases in Salcete, 52 succumbed to the disease. A total of 230 persons died of the disease during the year.[89]

Influenza

The growth and movement of the population in Goa was greatly affected by influenza of 1918. This epidemic had spread worldwide. The first case of influenza in Goa was reported in 1917 in Bardez taluka. The outbreak did not attract any particular attention of the Government as cases in the early period were not fatal. Able-bodied workers suffered the most on account of influenza. The attack rate was high among the young, old and expectant mothers. Pregnant mothers who suffered of influenza either died, miscarried or delivered premature babies. The highest number of women who are reported to have miscarried due to influenza were in Quepem (80%) followed by Bardez (73%), Bicholim (25%) and Pernem 13%.[90]

Influenza was little known in Goa until 1918. There were few cases in the late nineteenth century. The disease, just like some other contagious diseases, was carried from British India. Three hundred Goans fled from Bombay to Goa, during this epidemic. It coincided with acute shortage of provisions. In Siolim (Bardez) eight to ten persons died daily. The inhabitants of this territory in panic would run away at the mere sight of a dead body being carried away. The Government did not implement immediate measures to control or prevent the spread of the disease. In October 1918 a notification was issued advising the sick to refrain from sneezing in public and to make use of handkerchief to cover their mouth.

However, the military commander at Sanguem opened a ward to treat the sick suffering from influenza. During this influenza free medicine was supplied to the poor at the *Hospital Regimental*. Taleigão the Administrator of Ilhas ordered the local pharmacy to supply free medicine to the poor. All funerals were to be held privately. Free machilas were provided to the two physicians in charge of epidemics.[91] Influenza in epidemic form appeared again in 1959 all over Goa and rest of the continent. A list of important epidemics in the sixteenth to twentieth centuries in Goa is given in the Appendix 4-F.

Meningitis

Meningitis has been ravaging several developing countries of Africa and South America in present times. Meningitis is transmitted in its bacterial form by one of the three main group of meningoeocus. The disease usually causes inflammation of meninges, the membrane covering the brain. The bacteria is normally transported in the nasal cavity of the patient, and can be spread by sneezing. The disease attacks small children, who often died within 24 hours.

The first case of meningitis appeared in Goa in the beginning of this century. The disease was brought from Portugal by the Portuguese sailors, where a powerful epidemic broke out in 1902-1903. Meningitis took epidemic proportions in the second decade of this century. This time the disease was transmitted by emigrants of Africa. The disease attacked children, between the age group from 2 to 18 years in Velim and Assolna (Salcete). From Salcete the disease spread to Quepem. In 1919 a total of 151 children suffered from meningitis and about 38 died of the disease. Around 859 children succumbed to the disease from 1921 to 1927. Forty seven children succumbed to the disease in 1928 at Salcete.[92] In 1930, 29 cases were registered and 16 died of the disease.[93]

Dobó

Dobó, a disease of liver was common in Goa around 1930s. The disease was unknown outside India. It was called *Dobó* (box) because the liver turned hard. Infants in their teething period fell victim to the disease. The disease prevailed among children of *Bhat* (priestly) class, probably because of deficiency in their diet. *Dobó* was rare among Christians and Muslims in Goa.[94] Cow's urine mixed with equal parts of sugar and salt, concoction of wild egg plant mixed with *papar khar*, egg plant or *papod*

Diseases and Epidemics

khar boiled in a copper vessel and ground with cow's urine and jaggery, were some of the medicine prescribed by the native practitioners for *Dobó*. The symptoms of the disease were fever, depression, lack of sleep and enlargement of liver.

Pempigus

High fever, delirium, convulsions followed by transparent irregular boils were symptoms of *Pempigus*. The boils léft ash grey scars. *Pempigus* erupted in epidemic form in 1937 at Chicalim (Bardez). The disease was carried by a young boy from Bombay. The incubation period was from 10 to 15 days. Out of 34 registered cases ten died of the disease. *Pempigus* led to other complications such as pneumonia.[95]

Poliomyelitis

Poliomyelitis existed in Goa for a long time. It took epidemic proportions between 1937-1941.[96] After this period there was decline in polio cases. The victims belonged to the age group of 0-4 years. The highest incidence was in Bardez probably due to emigration, better means of transport and high density of population.

Other diseases

In 1922 diseases such as dysentery, whooping cough and chickenpox took epidemic form.

Uterine problems were prevalent among women. In rural areas snake bites were common. Many people died of snake bites and rabies.[97] A large numbers of people were reported to be suffering from leprosy.

Alcoholism and intoxication were other health problems throughout the period. Alcoholism prevailed among people of all classes.[98] *Tavernas* (liquor shops) were found in every nook or corner. The Church tried to curb this vice by imposing certain checks but the people continued with the vice.[99] *Liga Economico-Social da India Portuguesa* established in 1930s also fought against excessive drinking and smoking. Drugs like opium and bhang were openly sold in Goa until 1927.[100] These drugs were consumed by people of all classes. In the seventeenth century opium was supplied by employers to increase the working capacity of their labourers. For example, in the gunpowder factory and in the galleys.[101] There is an interesting description of the Portuguese ladies using *Dutro* to inebriate their husbands to allow them freedom with their lovers. This consumption of drugs led to acute and chronic intoxication. Men, women and sometimes even children smoked tobacco which was grown in this region:[103]

The inhabitants suffered also from problems of stress and strain, possibly connected with emigration that was highest in Bardez. *Rois de Christandade* gives us some statistics about the mentally ill among the Catholics of Goa.[104] In 1915 the highest number of mentally ill were found in Bardez.[105] This taluka had 156 mentally ill people among the Catholics. Two villages in Bardez that is Aldona and Ucassaim had the highest number. Salcete had 104 persons with mental problems. Old Conquests had a total of 341 mental cases and New Conquests just 36.[106] These figures are not very reliable. Many times the statistics included the deaf and the dumb together with mentally ill people besides Goa during this period had no trained psychologist who could diagnose such cases.

Several other diseases existed in Goa. Diphtheria, whooping cough, liver diseases, kidney problems, skin diseases and pneumonia were common health risks. Some school health studies have cited that majority of school children had health defects of some sort.[107] Most commonly they suffered from hookworms, malnutrition, anemia and caries. Tetanus known among the natives as *Sotvi*, was responsible for high mortality rate among infants followed by diarrhoea.

IV. PREVENTION AND CONTROL OF COMMUNICABLE DISEASES

Malaria

Before preventive measures were instituted malaria was one of the biggest public health problem. The disease was endemic in some parts of Goa, and accounted for 60,000 deaths a year before 1950.

Quinine tablets were for the first time in 1869 distributed in urban areas to prevent malaria. Regulations to prevent and control recurrent epidemics, including malaria epidemics, were issued on 14th March 1913.[108] It required that every house in the capital city and in Margão, Mapuça and Vasco should clean stagnant pools of water around them. Inspection of these houses was to be carried by personnel of Heath Services every week. All wells were to be covered and a pump attached to them. These regulations were evolved without considering the financial aspect. Large sums were required to implement these measures.

Diseases and Epidemics

Margão alone had 1,000 wells, a minimum of Rs. 215 was required to cover and provide pump for each well. However, no funds were provided by the Government.[109] In 1920s Dr. Froilano de Mello and Luis Bras de Sa from the Health Services discovered 18,000 unused wells in Old Goa and they were successful in closing these wells which were sources of malaria.

In the late 1940s the first anti-malaria campaign was launched on war footing in Old Goa.[110] Several unused wells were closed down, marshy areas were filled up. D.D.T. was sprayed and quinine tablets were distributed to the inhabitants. Large sums were spent to improve the sanitary conditions of the old city.

In early 1950s large scale malaria control programme was started in Goa. Two doctors from Goa Dr. Pandorinath A. Borcar and Dr. Francisco T. da Silva were sponsored by World Health Organisation to Malaria Institute in New Delhi to receive training in Malaria control.[111] Later they were sent to Bombay for further training. On their return they were posted in Sanguem and Canacona. Extensive surveys were carried out in these places to investigate the incidence of malaria. From October to June every house was sprayed three times with D.D.T and paludin tablets were distributed among the inhabitants. The eradication programme was then extended to Quepem. As result of these measures malaria almost disappeared from these areas. Recently malaria has come back in the capital town of Goa.

Smallpox

Until the mid nineteenth century no preventive measures to prevent smallpox were implemented. If any measures were introduced at all it was done after the outbreak. Repeated attack of smallpox during the second half of the nineteenth century forced the State to make vaccination compulsory in 1883.[112] Similar orders were repeated in 1893, making vaccination compulsory among primary school children.[113]

The vaccination campaign does not seem to have succeed. A number of factors worked against it. Chief among these was the difficulty of keeping the lymph potent for long enough period to dispatch to remote areas and use it in time. There were also faulty techniques of the vaccinators. The officials were reluctant to assert their authority in a field where people's attitudes were closely entwined with religion and tradition. The vaccinators were poorly paid.

Smallpox vaccine was not well received by Goans. In fact, in the middle of the nineteenth century several individuals from Bicholim sent a petition to the Government requesting to allow them to follow their own practices, as they found the vaccine not efficacious. A certain section of the population also believed that smallpox was cause by goddess Devi and vaccination would annoy her. The goddess in turn would maim or kill people.

In 1891 the Government opened a ward in Mormugão to isolate victims of smallpox.[114] Similar isolation wards were started at Colem and Reis Magos in the later period.

Vaccination was normally ordered after on outbreak of the disease, as for instance at Ponda in 1889 and Pernem in 1892. Since several cases of smallpox were detected in 1906, the Government asked physicians and heads of the family to inform about the occurrence of smallpox in their locality.[115] Vaccine was ordered from the Belgaum.[116] Doctors entrusted with vaccination work received a salary of Rs. 40 and a remuneration of Re. 1 when they moved out of the headquarters.[117] The Government fixed vaccination timings in various talukas.[118] The response of the people was poor. In 1908 the Government, repeated its order to taluka administration to fix a day for vaccination preferably on a Monday.[119] The place of vaccination had to be away from the church.

Smallpox vaccine was made again compulsory in 1914 to all children seeking admission in Government primary schools[120] and two years later to all ship crew leaving Mormugão harbour.[121] Earlier vaccination was made compulsory to all those who wished to migrate to British India.[122] Incentives were provided to vaccinators.[123] A fine of Rs. 50 was imposed on those who refused the vaccine. In 1927 smallpox vaccination was made compulsory for all individuals from eight months of age onwards. The same individuals had to be revaccinated at the age of seven. In addition vaccination was compulsory before marriage and taking up a Government job.[124] A total of 46,300 persons were vaccinated in 1928.[125] In 1933 about 11,064 persons received vaccine in Bardez. In 1941 altogether 60,343 persons received vaccine in Goa.

Smallpox did not disappear till quite after sometime, because people often concealed cases of smallpox from the authorities fearing they would be sent to isolation hospitals in Colem, Reis Magos, Mormugão and Margão. The concealment was never complete because uneducated people believed that *neem* leaves hung at the entrance of the room prevented the spread of the disease and the leaves had beneficial effect on the patient.

Diseases and Epidemics

Cholera

From mid-nineteenth century the Government began to introduce measures to prevent and control cholera. Earlier various measures such as firing in the air with gun, fumigation with gunpowder and tar as well as cleaning the affected areas with cattle were resorted to. These measures were ineffective.[126] At the end of the nineteenth century the Health Services were granted permission to appoint doctors to care for cholera victims. For instance in 1893 a doctor was appointed to take care of cholera patients in Taleigão and to provide medicine from *Hospital Regimental* to the poor victims.

Soon after a ban was imposed on people entering Goa on the northern side from British India to prevent the spread of cholera.[127]

Recurrent cholera attacks in the late nineteenth and early twentieth century led the Government in 1907 to adopt several measures. It instructed the State Health Board (*Junta de Saude*) to introduce therapeutic and prophylactic measures.[128] The inhabitants were banned from washing their clothes around the wells and from consuming water from the wells used by cholera patients.[129] Patients who were poor were provided with free diet at the expense of the State. In some talukas the doctors were provided with free transport facilities during epidemics.[130] Quarantine regulations were enforced.

Many physicians were reluctant to help the victims of cholera. In 1908, the Administrator of Ilhas was asked to report the names of those physicians who refused to work during epidemics. Such doctors would not be considered for Government services.[131] Jobs in the Health Services were in great demand in those days. During this period vigilance committees were appointed in the villages to introduce preventive measures and to render help to the cholera victims.

Cholera inoculation was introduced in Goa very late in the year 1927. It was made compulsory for passengers entering Goa from British India and to those who provided assistance or kept company to the cholera victims.[132]

Plague

Several plagues occurred in Goa from 1900 to 1918. The following measures were adopted during the plague of 1908 in Panjim.[133]

(i) A team of health workers were appointed to undertake the task of

cleaning areas inhabited by merchants who lived in ill ventilated places.
(ii) Houses and compounds were regularly inspected by a physician appointed by Health Services.
(iii) Streets and houses were fumigated with patrol and chemicals. In some houses tiles were removed.
(iv) Dead rats and cases of fevers were to be reported to the authorities.
(v) Windows were opened in houses lacking ventilation. Passengers entering Goa from British India were to be inspected at the border and if necessary preventive measures were to be introduced to contain plague which was wide spread in Bombay. [134]

It is interesting to note that blacks were generally employed by the Government to take care of those suffering from bubonic plague in isolation wards. As already mentioned a plague broke up in Margão in the year 1916. During this period houses and shops were inspected daily to search for dead rats. These houses were disinfected and new windows were opened for proper ventilation. Inhabitants of Margão were not allowed to change their residence, without prior notice to the Health authorities. Several roads and lanes were opened and cleaned. Finally cowsheds were shifted away from the town.[135]

Meningitis

Inoculation against meningitis was introduced soon after the disease took epidemic proportions in Velim and Assolna. About 60 children were vaccinated in 1927. The following year 399 children received vaccine in Salcete. In Velim the number of children who underwent vaccination was about 200. [136]

The second Sanitary Conference held in 1934 decided to start a full-fledged Government aided association to tackle problems related to T.B. "Assistencia aos Tuberculosis da India Portuguesa" was founded in 1941. A clinical and radiological survey of the population was carried out.

The sudden spurt in mining industries caused overcrowding and pollution of mining areas. The labor population was affected by diseases including T.B. In early 1950's two health officers were sent for training in T.B. at the National Institute at Bangalore. The B.C.G. programme was started at the end of 1950's. T.B. and B.C.G. vaccines were brought from Portugal every fortnight. Vaccination was carried out, after the person underwent Montroue Test. This scheme was looked after by the Health

Diseases and Epidemics

Services.

Epidemic diseases began to disappear during the fourth decade of the present century probably due to introduction of inoculations and greater awareness among the people regarding hygiene. Cholera ceased to be common by 1945 due to regular inoculations. Plague disappeared from Goa. Preventive measures helped to eradicate malaria in Canacona, Sanguem and Quepem. However, in recent years a more virulent variety has made its appearance in Goa and specially in the capital city.

REFERENCES

1. *The voyages of John Huyghen van Linschoten to the East Indies,* eds., A.B. Burnell and P.A. Tiele, II, London, 1885, pp. 235. (Henceforth Linschoten).
2. *Nicolau Manucci's Storia de Mogor,* ed. N. Irwine, III, Calcutta, 1966, p. 265. (Henceforth Manucci).
3. *Archivo de Pharmacia e Sciencias Accessorias da India Portuguesa,* Nova Goa, 1870, p. 19.
4. Conde de Ficalho, *Garcia da Orta e o seu tempo,* Lisboa, 1886, p. 52.
5. Gaspar Correia, *Lendas da India,* Tomo IV, Lisboa, 1864, p. 289; Coutinho, Fourtunato, *Le règime paroisial des diocèses de rite latin de l'Inde des origines (XVI siècle) nous jours,* Louvain, 1958, p. 36 : Says that during the epidemic of 1543, the Diocese of the city of Goa was divided into four parishes. This was necessary to bury 15 to 20 persons who died daily due to cholera.
6. J.N. da Fonseca, *An Historical and Archaeological Sketch of the city of Goa,* New Delhi, 1986, p. 149.
7. *Documenta Indica,* ed. Josef Wicki, vol. VIII, Rome, p. 319. (Henceforth DI); Teotonio de Souza, *op. cit.,* p. 116. Many potters left the city for more healthy place. The missionaries of St. Paul College too shifted their residence. (Sebastião Gonsalves, *Primeira Parte da Historia dos Religiosos da companhia de Jesus,* Coimbra, 1957-62, p. 98.).
8. *DI,* VIII, p. 318. During this cholera attack two to three persons were often buried in the grave because there were instances when the entire family were victims of the disease.
9. ARSJ: Goa 33, II, fls. 500, 718.
10. HAG: Ms. 1498 – *Ordens Regias* no. 2, fls. 11-12.
11. Gaspar Correia, *op. cit.,* p. 447, The children of the king of Ceylon were studying in Goa with the missionaries.
12. Linschoten, *op. cit.,* pp. 235-236.
13. Archives du Royaume Belgique, Bruxelles – Archives Jesuitiques, n° 1427, fl. 131. Many Portuguese left the city during this epidemic for more healthy places.
14. Agostinho de Santa Maria, *Historia da Fundação do Real Convento da Santa Monica da cidade de Goa,* Lisboa, 1699, p. 289.
15. ARSJ: *Goa 34, II – Goana Historia* 1648-1649, fls. 290 and 409v.
16. Linschoten, *op. cit.,* II, p. 240.
17. Thevenot and Careri, *Indian Travels of Thevenot and Careri,* ed. Surendranath Sen, New Delhi, 1949 (reprint), p. 161.
18. HAG: *MR.* 121 B fls. 692 V-194. Lack of medical facilities also were responsible for

mortality on board the ships. Barbers often did the work of surgeons. Many times the ships appeared to be floating hospitals.

19. Luis de Pina, *Subsidio para a Historia da Medicina Portuguesa Indiana no seculo XVII,* Porto, 1931, p. 9. He says that enema, bleeding and purgative were the main medicine used by the Portuguese to cure diseases.
20. Diogo Couta, *Asia,* decade 9a., Lisboa, 1786, pp. 50-51.
21. It was also known as Spanish or French disease.
22. Conde de Ficalho, op. cit., p. 181. Travellers Linschoten, Pyrard, Petro de Valle, Mandeslo also mention about widespread prostitution and free life style of many women in Goa.
23. João de Barros, *Asia,* (segunda decada), Lisboa, 1945, pp. 242-243. In the beginning non-Christians were shocked when they saw their daughters being taken away by the Portuguese as their wives but later were contented when the girls were well married. The Portuguese husbands treated them well.
24. *Ibid.,* p. 243; A.B. Bragança Pereira, Arquivo Portugues Oriental, I, c xivi.
25. Bragança Pereira, *op. cit.,* p. 509.
26. Bragança Pereira, *op. cit.,* p. 736.
27. J. Barros, op. cit., pp. 242-243. Nair women married within their caste.
28. *A.P.O.,* Fasc. IV, p. 52.
29. Teotonio de Souza, "A Pious Hindu Commemorates in marble the activities of the Paulists in Kumbarjua", *Goa Today,* February 1977, p. 14.
30. Manucci, *op. cit.,* III, p. 265.
31. *A.P.O.,* Fasc. III, p. 324.
32. J.M. do Carmo Nazareth, "Os religiosos da India e as Bexigas" *O Oriente Portuguez,* V, Nova Goa, 1908, p. 358.
33. HAG: *MR.,* 81, fl. 220; HAG; *MR* 114, fl. 77v: In November 1742 about 60 soldiers died in the Royal hospital, at times seven people would die in a day.
34. HAG: *MR.* 121 B. fl. 691.
35. HAG : *MR.* 131 B. fl. 379v.
36. HAG: *Mr.* 143 A, fls. 333 and 337.
37. Dr. Costa Portugal was the Chief Physician in Goa, details about him are given in chapter VII.
38. Germano Correia, *Colera-morbo na India Portuguesa, desde a sua conquista ate actualidade – Estudo nasografico, epidemiologico e climato-sanitario,* Nova Goa, 1919, p. 13.
39. HAG : *MR.* 173, fl. 150.
40. HAG : *MR.* 196, fl. 131.
41. HAG : *MR.* 196, fl. 131; Miguel Vicente d'Abreu, *O Governo do Vice-rei Conde de Rio Pardo no Estado da India Portugueza desde 1816-1821,* Nova Goa, 1869, p. 140.
42. *Arquivo de Pharmacia e Sciencias Medicas da India Portuguesa,* 15th March 1863, pp. 105-111.
43. Boletim do Governo de Estado da India, (Henceforth B.G.), 15th March 1945.
44. B.G., no. 26, 28th June 1845, p. 3.
45. B.G. no. 26, 28th June 1845, p. 3.
46. B.G. n° 32, 4th August 1854.
47. Appendix 4-A.
48. Filipe Nery Xavier, *Collecção de Bandos e outras differentes Providencias que servem de Leis Regulamentares.* II, Nova Goa, 1850, p. 205; HAG; *Ms.* 966 – *Cartas Ordens e Portarias:* contains orders appointing two doctors to handle the cholera

Diseases and Epidemics

epidemic at Dongrim (Ilhas). These two doctors were jointly paid by the Health Board and village *communidade*.
49. Appendix 4-B.
50. *Relatorio do Administrador do Concelho de Nova Goa 1870", *Archivo de Pharmacia e Sciencias Accessorias* Nova Goa, Imprensa Nacional, 1870, p. 16.
51. Germano Correia., *op. cit.*, p. 64.
52. *Ibid.*, p. 90.
53. *Ibid.*, p. 178.
54. HAG: *Correspondencia Diversa 11670*, fl. 124. (Henceforth C.D.).
55. HAG: *MR.* 161 C, fl. 858.
56. HAG: *MR.* 190 C, fls. 747-748.
57. *B.G.*, N°44, 31 de Outubro 1851.
58. *Estatistica Medica dos Hospitals das Provincias Ultra marinas referida ao ano 1869*, Lisboa, 1883, p. 31.
59. *Estatisca Medica dos Hospitals das Provincias Ultramarinas referida ao ano 1876*, Lisboa, 1883, p. 201.
60. *Diario do 3°. Conde de Linhares, Vice Rei da India*, II, Lisboa, 1943, p. 261. The British in India also resorted to bleeding to cure fevers.
61. "Relatorio do Serviço de Saude do Estado da India Portuguesa – 1879* (*Primeira parte)*, Nova Goa, 1880, p. 20.
62. HAG: *MR* 197, fl. 280.
63. HAG: *Ms.* 966 – *Cartas, Ordens e Portarias,* fl. 135.
64. HAG:*CD* 11668, fl. 138. Prostitutes and others resorted many times to abortion carried out with the help of various types of native medicine. One of the common methods used for abortion was to give a purgative to the pregnant woman.
65. Appendix 4-E.
66. *Proceedings of 1a. Conferencia Sanitaria 1914,* Nova Goa, 1917, p. 824.
67. In June 1897 the local Government asked the Health Services to inform the number of cases and the names of areas affected by bubonic plague. (HAG: Ms. 11670 – CD, fl. 126.).
68. Germano Correia, *op. cit.*, pp. 214-227.
69. Germano Correia, *Nosografia da India Portuguesa,* Nova Goa, 1919, p. 245.
70. *Ibid.*, p. 257. The annual report of Health Services from June 1919 to June 1920 reports that many times fishermen on their way back from British India would throw their crew members infected with cholera in the sea.
71. Information about Dr. Wolfango da Silva is given in chapter VII.
72. F.A. Wolfango da Silva, * Relatorio sobre a epidemia de peste Dezembro 1901 a April 1902," Nova Goa, 1902, p. 12.
73. Appendix 4-D.
74. F.A. Wolfango da Silva, "Relatorio sobre a epidemia de peste Dezembro 1901 a April 1902", Nova Goa, 1902, p. 12.
75. F.A. Wolfango da Silva, "Relatorio sobre a epidemia de peste Dezembro 1901 a April 1902," Nova Goa, 1902, p. 12.
76. *Loc., cit.*
77. *Arquivos da Escola Medico Cirurgica de Nova Goa.* Bastora, 1942, p. 177.
78. Wiseman Pinto, "O Beriberi e endemico em Goa" *Arquivo da Escola Medico – Circurgico de N. Goa* 1928, Bastora, 1929, p. 206.
79. Proceedings of the 1st Sanitary Conference 1914, Nova Goa, 1917, p. 762.
80. Details about Dr. de Mello are given in chapter VII.
81. Viriato Almeida, "Tuberculose" 1ª Conferencia Sanitaria 1914, II, Nova Goa, 1917,

p. 813.
82. *Ibid.*, p. 818.
83. "Relatorio de Servicos de Saude 1933", *Boletim Geral de Medicina e Farmacia*, Bastora, 1934, p. 18.
84. *Arquivos de Escola Medico – Circurgica de Nova Goa*, Bastora, 1942, p. 168.
85. *Arquivos da Escola Medico-Circurgica de Nova Goa – 1942*, Bastora, 1942, pp. 168-171.
86. A.C. Germano S. Correia, *India Portuguesa – Prostituição Profilaxia Anti-venerea – Historia Demografia Etnofrafia Higiene e Profilaxia*, Bastora, 1938, p. 74. In 1938 the highest number of Prostitutes were found in Ponda followed by Sanquelim. There were about 144 known prostitutes in the age group of 15 years.
87. Appendix 4-E.
88. *Arquivos de Escola Medico-Cicurgica de Nova Goa*, 1929, p. 487.
89. "Relatorio de Serviços de Saude", *Boletim Geral de Medicina e Farmacia*, 1934.
90. Pedro Correia Afonso, "0 Problema da Mão d'Obra Agricola na India Portuguesa", 70. *Congresso Provincial*, Nova Goa, 1927, p. 32.
91. "Serviços de Saude de Estado da India", Nova Goa, 1926, pp. 30-31.
92. Froilano de Mello, "Le Service de Santé á L'Inde Portuguaise", *Arquivos de Escola Medico-Circurgica da* Nova Goa, 1930, p. 660.
93. Report by Taluka Health Officers of Goa 1930, *Boletim Geral de Medicina e Farmacia*, April-June 1931, p. 93.
94. F.X. de Sequeira Nazareth, "Dobó ou Dobá", *Arquivos da Escola Medico-Circurgica de Nova Goa*, Bastora, 1930, p. 477.
95. L.J. Bras de Sa, "A epidemia de Pempigus numa aldia de Bardez", *Arquivos de Escola Medico-Circurgica de Nova Goa*, Bastora, 1938.
96. L.J. Bras de Sa, "Algumas notas epidemiologicas sobre a poliomielite em Goa", *Arquivos da Escola Medico-Circurgica de Nova Goa*, Bastora, 1942, p. 222.
97. The Government appears to have been concerned with incidence of snake bites. In 1910 it directed the *regedor* and other local authorities to send monthly report about mortality rate due to snake bites and bites of other animals so that appropriate measures could be taken to contain the cases. (*Legislação relativa ao Estado da India*, 1910, Nova Goa, 1911, p. 160, henceforth LREI.).
98. PP: *Visita Pastoral*, vol. 7-8, fl. 13. (Henceforth VP); VP, vol. 16-17, fls. 83v-84; VP, vols. 13-15, fls. 21-22.
99. PP: *VP*, vol. XII, fl. 186. In 1772 two brothers from Quelossim (Cortalim) were accused of over drinking. They were fined six xerafins each. During Pastoral visit of 1772 a man from Moira was accused of excessive drinking.
100. LREI, 1927, Nova Goa, 1928, pp. 22-23; B.O. no. 10, 4th February 1927. In this year the Government banned the sale of ganja, bhang and other intoxicating drugs. Persons found selling or buying drugs were to be fined Rs. 500. However, drugs could be sold for medical use through the Health Services.
101. HAG: *MR*. 85, fl. 59v.
102. Pyrard, *op. cit.*, p. 87.
103. HAG: *MR*. 159 C, fl. 691v.
104. The bibliographical essay in this work gives detailed information concerning these *Rois*.
105. *RC*, 1906-1917.
106. PP: *RG*. 1773-1941.
107. *Proceedings of 1a. Conferencia Sanitaria*, 1914, Nova Goa, 1917, pp. 510-544.
108. B.O., n° 21, 14th March 1913.

Diseases and Epidemics

109. Proceedings of 1st Sanitary Conference 1914, Nova Goa, 1917, p. 598.
110. Victor Dias, *Velha-Goa e o seu saneamento*, Fasc. I, Cidade de Goa, 1940.
111. Fatima Gracias, "Quality of Life in Colonial Goa: Its hygienic Expression (19th-20th Centuries) in Essays in *Goan History*, ed. Teotonio R. de Souza, Delhi, 1989, p. 201.
112. B.O. no. 32, 11th February 1883.
113. HAG: *CD.* 11668, fl. 110.
114. *Ibid.*, fl. 10.
115. HAG: *CD.*, 10471, fl. 39.
116. HAG: Ms. 11668 – CD, fl. not numbered. Vaccine brought from Belgaum was to be supplied in areas situated along the railway lines.
117. *Ibid.*, fl. 43.
118. The expenses were to be met by respective Municipalities. (LREI, 1906, Nova Goa, 1907, p. 22).
119. *Ibid.*, fl. 86.
120. HAG: Ms. 10550 – *Administração Civil – Saude e Benificiencia*, fl. 5.
121. *Ibid.*, fl. 81.
122. *Ibid.*, fl. 109. In 1908 the local Government had received reports from Bombay that several victims of smallpox were of Goan origin.
123. Their remuneration was increased in 1916 to Rs. 3 per every ten vaccinated persons.
124. LREI, 1927, Nova Goa, 1928, p. 77. A fine of Rs. 5 was to be imposed to those who failed to follow the order.
125. *Arquivos da Escola Medico-Cirurgica de Nova Goa*, 1942, p. 177.
126. In 1858 the Governor of Estado da India approved several measures submitted by the Health Board to eradicate cholera and to provide assistance to the victims of the disease with the help of Administrators of the New Conquests.
127. HAG: Ms. 11668 – CD, fl. 116.
128. *Ibid.*, fl. 131.
129. HAG: Ms. 10471 – CD, fl. 79. Patients who were poor were provided free diet. These expenses were to be met by the Department of Accounts.
130. HAG: Ms. 10471 – CD, fl. 79.
131. *Ibid.*, fl. 80.
132. B.O. no. 83, 16th October 1931.
133. B.O. no. 65, 21st August 1908.
134. HAG: Ms. 10471 – CD, fl. 84.
135. Antonio Augusto do Rego, "*Relatorio da Canpanha Anti-pestosa em Margao e em varias aldeias de Salcete*", Nova Goa, 1918. A ward to isolate patients suffering of suspected plague was opened in Margao during this period much against the wishes of the inhabitants.
136. *Arquivos da Escola Medico-Cirurgica de Nova Goa*, 1930, Bastora, 1930, p. 660.

5

HOSPITALS AND EXTENSION SERVICES

Hospitals were few in Goa during the colonial period. They were situated in urban areas and mainly in the city of Goa in the early centuries of Portuguese rule. Hospitals were established to cater primarily to the needs of the ruling class. They were run usually by social agencies and missionaries. In this connection, it must be mentioned that Christian missionaries played an important role in the medical field in Goa.

The standards of the hospitals were low as a rule. These hospitals were small in size, very often with less than fifty beds. They were housed in unsuitable buildings and inadequately staffed. Hospitals had few or no facilities for special care and lacked proper equipment as well as trained technical personnel. Their dispensaries and kitchens were poor. They had no running water, septic tanks or electricity for a long time. Medicine and all equipment had to be imported from Portugal, Spain, China, British India and other parts. They were not easily available in Goa and because of long journeys many drugs reached Goa in adulterated conditions.

In rural areas, the inhabitants depended on local medicine men and quacks. Many could not avail themselves of hospital facilities in urban areas because the distance was a formidable barrier on account of inadequate or non-existent transport facilities.

Specialized hospitals were even fewer in number. They were established by the Government in the twentieth century for lepers, tuberculosis patients and the mentally ill. All these hospitals were situated in Old Conquests. These hospitals were places for detention of persons considered dangerous to the community, rather than institutions for the treatment of the sick.

Maternity homes and private nursing homes were non- existent before this century. When they were established, women even in urban areas were reluctant to avail themselves of the facilities. Superstitions, ignorance, easily available cheap quacks may have contributed to this attitude. Majority of the nursing homes were established between 1930-1948 in Salcete and Bardez. Isolation wards were also established in Margão, Marmagoa, Colem and Reis Magos for the victims of epidemics.

Hospitals in Goa had limited number of trained doctors in western medicine. Portuguese physicians who came to India were inexperienced in tropical diseases. Besides, Goa did not attract the cream of Portuguese medical profession. The great paucity of specialists and surgeons made it difficult to get competent treatment but for routine ailments. Lack of proper facilities led the patients to seek medical facilities at faraway Vellore, Bombay and Miraj.

Indigenous practitioners of medicine were allowed to practise in the Royal Hospital in the early seventeenth century when physicians trained in western medicine were banned from practising in the hospital. The ban was imposed due to high mortality. This high mortality was the result of incompetence on the part of Portuguese physicians. Pyrard, a French traveller, who visited Goa during this period remarks that 1,500 patients died every year in the Royal Hospital.[1] The mortality rate was high taking into consideration the fact that the hospital catered only to the needs of the Portuguese. Then again between 1782-1801, Goa had no trained doctors on account of their scarcity in Portugal.[2] The establishment of Goa Medical school helped to meet the need of doctors at least in the Old Conquests.

Until the twentieth century Goa had no trained auxiliary personnel, including nurses. The shortage of trained nurses and consequent reliance on poorly qualified persons or relatives of the patients for nursing services often meant that the rules of hygiene were not observed. Since toilet facilities were inadequate and wards were overcrowded, infections quickly spread from one patient to another. Because of these and other conditions, the case fatality ratio was high, lending substance to the popular belief that hospital was the place where one is bound to die. Hospitals in Goa suffered from financial and physical limitations.

The two hospitals situated in Ilhas taluka, namely *Hospital Regimental* and *Hospital da Misericordia* were always overcrowded with patients. To prevent such situation the Government issued orders in 1906 to all taluka administrators other than of Ilhas to avoid sending patients from their jurisdiction to the above mentioned hospitals.[3]

A total of 2,879 patients were treated in various hospitals and homes for the aged in 1927. In 1942 the number of patients in various hospitals rose to 4,294.[4]

Goa had four full-fledged hospitals in this period. All these hospitals, excepting one, were run by private institutions aided by the State. At the fag end of the Portuguese regime there were few regional or cottage hospitals in some talukas with a strength of 40 beds.

This chapter has two parts. The first is concerned with institutional care in urban and suburban areas, that is, in the city of Goa and the surrounding areas. The second part considers the institutional care in rural areas.

HOSPITAL FACILITIES IN URBAN AND SUBURBAN GOA

The Royal Hospital

The first European hospital in India was the Royal Hospital (*Hospital Real*) in the city of Goa. The hospital was founded by Afonso de Albuquerque for Portuguese whites to help them recover from the fatigue of long sea voyages, wars of conquests and infectious diseases prevailing in the city.

The Royal Hospital existed in 1511. We know of orders issued by Albuquerque to the Factor of the city of Goa, directing him to supply the hospital with a bale of sugar.[5] By another order issued on 14th October 1511 the hospital received 135 *barganis*, spent on six patients between 22nd September and 13th October 1511.[6]

To begin with, the Royal Hospital was a single-storied building covered with palm leaves near St. Catherine's gate. It was Albuquerque's favourite institution in India. The successive governors ran the institution effectively.

In 1520 statutes were framed for the hospital placing it on firmer basis and providing systematic rules for its efficient management. It directed the Factor to provide funds for the monthly expenses of the hospital. The daily requirements of the hospital were bought by a Purchaser (*comprador*) in consultation with the nurses after checking the surplus left over from the previous day. The Purchaser was responsible to the Factor of the city.[7]

To avoid pilferage of medicines from the hospital, all medicines prescribed by the physicians and surgeons had to be entered in a register and signed by the clerk.[8] It appears that the *boticario* continued to sell medicine to persons outside the hospital despite the restrictions imposed on such activity. In 1524 Dr. Pero Nunez, Superintendent of Public Exchequer issued fresh orders to the Factor not to allow sale of medicine outside the hospital.[9]

Two years later in 1526 a more detailed regulation was issued to end

Hospitals and Extension Services

irregularities, indiscipline and to introduce new amenities. The regulation made it clear that the Royal Hospital was to cater to the needs of the Portuguese working on the ships. The Portuguese suffering from incurable diseases were to be treated in the *Hospital da Misericordia* run by Holy House of Mercy in the city of Goa.[10]

Patients seeking admission in the Royal Hospital had to comply with certain formalities. For instance, they had to supply the hospital their personal case history. Every patient was provided a bed and clean linen. Soon after admission the patient was washed with water that had been boiled with certain herbs.

Linen and items of the clothing were supplied to the hospital by the Factor at the expense of the Royal Treasury. In case of an emergency, the regulation empowered the clerk to directly buy linen with the hospital funds. Old linen could not be discarded. It was used to clean and tie the wounds.

The regulation of 1526 created a post of a clerk (*escrivão*). This clerk was responsible for supervision of the hospital and for maintenance of accounts. The staff and patients were banned to carry away live fowls from the hospital kitchen to their homes.[11] It also forbade women and slaves to visit the sick. It was noticed that they often carried food to the sick from outside the hospital. The slaves of the Purveyor (*Provedor*) and those of the clerk had their meals in the hospital. The regulation banned such abuses.

A diet of meat and bread was provided to the sick. Much bread was wasted. Therefore, in 1526 the number of loaves supplied to the patients was reduced to four. Each loaf weighed six ounces.[12] Edible commodities such oil, butter, honey, sugar and rice were bought at wholesale prices.

The cleanliness of the hospital and care of the patient was attended to by nurses, barber, washerman, servants and slaves. The barber had to be present daily at 8 a.m. to bleed the sick on the advice of the physician. Servants were paid 8 *leaes* a month. The slaves who worked as scavengers were owned by the State. They received no salary for their work but only food and clothing. The hospital was provided with a native cook and assistant cook. Both were given free meals in addition to their salaries.

This hospital catered to the needs of the ruling class in the city of Goa. In 1542 the hospital was given a *pauta das mezinhas* (price list of medicine) which was valid for 30 years. Around this time the hospital building was renovated and enlarged with new varandas and a new pharmacy.[13] The Royal Hospital run by the Factor of the city faced serious problems of mismanagement and corruption. The subsidy of 3,500 *pardaos* from the Government was misused by the hospital authorities. Consequently, the Government persuaded the Holy House of Mercy to manage the institution.[14] The offer was accepted with much reluctance and an agreement was signed under the following terms.[15]

(1) The hospital would receive from April 1543 an annual grant of 3,697 *pardaos* to be paid quarterly out of Royal revenues from the island of Jua and Chorão.
(2) The hospital was exempted from Royal and ecclesiastical control.
(3) The administrator and the members of the Holy House of Mercy would have free hand in the appointments of personnel in the hospital.
(4) In case the assigned funds were insufficient, the Holy House of Mercy would have to spend from its own funds. The extra expenditure would be reimbursed later by the Government.
(5) In addition to the above, the hospital would receive annually (114 gallons) of wine, one barrel of vinegar and a quarter barrel of oil from Portugal all free of Custom duties.

The conditions in the Royal Hospital greatly improved under the new management. A distinguished *fidalgo* (nobleman) was elected every month by the members of the Holy House of Mercy to run the Hospital. This post of Superintendent (*mordomo*) was honorary. He was responsible for buying the supplies for the hospital at proper time.[16]

The Royal Hospital had a capacity for 40 beds. Their number would go up in June with the arrival of the annual fleet. Around 1545 the doctors working in the hospital neglected their duties and left the sick to the care of the slaves.

After a span of 30 years the Royal Hospital was granted in April 1573 a new *pauta*. The earlier *pauta* had not been changed for 30 years, except for minor changes at the time of the Viceroy Dom Constantino. The new *pauta* was approved by the viceroy in April 1573. Baltazar Rodrigues the *boticario* (in-charge of the pharmacy) of the hospital had asked for this revision.[17]

Between 1565-1584 the Royal Hospital received at least two sets of statutes. Viceroy D. Antão de Noronha provided a standing order in 1565. This regulation increased the subsidy from 4,000 *pardaos* to 6,666 *pardaos*, 200 *reis* to face the increased cost of living. The subsidy was to be spent on the diet of the patients, payment to the staff, oil, wine and olives from Portugal. The Purveyor, purchaser and the nurse were paid

1,000 *reis* each.

Around 1570 the conditions in the Royal Hospital began to deteriorate. Poor medical care, lack of hygiene and scarcity of funds were responsible for the situation. The Jesuits who were asked to manage the hospital often carried beds full of bugs to clean them up at the sea.[18] They went around collecting clothes for the patients in the hospital. It appears that the Government had lost interest in the institution, probably because it was preoccupied with the political situation in the land. Furthermore, the hospital was too small to accommodate the growing number of patients. About 500 patients were treated annually. Many times due to lack of space the sick were accommodated in verandas and adjoining houses. In addition to the sick, Portuguese men who lacked sufficient means of livelihood also sought shelter in the hospital. This was contrary to the orders issued earlier by the Viceroy D. Vasco de Gama permitting admission only to the sick.

In 1583 when the Jesuits were about to take over the Royal Hospital from the Misericordia they were asked to prepare a new regulation for the same. The regulation approved in 1584 was a lengthy one. It defined the functions of the members of the staff and specified the time for the purchase of various commodities. It laid much importance on spiritual well-being of the staff and the patients. The legislation also laid stress on cleanliness as an important factor in the maintenance of health.

The staff as well as the patients were ordered to attend Mass daily at 5 a.m. Soon after the Mass, the physician accompanied by Superintendent (*mordomo*), nurse, *boticario*, *escrivão* (clerk) and helpers had to pay a visit to the wards. Prescriptions of the physicians were to be entered in a book by *boticario*. Medicine to the sick was dispensed by the nurse. At the same time the surgeon paid a visit to the ward of wounded patients. Finally the staff gathered at the admission counter to admit new patients.[19]

It was believed that confessions were necessary to cure various illnesses. Even then, the psychosomatic connection seems to have been noted. Therefore, no patient was admitted unless he confessed to a priest appointed for such purpose. For this reason the patient was kept in a veranda until he confessed. However, this rule did not apply to patients in serious condition or the high officials. They were directed to confess the following day.

Breakfast was served at 9 o'clock. After breakfast the sick rested till one o'clock, that is when the physicians and surgeons paid their second visit to the sick. Patients who recovered were discharged in the afternoon. When the dinner was served to the patients at 5 p.m. the nurses had to tidy up the wards. Three servants and a room boy spent the night with patients. All nurses on duty had to report to the hospital in the early hours of the morning.

Bed linen was changed once a week on Saturdays, and if necessary more often. Table linen and clothes of the patients were changed on Sundays and Thursdays. Clothes from the surgery ward were washed and dried separately by *mainatos* (washermen). Any loss of clothing had to be reported to the *mordomo* by the nurses. The wards were cleaned thrice a week. Drinking water was carried in vessels from Banguenim spring. The hospital was white-washed thrice a year when the sick were due to arrive from Portugal, for Christmas and at Easter time.

Purchases were made when commodities were cheap. In the months of September and October the hospital was provided with goods from Portugal such as barrels of *xeiçal* or *caparica* wine for the sick, oil, vinegar, olives, saffron, paper, pens, preserved food and chamber pots. Goods were imported from Ormuz in October and November including dry fruits, saffron, bottles of rose water and dates. In April and May the *mordomo* bought goods from China, Maluco and Malaca such as *Pão da China (China* root) for venereal diseases, condiments and porcelain. From Bengal the hospital received rice for ward boys and the sick. Apparently, the ward boys were given cheaper quality rice. Finally, in July the hospital had to be prepared with things necessary for the sick due to arrive in the ships of *carreira*.

The *mordomo,* chosen for his good character, was the main official of the hospital. He performed several duties including purchasing of goods, maintenance of accounts, cleanliness and discipline. It was his duty to arrange for best doctors and to see that their instructions were implemented. No staff in the hospital could be appointed without his recommendation. The *mordomo* very often neglected duties, possibly because he was elected monthly, which did not allow sufficient time to implement changes. Nurses had to reside within the hospital since they had to report for duty very early and leave the wards late. As the health of the patients greatly depended on the care of the nurse, the nurse had to follow the instructions of the doctors carefully and maintain cleanliness as important factor for the good health. The regulation of 1584 was valid upto mid eighteenth century subject to minor changes at the time of Ayres de Saldanha (1600-1603).

The Jesuits managed the Royal Hospital since 1579. They tried several times to give up the administration due to differences with the Government over financial and administrative matters. Jesuit superiors

Hospitals and Extension Services 123

wished their men to give up in 1583, but the Portuguese King would not agree to it as he was satisfied with their work. Nevertheless, they gave up the administration offering various excuses. In 1591 they took up the task again at the request of the King.[20] At this time the hospital was sanctioned a grant of 11,630 *pardaos*. Five years later the Jesuits severed their connection with the institution, because the Government had stopped providing them with necessary funds for the expenses of the hospital. The institution was again handed to the care of the *Santa Casa da Misericordia*.

Viceroy Mathias de Albuquerque proposed a new building for the Royal Hospital. The proposal was accepted in 1593 by the Portuguese King with a recommendation that the new building should be built on the grounds of the existing one and if necessary adjoining land should be acquired. However, the plan could not be implemented immediately.

It appears that the Government was running short of funds to spend on the proposed hospital building. This prompted the Portuguese king to grant license to some merchants to undertake a trip to China.[21] The money realized from this license was to be used for the new building. Finally, when the trip materialized the hospital was granted only 4,000 *xerafins*. Since the funds were insufficient another trip to China was proposed by the local Government.

In 1595 the Viceroy Mathias de Albuquerque issued some instructions to the Royal Hospital. It was stated that these instructions had the same powers as regulation issued by the crown. The purpose was to introduce discipline. It put to end many ills resulting from the visit of the relatives and friends to the sick. Apparently, the visitors still carried food to the patients and fire-arms inside the institution without the knowledge of the authorities.

Visits to the sick were restricted to the father and brothers. Since many of them had no families in India, it is quite possible that the sick felt lonely and depressed. Any other visitor who tried forcibly to enter the premises was to be arrested and detained by the doorkeeper After he was charge-sheeted by the clerk he was to be sent to the *Ouvidor Geral do Crime*. The guilty would be exiled to Daman for two years. Ward boys who were found carrying food to the wards were to be warned for the first time and then sent to the galleys. In case they were below 15 years of age they were to be beaten up. Letters from women other then from mother or sisters were not allowed. Even letters from mothers and sisters were censored by the nurses. Any other women sending letters were to be fined 10 *pardaos*. These precautions were followed in order not to disturb the sick. It was feared that letters could disturb the recovery of the patient by making him depressed and restless.[22] The doorkeeper who failed in the performance of his duties was to be exiled to Daman for two years.

The Jesuits once more undertook the administration of the hospital in 1597 as they received assurances of great punctuality in the payment of the grants required for its maintenance. The new building of the Royal Hospital was completed in 1609.

Jesuits made the Royal Hospital famous. Foreign travellers who visited Goa in the late sixteenth century and early seventeenth centuries were full of praises and considered the hospital better than some good hospitals of Portugal, Rome and Malta. Linschoten, the Dutch traveller speaks in flattering terms about the hospital. He says that "these Hospitals in India are very necessary for the Portingals, otherwise they should consume away like miserable men, but by ye means they are relieved, whatsoever they have, eyther sickness, secrete diseases, pockes, piles, or such like, there they are healed". [23]

By far the most detailed and interesting account of the hospital is the one provided by Pyrard a French traveller. In 1609, Pyrard was a patient in the hospital. He states that the hospital was the best in the world. The new building overlooking the Mandovi river and the nearby islands of Divar and Chorão, occupied a large area with courtyards and pleasant gardens where the sick could breath fresh air. The corridors were decorated with pictures, portraying scenes from the Bible.

The hospital had separate wards for various illnesses. Each patient was given a bed placed at a certain distance from one another. Cotton mattresses were piled one on the top of the other. Bedsteads were low, painted in different colours. Sheets were made of fine white cotton or silk. Pillows were of white calico. Bed linen was changed daily. Patients were also provided with pajamas, towel, handkerchief, *chinelos* (slippers) bedside table, paper fan, jug of water, chamber pot and other articles.

The hospital was a model of cleanliness. Every room was swept, cleaned and fumigated with incense twice a day and the walls were whitewashed twice a year. The nursing facilities were highly praised. Immediately after admission the patient was shaved and given a bath. Physicians, bleeders, barbers, apothecaries and priests visited the sick twice a day. The apothecary lived on the premises and his shop was well-stocked. Servants were obliged to treat the patients with courtesy and appear before them in clean clothes.

The diet in the Royal Hospital was of a high standard, consisting of variety of viands, fish, vegetables and sweets. Breakfast consisted of bread with raisins, *alvo* (a sweet dish made of wheat) and *canjee*. For

Hospitals and Extension Services

lunch patients were served a full or half boiled or roasted chicken and sweets. Dinner at five p.m. consisted of meat, soup, vegetables such as lady fingers and rice. In addition, the patients were served on doctor's prescription a variety of fish, eggs, fruits and bread. Patients could dine with their visitors for whom extra food was provided. Food was fresh and none of the left-over were served again.

Bleeding was a panacea for all kinds of fevers. Fevers, dysentery and syphilis were common in the hospital. The hospital had no running water. Water was brought by slaves from the springs of Banguenim. Convalescents were shifted to a convalescent ward. The hospital had a separate room for those on the verge of death so that their death throes did not upset other patients. Priests stayed with such patients until their end to provide spiritual care.[24]

The Royal Hospital was endowed by the Portuguese rulers with 25000 *pardaos*. It received also gifts from the Viceroy and Archbishop. These funds were large, considering the fact that the expenses were not high and food was cheap.

In spite of good food, comforts and hygiene, the mortality rate was high in the Royal Hospital. As mentioned earlier more than 1,500 patients died every year. The mortality rate was high due to the dearth of competent physicians and this continued for a long time. The situation led the Government to forbid the Chief Physician from practising in the hospital between 1607-1613.[25]

This famous hospital began to decay in the second half of the seventeenth century. Tavernier who visited the hospital during this period complained of negligence, corruption and high mortality rate.[26] The sick were given little meat. Helpers demanded payment even to bring a glass of water. Tavernier adds that besides the above factors, the system of bleeding the patient was responsible for the decline of the hospital. Dr. Fryer an English traveller, corroborates the statement of Tavernier. Patients were bled as many as forty times during their stay in the hospital.

A practice that may seem odd to us today was prescribed in the Royal Hospital as post-operative therapy — the urine therapy. The patient was asked to drink three glasses of cow's urine for twelve days after an operation. This was meant to recover his healthy colour and energy. It was believed that the urine of a cow had medicinal value. A patient had to stay in the hospital for twelve days even if he drank no urine.

In 1645 the hospital was granted 1,000 *xerafins* for its expenses on the patients.[27] The Jesuits who managed the hospital collected 12,000 *xerafins* from medical care provided to the patients.[28] In 1667 they were forbidden to accept patients other than soldiers.[29]

The Jesuits decided to give up the administration of the hospital by the end of the seventeenth century on the grounds that it was not proper to their ministry. By a royal letter dated 1688 the hospital was handed over to the missionaries of St. John of God. After some years it was handed back to the Jesuits who had proved to be good in the field of medicine. The Customs House (Alfandegas) contributed to the Hospital with two thirds of its revenue on goods brought from Maluco, China, Pegu, Bengal and Ceylon.[30]

The Jesuits took over once again the Royal Hospital in the early eighteenth century. During this period the hospital had no trained doctors. Whenever someone was sick, regardless of the illness, his feet were burnt with glowing iron till the flesh was raw. The patients were bled by making a deep cross-wise incision on their backs with a knife. Brother C. Matter who managed the hospital did not succeed in getting rid of these practices. However, he was successful in his fight against the custom of giving a purge of whole and half-a-pint which caused either strong vomiting or the loosening of the bowels. He prescribed only 3 to 4 ounces and recommended gentle sweating potions.[31] In 1730 the chief physician and the surgeon were deprived of their food and house rent allowances at the instigation of Jesuit administrators.[32] The hospital received an annual income of 1,300 *xerafins* from the Government.

Hospital Militar

In 1759 the Jesuits were sent away from Goa. The hospital was taken over by the Government and renamed *Hospital Militar* (Military Hospital). It was first shifted to St. Rock College in the city of Goa and from there to Old *Palacio (Casa de Polvora)* at Panelim on suggestion of Viceroy Conde de Ega.[33] The hospital was moved out of the city because the city of Goa had become a very unhealthy place. Many times seven to eight patients died daily in the hospital.[34]

A sum of 22,000 *xerafins* was spent in 1765 to set up this hospital at Panelim. It appears that besides providing care to the sick and selling medicine to private *boticas*, the hospital also gave loans to the local merchants.[35] Altogether 235 servicemen died in 1786 in the Military Hospital including 22 native soldiers of Goa.[36]

The Military Hospital was mismanaged by the staff appointed by the Government. They appropriated for themselves what had to be spent for the care of the patients. The staff was also involved in vices like gambling. The hospital had no trained doctors for a long period. Drugs imported from Europe reached Goa in adulterated state for several reasons. European manufacturers often sold drugs banned in the country. Some drugs reached Goa after the expiry date, while others were affected by long journeys and the weather.[37]

No discipline was observed in the Military Hospital. Patients were free to eat whatever they desired and cooked according to their taste. Food was served from 3 a.m. to 10 p.m. There were no restrictions on the movement of the patients. Visitors could carry alcohol for the sick and spend the nights with them. Nurses were incompetent. They left their work in the hands of many ward boys. Patients were seen moving around in dirty clothes. The hospital lacked hygiene. The Government did not implement any measures to end these undesirable activities and enforce discipline until the beginning of the nineteenth century. The Military Hospital was handed over to an Administrator and a Director. This Director was also the Chief Physician of the State. As per the orders of the home Government complete hygiene in the hospital was to be maintained by cleaning the wards and toilets twice a day. Patients were bathed on admission, except those suffering from fevers. They were forbidden to carry arms or play cards in the wards.

Patients with sores and suffering from leprosy were not admitted in the hospital. The regulation asked every physician to maintain a case paper for the sick. A prescription of medicine had to be kept on the bedside table. Physicians were permitted to ask for second opinion. Autopsy could be carried out if necessary. Every ward had a nurse, two ward boys and a Negro slave to care for the patients. The chief cook was responsible for the diets. In case mistakes were repeated by the cook more than two times, the cook was to be dismissed. No staff and patients could leave the hospital without prior permission of the Director.[38] Food from outside was not allowed inside the hospital. The changes improved the conditions of the hospital. A table given below provides a comparative study of number of patients who died from 1801 to 1805 with those who died between 1791-1795.[39]

Year	Deaths	Year	Deaths
1801	97	1791	338
1802	158	1792	269
1803	129	1793	248
1804	162	1794	179
1805	126	1795	190
Total	672		1214

It seems that the Chief Physician often interfered in the administration of the Military Hospital. In an order dated 8th February 1821 the Governor Conde do Rio Pardo asked the Chief Physician to refrain from such activities. Any complaints against the lower staff had to be brought to the notice of the Administrator for necessary action.[40]

In addition to food and clothing the patient in the hospital were supplied with free shaving cream and soap.[41] Their relatives who kept them company were provided with food and soap.[42] It is not surprising that the expenses exceeded the income. From January to March 1828 about 4,925 *xerafins*, 1 *tanga*, 3 1/2 *reis* were spent on food and other items. Expenses varied according to the season. For instance, just before the monsoons expenses were high as provisions were made for rainy season. In 1827 a total of 2,153 patients were treated in the hospital.[43]

Military Hospital continued to face serious problems in the third decade of the nineteenth century due to corruption, mismanagement and multiplicity of regulations. The government decided to reorganize the hospital. A committee was appointed to study the problem and to recommend new regulations. The outcome was yet another set of rules in 1830 covering various aspects of the administration.[44]

A Medical Board consisting of Chief Surgeon and other staff was constituted to improve the service conditions. The Board had to meet weekly to appoint lower staff on the advice of the Chief Physician and to check that the staff received their salary in time. Military personnel proceeding on sick leave had to appear before the Board. The decision of the Board in this matter was final and binding even on the Central Government. For instance, in 1833 João de Souza, Captain of Garrison of Mozambique was sick in the Military Hospital of Goa. He was ordered by the Portuguese king to return to Portugal immediately in a ship known as *Princesa Real*. The captain who could not undertake the long journey approached the Board to declare him unfit. The Medical Health Board upheld the request and issued him the necessary certificate declaring him unfit to travel.[45]

The Military Hospital was run by an administrator, a distinguished official who was paid in addition to his salary, a gratuity of 120 *xerafins*. The regulation of 1830 made provisions for the following staff: One Chief Physician, one Assistant Physician, one Chief Surgeon and one Assistant Surgeons who were helped by nurses.[46] The Chief Physician recommended and checked medicine imported from Europe and other parts of Asia. He had to maintain a journal describing the illness and treatment prescribed to the patients. Physicians were bound by the regulation to visit

Hospitals and Extension Services

the wards daily in the morning. One of them together with the surgeon had to be on duty for six hours. Cleanliness and maintenance of surgical instruments was the responsibility of the Chief Surgeon.

The Military Hospital had different wards for fever, surgery, V.D. and convalescence. Interestingly fever ward was isolated from the others. The fever ward had a nurse for every 30 patients. Attached to the ward was a bathroom. The beds were arranged four feet apart from each other. Bed linen was changed weekly. Each ward was provided with separate linen that could not be interchanged. The walls of the wards were white-washed every six months. Its floor was swabbed with lime every fortnight. Wards were fumigated with nitric acid.[47]

The dead bodies of the patients were kept in a mortuary until they were certified dead by the Chief Physician. Their clothing was disinfected. In case a patient died of a contagious disease, his mattress was destroyed.

Diet for the patients was prepared by the Chief Physician. Officials had better diet then the soldiers. The hospital had eight types of diets.[48] The records of the hospital indicate that food was also provided for the lower staff. Physicians could prescribe upto 4 ounces of fenny and Portuguese wine to the patients. Food was tested before it was served to the patients.

The Military Hospital catered to the needs of the armed forces. The civilians employed in the Government agencies could also avail themselves of the facilities. From January to October 1830 a total of 2,230 military men and 175 civilians received treatment in the hospital.[49] In the year 1832 about 59 patients died in the hospital and of these thirty patients were Europeans, four were Portuguese born in Goa and the remaining were natives.[50]

Just as the hospital lacked proper medical care it also lacked water supply which was essential for the maintenance of hygiene. Water was scarce. It was carried from Banguenim. This water was used for drinking and in preparation of medicine. For other purposes the hospital used water from the wells.

Large sums of money were spent on edible goods. These commodities were imported from across the border. During a period of ten months among other food stuff more than 10,884 chickens, 292 *arrobas* of beef, 50 *khandis* of rice, 15,018 mangoes, 737 eggs, 40 *khandis* of wheat, 346 *arrobas* of fish, 11,900 pickled mangoes, 88 *almudes* of wine, 121 *almudes* of fenny were consumed in the hospital.[51] The income for the same period was 26,549 *xerafins*, 4 *tangas* and 11 *reis*. The expenditure of the hospital amounted to 24,216 *xerafins*.

Surgical instruments were imported from Portugal. In September 1831, the hospital sold medicine worth 447:3:291 including *salsaparilha*, *neem* syrup and crabs eyes.[52] In the year 1832 total of 28,733 *xerafins*, 3 *tangas* and 2 *reis* were spent on the salaries of the staff. The administrator drew a salary of 1,584 *xerafins*. The Chief Surgeon received 2,000 *xerafins* a year.[53] The income and expenditure chart for the 1838 shows that income was 20,819 *xerafins* and *reis*. The expenditure for the period was 19,985 *xerafins* and 9 *reis*.[54] The income for the following year was 27,348 *xerafins*, 3 *tangas* and 56 *reis* and the expenditure 23,673 *xerafins*, 3 *tangas* and 56 *reis*.[55]

The regulation of 1830 made it clear that the hospital was primarily for servicemen and ex-servicemen. Others including the natives could be admitted with prior permission from the Government. The number of patients who availed treatment at the Military Hospital in the year 1830 was 2,256.[56]

Medical care at this hospital continued to be poor leading to high mortality rate. The situation forced the Government to appoint a Committee to investigate the complaint made by one Alferes Xisto Antonio Barata Feio regarding poor care on the part of the staff. Among others the warden Fr. Mariano de Maria Santissima is mentioned. The committee felt that Fr. Santissima being a missionary should have shown greater zeal and dedication. The verdict of the inquiry was against the warden. He was dismissed from the job and his superior was informed. Two nurses, Fillipe Jose da Silva and Antonio Sebastião Carvalho, were also dismissed for neglecting their duties.[57]

The physicians and the surgeons in the hospital blamed the military authorities for the high mortality rate. They argued that military authorities sent patients in serious conditions to the hospital. Many were admitted only to die, while others had to undergo prolonged treatment resulting in extra expenses to the public treasury. Therefore, they made a plea to the Government to stop such practice.[58]

Subsequently, in January 1840 the Government passed yet another regulation for the Military Hospital. The main purpose of this regulation was to control expenses, define the duties of the hospital staff and provide better care to the soldiers. However, these changes increased the expenses of the hospital.[59]

A Council for Military Health replaced the existing Medical Board. The new Council consisted of Chief Physician, Chief Surgeon and one assistant surgeon of the hospital. It had to manage the hospital and

Hospitals and Extension Services

supervise the teaching of medicine in the hospital. Besides government subsidy, the hospital received income from a farm. The hospital still lacked many facilities including operation theater, running water, drainage system and a morgue. Perhaps these facilities could not be introduced due to paucity of funds.

In 1842 the Military Hospital was shifted from Panelim to the residence of Dom Joaquim Christovam de Noronha in Panjim for reasons of convenience. It is here that formal teaching of medicine was started. The building still exists and houses one of the departments of Goa Medical College.

The hospital had capacity for 90 beds distributed in seven wards. All wards except two were on the first floor. The two wards on the ground floor were reserved for natives and prisoners. Interestingly, there were separate bathrooms for Christian and Hindu patients. It had no running water and drainage system. Drinking water was brought to the hospital from a spring in the city.[60]

Between 1840-1844 a total of 9,016 patients were admitted, of these 7,189 left the hospital cured and 185 died of various diseases including dysentery and fevers.[61] During the second semester of 1849 about 300 patients were treated for all kinds of fevers.[62] The hospital experimented with different types of herbal medicine. *Salsaparilha* was used for skin problems, venereal diseases and rheumatism.[63]

Hospital Regimental/Escolar/Central

Hospital Militar was handed over in December 1851 to *Conselho Administrativo de Regimento d'Artilheria* and was renamed *Hospital Regimental*.[64] From 1863 to 1867 a total of 20,938 patients were admitted in *Hospital Regimental*. The death rate amounted to 240. About 115 patients were treated in June 1864 for malarial fevers.[65] Their number went up in August of the same year.

Venereal diseases were common in Goa at the end of the nineteenth century particularly among the soldiers and prostitutes.[66] A clinic was started for such victims in 1896 attached to the *Hospital Regimental*. The clinic was managed by a doctor, nurse and servants. Nearly 25 people were treated for syphilis at the clinic in the first year.

A report from the Health Services dated 1920-1921 states that the hygienic conditions of the Hospital were poor.[67] By the third decade of this century *Hospital Regimental* was known as *Hospital Central Hospital Escolar*. This institution was always overflowing with patients from

Goa and neighbouring areas.[68] The hospital had facilities for 75 beds but many a time it accommodated even 115 patients at a time. They had to sleep on the floor due to lack of beds. A total of 1,817 patients were treated in the hospital during the year 1945. This number in 1959 had gone up to 2,950 patients.

St. Lazarus Hospital

Lepers were seen moving in the streets of the city of Goa in the early sixteenth century with no one to take care of them. In those days leprosy was an incurable disease. Persons suffering of the disease were ostracized by the society. This state of affairs forced the authorities to start in 1530 an isolation hospital on the eastern boundary of the city of Goa dedicated to St. Lazarus.[69] The hospital was subsidized by the Goa Municipal Council (*Senado de Goa*) and the Holy House of Mercy. Later patients suffering from other contagious diseases such as smallpox were also isolated in the hospital.[70]

Hospital For The Poor (*Hospital dos Pobres*)

Institutional medical care of the native inhabitants of the city of Goa was organized by missionaries and social agencies.

The Confraternity of Holy Faith which was founded in 1541 made provisions for setting up a hospital for the poor. The Jesuits executed what was envisaged by the Confraternity. The hospital existed around 1546.

Fr. Paul Camarte of the Society of Jesus bestowed great care on the *Hospital dos Pobres*. This was the first institution to cater to the needs of the native inhabitants of all creeds. Initially, the hospital was started for native Christians,[71] but in course of time non Christians were also admitted.[72] The institution was well organized and clean. It could accommodate 40 patients at a time. There were separate wards for men and women. Fr. Camarte was helped by other Jesuits and eight servants. It had a full time barber who shaved, bled and applied sucking-glass to the patients. The hospital used imported *Pão da China* to cure wounds and running sores. The hospital had a good kitchen, where food was cooked for the sick with great care. The funeral of those who died in the hospital was performed by the Jesuits.

No hospital existed outside the city of Goa. The Jesuits who were given the charge of Salcete in south Goa, shifted their *Hospital dos*

Hospitals and Extension Services

Pobres from the city of Goa to Margão. This shift took place after 1568. There are differences of opinions about exact date.[73] Later it was moved to Rachol, a village in Salcete.

The inhabitants of Salcete and other neighbouring areas flocked to the hospital to find cure at the hands of Bro. Afonso a well known practitioner of western medicine.[74] The 30-40 bed hospital was renowned as charitable institution. When the armies of Adil Shah overran Salcete, they burned and destroyed churches and schools but left the hospital intact. In 1630 the subsidy of 300 *pardaos* was raised to 600 *pardaos* on account of inflation.[75]

The Jesuits had also an infirmary attached to their College of St. Paul in the city of Goa. At the start of the eighteenth century the College infirmary consisted 17 single rooms and one hall. Each patient had his own special Indian attendant. An average of 20 to 24 patients were housed in the infirmary. To cover the great expenses they started a coconut plantation.[76]

Hospital of all Saints (*Hospital de Todos os Santos*)

Hospital of All Saints for the Poor commonly known as *Hospital da Misericordia* was started by Holy House of Mercy *(Santa Casa da Misericordia de Goa)*. It is difficult to pin-point the exact date of the establishment of this hospital. The hospital existed in the early decades of the Portuguese rule. The institution catered to the needs of the Portuguese mestiços and the native Christians who suffered from incurable diseases. The subsidy it received from the Government was too small to meet the expenses.

In the early seventeenth century Hospital da Misericordia which was housed not far from St. Paul's college in the city of Goa was shifted to a new building. In 1612 the hospital was presented with a set of regulations to improve the condition of the hospital.[77] This regulation of 1612 made provision for a superintendent, physicians, surgeons, nurses, chaplains, barber, bleeder and clerk. The Superintendent had to manage the hospital, procure provisions and maintain the accounts.[78] The physician who was paid 15 *xerafins* a month had to examine the patients before admission and provide treatment during their stay in the hospital. The dispensing of medicine was supervised by the physician. The surgeon was paid 12 *xerafins* a month. He did not have much work as very few operations were performed. However, the surgeon had to reside within hospital premises.[79]

Nurses were expected to be cordial. Their duties included the maintenance of cleanliness and supervision of the lower staff. Servants on night duty were asked to sleep in the wards so that they would be available in an emergency. The staff of the hospital was expected to seek prior permission of the Superintendent to leave the premises. Visitors were allowed during the day time. They were strictly checked in case they carried alcohol into the wards.

The overall supervision of the *Hospital da Misericordia* was entrusted to a Board consisting of Superintendent, Director of the hospital and the assistant physician. The Board met on 5th of every month to discuss the problems of the institution and to appoint the lower staff whenever required. Some of the personal needs of the sick were taken care of by the barber who visited the hospital once a week and by a washerman who came every 10 days.

There were separate wards for male and female patients. Women were not permitted to visit male ward and vice versa. The legislation of 1612 banned rearing of pigs, hens and pigeons in the hospital compound. It appears this was the practice earlier. It was considered unhygienic.

In 1630 the hospital received new set of statutes. According to this order, the Superintendent was elected every month. The *Fidalgos* resented the nature of the appointment. The Superintendent was now obliged to accompany the physicians and the surgeons on their rounds of the wards.

He was entrusted with several duties such as buying provisions to the hospital, making payment to the staff, keeping accounts and issuing instructions to the apothecary and the cook. The Superintendent was instructed to use only old bedsheets to cover the dead bodies.

Food served to the patients was wholesome and clean. No patient was allowed to carry food, cash or any other article inside the hospital. Any belongings were to be deposited at the reception. The new regulation forbade the admission of Portuguese and the slaves in the hospital. The former had a hospital exclusively for themselves in the city of Goa. Slaves who found their way in the hospital were to be returned to their master by the Superintendent.[80] The statutes fixed the salary of the hospital staff. Male servants were paid 4 *bazarucos* each in addition to food. The doorkeeper received 8 *xerafins* and a bleeder was paid 5 *xerafins* a month.[81]

In 1681 *Hospital da Misericordia* was merged with *Hospital de N.Sra. de* Piedade. Few years later *Hospital da Misericordia* faced several problems due to paucity of funds. Expenses exceeded the income. To stop

Hospitals and Extension Services

extra expenditure the hospital stopped providing the patients with bread, chicken, confectioneries and tobacco. The strength of the hospital beds were reduced to 12 beds with only a male and female nurse for respective wards. The post of the sacristan was abolished. These changes were effective from 1775.

The building in which the hospital was accommodated began to decay around 1822, as a result it was transferred to the old house *Real Estanco do Tabaco* and from here to the convents of St. John of God and Santa Barbara. In the year 1851 *Hospital da Misericordia* was shifted from the convent of Santa Barbara in the city of Goa to Ribandar. The building still exists and a hospital is run by the Government. The hospital was shifted from the city of Goa as the place had become unhealthy. The building in the city of Goa was surrounded by thick trees. It could accommodate only eight patients. The hygienic conditions of the hospital were poor as the staff took no interest in the cleanliness of the place. Besides many malpractice took place in the institution. For example many times the apothecary would replace drugs in good conditions supplied by *Santa Casa* with adulterated ones bought at low prices so that he could resell at higher rates. The hospital spent a total sum of 5,555 *xerafins* annually with just eight patients.

Another regulation was introduced in the *Hospital da Misericordia* in the early twentieth century. The regulation of 1902 made arrangements for the treatment of 40 patients. Twenty of these patients would receive free treatment if they submitted a certificate issued by the Parish priest or *Regedor* stating that they were economically backward. The rest of the patients were to be charged 10 *tangas* daily, besides a deposit of Rs. 30 at the time of admission. A concession was made to the members of the Holy House of Mercy and their families.[82] The regulation provided for two wards for surgery, one for medicine, one for contagious diseases and one for the mentally ill. One of the two private rooms reserved for women from the two institutions run by Holy House of Mercy namely *Recollhimento de N. Sra. de Serra* and *Santa Maria Magdalena*.

A case paper was attached to every bed.[83] This system does not exist even today in many hospitals in Goa. Besides their routine duties the nurses had also to dress the corpse and ready it for burial. The cook of the hospital had a rather odd duty of carrying the dead to the cemetery. This was probably in case of destitute patients. To meet the needs of the increasing number of patients a post of assistant physician was created. This physician was responsible for maintaining case papers of the patients. He could ask for a second opinion on critical cases or cases requiring surgery. The assistant physician had to reside in the hospital premises or in the *Recolhimento de Serra*. Earlier physicians used to stay away from the hospital and could not reach the sick in time due to poor transport facilities. In 1902 the hospital had a housekeeper directly responsible to the Director. The housekeeper was helped by a number of servants. The hospital had a chaplain and a sacristan who worked as doorkeeper.

In the early twentieth century a ward *Enfermaria Anibal Mendes* was opened in the *Hospital da Misericordia*. The ward was established to treat patients suffering from tuberculosis. It was under the care of a doctor and four nurses.[84] A total of 1,149 patients were treated in the *Hospital da Misericordia* during the year 1941.[85]

Hospital of Our Lady of Piety (*Hospital de N. Sra. de Piedade*)

Conde de Linhares the Viceroy of Goa (1629-1635) started this hospital around 1631.[86] The hospital was run by Carmelite missionaries. For reasons of economy and convenience this hospital was merged with *Hospital da Misericordia* in 1681. This institution received a sum of 840 *xerafins* from the Municipal Council of Goa. This came from the interest on 12,000 *xerafins* left behind by Conde de Linhares by way of an endowment to the Hospital of Our Lady of Piety. In addition the hospital received a rent from the houses occupied by tailors in the city of Goa. These houses belonged to the State.[87]

There are also references to two other hospitals in the city of Goa. One was managed by the Dominican missionaries. It was established in mid seventeenth century to help destitutes suffering from the effects of the famine of 1630. A list of medicine and expenses in the Goa Archives indicates that there was hospital attached to the Convent of St. John of God in the city of Goa between 1732-1733.[88]

Lady West who visited Goa in December 1824 along with her husband Sir Edward West (King's judge under the East India Company) mentions in her diary a hospital on the way to Cabo. This hospital according to her was kept in repair by the English East Company. Further she writes that many soldiers were treated there 7 years earlier. No other information to support this statement has been found so far.[89]

INSTITUTIONAL CARE IN RURAL GOA

Rural Bardez had few Hospices aided by private individuals. Franciscan missionaries established Hospices in some villages of Bardez. These hospices were probably established to provide care to the old missionaries of the Franciscan society.

One of the Hospices known as *Hospicio dos Desamparados* was situated at Monte de Guirim. There was a Hospice for the deaf and needy at Pomburpa. Hospice of O.L. of Health Valverde, was maintained with donations left behind by Baltazar de Souza. The hospice existed as late as 1797.[90] In 1804 this hospice run by Franciscans was used as convalescent home for the Friars of St. Francis Friary and St. Bonaventura's College.[91] Franciscan missionaries had another Hospice at Penha de França run with the funds kept by Ana Azavedo which in 1776 amounted to 444 *xerafins*.[92] It appears that the Franciscans also managed the Hospice of O.L. of the Angels at Rachol an old garrison town of Salcete. This hospice existed in mid-eighteenth century. In January 1829, the hospice had only one inmate Bro. Jeronymo de S. Francisco.[93]

Asilo dos Milagres

Perhaps the first institution in Mapuça in the nineteenth century to offer free treatment to the poor was *Asilo de N. Sra. dos Milagres*. The institution established in 1875 by some priests was housed in two buildings.[94] One for the invalids and the second one situated in an isolated locality housed the lepers, and later tuberculosis patients.[95] In 1915 the Leprosarium of Asilo dos Milagres had 40 patients. Attached to the Asilo was the *Dispensario Dr. Daniel Gelasio* In this clinic the needy received free medicine. The foundation stone of Asilo Hospital was laid on 16th April 1923.[96] Asilo was maintained with the help of lotteries.

Hospicio do Sagrado Coração

Hospital for the Poor in Salcete run by the Jesuits ceased to exist after the Jesuits left Goa in 1759. It appears there was no other hospital in Salcete, except the *Hospicio of O.L. of Angels* until 1867.

In the year 1867 Fr. Antonio João de Miranda started a ten bed *Hospicio do Sagrado Coração* in Margão.[97] In course of time the 4 room Hospice was expanded with the help of lotteries. A total of 1,172 patients received treatment in 1941. The right to issue lotteries was discontinued in 1947.

In 1959 the Hospicio revised the fees charged to the patients. A patient in a first class room was charged 18 *escudos* in addition to the expenses incurred on medicine, food, doctors and surgeons. A patient admitted in room was charged 12 *escudos* besides the above mentioned expenses. Similarly patients in the wards with reserved bed paid 3 *escudos* and 50% of expenses incurred on medicine and food. Poor patients were charged 3 *escudos* but were provided with free food, medicine, surgery and facilities for testing blood.

Women admitted for delivery were charged extra. In a first class room they paid 30 *escudos* in a second class room 18 *escudos* and in a third class room 12 *escudos*. Fifty percent of this income was paid to the midwife as allowances.

Asilo de S. Francisco Xavier da Ilha de Divar

This Asilo was set up on 13th January 1884 by Simão Vicente Quadros with the help of donations collected from British India and a lottery. This institution was closed down by 1930.[98]

Asilo de N. Sra. de Piedade

Asilo de Sra. de Piedade was situated at Quepem. It was established to take care of the poor patients of Quepem taluka. In 1930 the institution had a fund of Rs. 1,500 and was managed by a committee consisting of Fr. Luis Filipe Ataide, Abilio Sousa, Anastasio Mascarenhas and Manuel de Piedade Monteiro.[99]

Hospicio do Clero

The foundation stone of this Hospicio at Margão was laid on 15th November 1925.[100] It came into existence due to the initiative of Fr. Manuel João Socrates de Albuquerque who was concerned about the plight of the old priests. The idea came to him when he visited an old priest at *Albergue* in Margão and saw its conditions. *Hospicio do Clero* was provided with rules on 18th October 1928. This institution had rooms for the aged priests who wished to live there, holiday room for those priests who wished to have a change of environment and a ward for the sick. It is situated opposite *Hospicio do Sagrado Coraçáo*.

ISOLATION HOSPITALS

In the early twentieth century Goa had no special hospitals to isolate and

Hospitals and Extension Services 139

treat patients suffering form tuberculosis, leprosy and mental illness.

Tuberculosis was a disease rare in Goa till the end of the nineteenth century. The rapid spread of the disease after the beginning of the twentieth century was due to emigration of Goans to British India and the introduction of railways in Goa.

The disease prevailed in Bardez and Salcete. The disease accounted for large number of deaths. Tuberculosis was incurable in those days. In the absence of an isolation hospital, patients were isolated in their homes in a room away from family quarters or in an out-house. *Santa Casa da Misericordia de Goa* had a ward *Enfermaria Anibal Mendes* for T.B. patients attached to its hospitals in the early years of the present century. This ward catered mainly to the needs of the mestiços and the Portuguese. It was situated behind *Hospital da Misericordia*. The ward had a 24 bed accommodation which was later increased to 40 beds. The ward was always overcrowded.

The first sanatorium was established in the early 1940s at Margão. This sanatorium dedicated to S. Jose was attached to *Hospicio do Sagrado Coração* a second sanatorium was started in 1949 at St. Inez, Panjim.[101] However, another source states that it was started as early as 1947.[102] This sanatorium was run by *Provedoria de Assistencia Publica* with the help of two doctors, 3 nurses, one mechanic to look after X rays machine and 3 servants. The dispensary was only one of such kind in Ilhas. The dispensary *Virgem Peregrina* is today a full-fledged T.B. Hospital with separate wards for men, women and patients in advanced stage of the disease.

The mentally ill in the nineteenth century, were either treated at the Military Hospital or sent to special institutions in British India.[103] Many times as late as 1922, due to lack of accommodation at the Military Hospital the mentally ill were jailed.[104] The British Government in India demanded exorbitant sums from the Portuguese Government to provide treatment for mentally ill from Goa in their institutions. This factor prompted the local Government to help two institutions in Goa namely *Hospital da Misericordia* and *Hospicio do Sagrado Coração* wards were too small to meet the needs of the inhabitants. *Hospital da Misericordia* could accommodate only 8 patients. Furthermore, the mentally ill patients disturbed the peace of other patients in the above mentioned institutions. This problem forced the Government to plan for an Asylum in the island of Rats. But the plan could not be implemented due to paucity of funds.[105] Finally it was not until 1930 that the Government set up an Asylum for the mentally ill at Chimbel (Ilhas).[106]

Asilo dos Alienados

Asilo dos Alienados (Asylum for the Mentally ill) was started at old *Recolhimento* of Chimbel to accommodate 20 patients. Sixteen beds were reserved for the economically backward classes. The institution was managed by *Santa Casa da Misericordia*.[107]

Asilo dos Alienados received its first statutes in November 1930.[108] The institution was maintained with a grant of Rs. 4,000 from the State and a subsidy from three institutions of charities: *Santa Casa da Misericordia de Goa*, *Hospicio da Sagrado Coração*, Margão, *Asilo dos Milagres*, Mapuça. The first two contributed with equal share of Rs. 10,000 each and the last one Rs. 4,000 The expenses could not exceed Rs. 25,000.

In those days no trained psychiatrists were available in Goa. The treatment in the Asylum was poor. The staff often resorted to physical force as a means to treat and control the patients. Even though the regulation of 1930 specified that great cleanliness should be maintained in the institution little attention was paid to such details.[109] The need for female nurses to care for female patients was satisfied in 1935 with the creation of two posts of female nurses.[110] In November 1947 the Asylum was handed over to *Provedoria de Assistencia Publica*.

The Mental Asylum received another set of rules in 1948. The number of the staff was increased. Doctors were instructed to visit the patients daily. Maintenance of cleanliness, supervision of food and dispensing of medicine was the responsibility of the warden. He was in charge of opening and closing the cells at fixed times. In those days the mentally ill were kept under lock liked caged animals. A special watch was kept on those with suicidal tendencies.

The staff of the Asylum was paid a fixed salary and a monthly pension in case they were injured by a patient. This pension was transferable to their families in the event of death.[111]

In the early 1950s the facilities at the Asylum continued to be unsatisfactory. Patients were given bare minimum. They slept on the floor with a mat and a pillow. The Asylum lacked sanitation, running water, drainage system and bathrooms. The patients had their bath by the well side. The diet varied in accordance with inmate's status. The Europeans were given a better diet. The natives were given rice curry and fish. Tea was served without milk. Besides medication, no other treatment was provided to the sick.

In 1958 *Asilo dos* Alienados was renamed *Hospital Abade Faria* and

Hospitals and Extension Services

handed over to the Health Services.[112] The Asylum was shifted to Panjim. A neuro-psychiatrist Dr. Adelia Costa was given the charge of the institution. Under her many changes were introduced to meet the needs of 250 patients. Hygiene and general sanitation was greatly improved. Patients were now provided with a bed, mattress, pillows and linen. Bed linen was changed as often as necessary. Patients were given baths more frequently. Their families were encouraged to take home those patients who had improved in health and were capable of leading a normal life. To help these patients an out-patient department was opened so that they could come for consultations and treatment. The out-patient department was open thrice a week and on average 70 patients were attended every week. Electroencephalograph was introduced to treat those patients who did not respond to medication.

The hospital in its new premises had five sections: occupational therapy section, asylum section, dispensary, section for infectious diseases and a section for neurological patients. The hospital received a total sum of 6,60,000$00 in 1959 from the exchequer. During this period additional staff was appointed including 3 assistant doctors, 2 male nurses, 2 female nurses, 2 assistant nurses and a technician in charge of encephalography.

The year 1930 marked the establishment of another isolation hospital for the victims of leprosy.[113] Earlier leprosy patients were sheltered at *Asilo de N. Sra. dos Milagres*. The *Leprosaria Central* at Macazana; in Salcete was the brain child of Dr. Froilano de Mello, a distinguished Goan doctor who was the Director of the Health Services. The institution was started with funds provided by the State to the tune of Rs. 27,677 and donations collected by Dr. de Mello through various cultural activities. Expenses on food were to be met by *Santa Casa da Misericordia* and *Hospicio de Sagrado Coraçao*. These two institutions had the privilege of issuing lotteries. Three blocks with 3 wards each could accommodate a total of 150 patients. Surprisingly, Hindus suffering of leprosy refused to share a ward with Christian patients. Therefore a separate ward was started for the Hindus. Because the lepers were shunned by the society and stigma was attached to the disease the patients preferred to stay in the institution often cured. In 1959 the Health Services took over this hospital.

Private Nursing Homes

Private nursing homes mushroomed in Salcete and Bardez in the third and fourth decade of the present century. Some of these nursing homes were situated in villages. They were the outcome of enterprising efforts of some Goan doctors.

The first maternity home in Goa was started by Dr. Luis Alvares in Margão. Dr. Alvares a graduate of Grant Medical College, desired to set up a hospital similar to the ones existing in Bombay. On account of financial constraints he had to be content with a modest maternity home. In those days Goan women, even of upper strata were reluctant to avail themselves of the hospital facilities for their deliveries. On account of this attitude Dr. Alvares Maternity Home was limited to perform minor surgeries for many years.

This *Consultorio Dr. Luis Alvares de Cirurgia e Obstetrecia* was founded in 1924 with 3 private rooms and a ward to accommodate nine patients. It was expanded in 1942 with a new ward for men and the appointment of additional staff. The nursing home was renamed *Casa de Saude do Dr. Luis Alvares* and still exists under the same name.

In the early 1930s Dr. Simon T. Paul hailing from British India started a nursing home at Gogol (Margão). Dr. Paul with a team of two doctors and an untrained anesthetist and two untrained nurses performed surgeries in the branch of Gynaecology. In 1941 *Centro Maternal Miguel Gracias* was started in Margão by Dr. Antonio Gracias with 15 beds. Today the rebuilt nursing home has a capacity for 30 patients.

Probably the first nursing home in a Goan village was started by a husband-wife team of doctors, João Costa Pereira and Adeline de Souza, both graduates from Grant Medical College, Bombay. They established their nursing home in 1931 at Sirlim in Chinchinim (Salcete) with 10 beds. The nursing home was shifted to Margão in 1961. The new premises could accommodate 32 patients. It had six private rooms and four nurses. E.N.T. and eye surgery were performed . Incidentally Dr. Costa Pereira was one of the first Goan E.N.T. surgeons to practice in Goa.

Orlim in Salcete had two nursing homes in late 1930s. The first was opened by Dr. Silvano Rebello in 1937. This nursing home closed down within ten years. The second nursing home *Hospital de N.Sra. de Conceição* was started by Dr. Samiro Vas. The hospital was housed in three cottages close to one another and could accommodate 35 patients.

Soon after World War II rural Salcete had one more nursing home at S. Jose Areal. It was started with only 8 beds. Later the number was raised to 30 beds. Dr. Feleciano Reis Falção, the founder of this home was assisted by two untrained nurses and a servant. A special feature of this *Casa de Saude* was that both major and minor surgeries were performed with local anesthesia.

It is clear from the information gathered that there were at least four nursing homes in Bardez during the last decade of the Portuguese rule in Goa. However, *Anuario Estatistico da India Portuguesa* (1956) states that Bardez had only 2 nursing homes. One of these was a nursing cum maternity home.

Perhaps the first private maternity home in rural north Goa was the one established by Dr. Antonio Menino Machado at Saligão (Bardez). This maternity home named *Clinic Ave Maria* had four private rooms and a ward. Dr. Machado worked in his clinic until his death on 8th March 1965. The clinic remained closed for several years. The nursing home is now sold to another doctor and is under renovation.

Dr. Olencio da Gama Pinto started in mid 1930s a four bed nursing home at his residence at Anjuna (Bardez). In a tiny village of Porvorim, Dr. Antonio Pinto do Rosario started a maternity home with 10 beds and a single nurse. The following year Dr. Olavo Ribeiro opened a hospital to accommodate 20 patients. *Remanso* was another nursing home established soon after by Dr. Francisco Correia at Mapuça. These institutions continued to function upto 1961 and many of them still exist.

Panjim had only one nursing home in 1957. The nursing home was established by Dr. Bhandari with 15 beds. Apparently this was the first private nursing home in Ilhas taluka.

Most of the nursing homes in Goa were small in size They lacked proper equipment, trained nurses and auxiliary personnel. They had no running water, proper drainage system and electricity. These nursing homes received no aid from the Government. In 1920 a demand was made through a local newspaper *Vidiaprassar* to establish nursing wards in all talukas of New Conquests. No measures were taken in this direction by the state authorities.

A government order dated October 1959 granted a sum of 6,000$00 to the two regional hospitals at Ponda and Sanguem. Similar hospitals existed at Pernem, Satari and Canacona.

EXTENSION SERVICES

Extension medical services were those available outside hospitals in the form of Health Services, apothecaries, dentists, midwives and others. These facilities left much to be desired and barely met the needs of the majority of the local population.

Soon after the Portuguese captured Goa, they introduced the western system of medicine. This medicine was available to the ruling urban class. However, in 1519 a royal *alvara* decreed that the Chief Physician of the State should provide free medical aid to the poor converted Christians of the city of Goa. Apparently, the purpose of the order was to give certain privileges to the newly converted people and at the same time to act as an incentive to the would be converts.[114] From the beginning the Portuguese rulers appointed a Chief Physician. However the Portuguese doctors who came to Goa were few and inexperienced in tropical medicine. Goa as mentioned earlier did not attract the cream of Portuguese medical profession. This set of professionals held a complete sway over the health services. At the same time the colonial rulers created conditions that led to the decay and degeneration of the traditional native health practices, particularly the ayurvedic medicine that prevailed in Goa when the Portuguese arrived. Scarcity of doctors forced the Government to grant licenses to various individuals with some experience, to practise as doctors. Those who wished to obtain certificates had to pay 100 *xerafins* in addition to what they paid privately to the Chief Physician.[115] The practice of granting licenses was stopped in 1838. During later period graduates from Bombay, Calcutta and Madras Universities were permitted to practise in Goa.[116]

Various factors compelled the Portuguese to start formal education in medicine in 1842. Physicians who graduated from this school were general practitioners. There was acute shortage of specialists. Majority of native population resorted to indigenous medicine. The sick were treated at home.

Apothecaries and male nurses often practised as doctors due to dearth of trained physicians. They were in great demand and are reported to have cured complicated diseases. There were constant conflicts between them and the existing physicians, probably because the former encroached on latter's field of activity, thus contributing to damage their material interest. This resulted in many injunctions from the Government against apothecaries, evidently at the instigation of the physicians. Shortage of apothecaries around 1864 forced the Government to grant permission to certain individuals to open drugstores (*boticas*) in the villages.

New Conquests had no trained doctors, in the first half of the nineteenth century excepting the military surgeons at Ponda, Bicholim and Pernem. In mid nineteenth century Goa had a total of 135 doctors. The medical personnel clustered around towns. A number of factors contributed to the lack of physicians in rural areas. City life was more attractive. Rural areas lacked amenities of city and towns. Due to the growing

Hospitals and Extension Services

shortage of trained doctors in Goa graduates from Bombay and Calcutta universities were permitted to practise in Goa. This measure did not solve the problem. In fact the situation deteriorated after 1838 when the Portuguese Government stopped granting license to the native practitioners.

In 1895 a post of *Delegado de Saude* (Health Officer) was created for every taluka.[117] They had a number of functions to perform, such as to provide free medical treatment to the poor, submit monthly reports about the health conditions in their taluka, inspect pharmacies and restaurants from time to time and carry out preventive measures against diseases that erupted in an epidemic form. [118]

Embarbacem with 26,118 inhabitants had only one doctor in the early twentieth century. Goa had 186 doctors and out of these 178 practised in the Old Conquests and only 8 in the New Conquests. In 1910 the Government was planning to abolish the post of Health Officer of Agonda created in 1907. The inhabitants of Agonda, Sinquerim and Nerul sent a petition to the Government not to take such step as these areas lacked medical assistance.[119] Another doctor was appointed at Curpem (Sanguem taluka) in 1908.[120] In 1917 a doctor was appointed at Mardol (Ponda).[121] In 1921 Sanguem had two trained doctors for a population of about 20,000 whilst Satari during the same period had one doctor for 17,313 inhabitants. The situation did not improve much in the early 1930s in Sanguem taluka. It had only 3 doctors — one Health Officer, one *Medico do Partido* de Curpem and another private practitioner.

By 1945 Velhas Conquistas with a population of 2,98531 inhabitants had 312 doctors who practised privately. It meant 948 inhabitants per doctor. New Conquests had 36 doctors for a population of 2,06,750. That is about 5,743 inhabitants per doctor. The number of physicians and pharmacists went up.

The Health Services were looked after by a Director who was assisted by an Inspector of Medical Services, two pharmacists, the teaching staff of the medical school and the health officers. Medical school was linked with Health Services right from its inception. In 1945 the school was separated from the Health Services. It became an autonomous body.

There was a shortage of trained nurses and midwives for a long time. Girls from higher classes hardly ever joined this profession. Work outside the home was commonly regarded as unsuitable for any women other than those of the lower classes. Fortunately this attitude changed in course of time. Between 1917-1926 a total of 50 women were trained as midwives. Nursing was not well developed under Portuguese rule. The conditions of the nurses were deplorable. They received low pay. Nurses were usually drawn from low class because of the nature of their work. In the later part of the Portuguese regime eight sanitary posts in charge of male nurses were opened in mining areas of New Conquests.[122] Trained midwives were posted at the headquarters of some talukas of New Conquests to help women at times of delivery.

Just before 1961 Goa was divided into twenty sanitary jurisdictions namely the Port Health area of Marmagoa, 15 *Delegacias de Saude*, (Health Centres) and 3 *Sub-Delegacias* (Sub-Health Centers). The capital town had a Health Center as well as sub-Health Center. The Health Center looked after the Health Services of Ilhas and sub-Health Center took care of inspection of ships and the Sanitary Police. Although urban areas were provided with some medical facilities, rural areas were completely neglected by the Government. There was still paucity of doctors and other medical facilities.

There were four general hospitals, one in Panjim and the remaining in Ribandar, Margão and Mapuça. The Goa Medical School was attached to *Hospital Central* in Panjim. In addition there were regional hospital at Ponda, Sanguem, Satari and Pernem, a TB sanatorium in Margão, two TB dispensaries, a Mental Hospital in Panjim and a Leprosy Hospital with 150 beds at Macazana.

Since 1961 the medical scene has changed. The number of trained doctors has increased and almost every village has a health center. Many villages have cottage hospitals where medical aid is available free of charge to the poor. Several small clinics have been set up in rural areas by the Government and private doctors.

REFERENCES

1. *Viagem de Francisco Pyrard de Laval,* ed., Magalhães de Bastos, Porto, 1944, p. 15. Only Portuguese who were *Christãos velhos* were admitted. Women and servants were not treated in the hospital.
2. HAG: Monções do Reino. 177 A, fls. 211-212. (Henceforth MR.)
3. HAG: *Correspondencia Diversa.* 10471, fl. 55. (Henceforth CD.).
4. *Arquivos da Escola Medico-Cirurgica de Nova Goa, Bastora,* 1942, pp. 160-174.
5. Antonio da Silva Rego, ed., *Documentação para Historia das Missões do Padroado Portugues do Oriente India,* II, Lisboa, MCMXLVII, p. 42. The hospital was dedicated to the Holy Spirit.
6. R.A. de Bulhão e Pato, *Cartas, seguidas de documentos que as elucidam,* Tomo VI, Lisboa, p. 465.
7. HAG: Ms. 3027 – *Provisões. Alvaras e Regimentos,* fls. 98v.-99.
8. J.H. Cunha Rivara, ed., *Archivo Portuguez-Oriental,* Fasc. V, pp. 71-72. (Hence-

Hospitals and Extension Services 147

forth A.P.O.).
9. APO., Fasc. 5, pp. 71-72.
10. HAG: Ms. 3028 – *Provisões. Alvaras e Regimentos*, fl. 119.
11. *Ibid.*, fl. 201.
12. *Ibid.*, fl. 201.
13. Georg, Schurhammer, *Francis Xavier : His life, His times, 11, Rome*, 1977, p. 201.
14. Around this time the building of the hospital was renovated and enlarged with new verandas and new pharmacy. (Georg Shurhammer, Francis Xavier : His Life, His Times, II, Rome, 1977, p. 201).
15. Georg Schurhammer, *Francisco Xavier : His Life, His Times*, II, Rome, 1977, p. 202.
16. *Ibid.*, p. 204.
17. *Achivo Portuguez-Oriental*, Fasc. V, pp. 877-883. (A.P.O.)
18. *Documenta Indica*, VIII, ed., Josef Wicki. (Henceforth (DI).
19. A.P.O., Fasc V, fl. 1007.
20. A.P.O. Fasc III, p. 333.
21. *Ibid.*, p. 433.
22. *A.P.O.*, Fasc III, fls. 547-550.
23. *The voyage of John Huygen van Linschoten*, vol. II, ed., A.C. Burnell an P.A. Tiele, London, 1885, p. 237.
24. Pyrard, *op. cit.*, p. 11.
25. Nicolau Manucci's *Storia de Mogor*, vol. III, ed., W. Irwine, Calcutta, 1966, p. 269 writes that after the death of a patient a special auction was held within the hospital of all the belongings of the deceased. They were sold for much less then they were actually worth. The Jesuits sent the goods to the north so that they could be sold for higher prices.
26. *Jean-Baptiste Tavernier Travels in India*, vol. I, ed., William Crooke, London, 1925, p. 160.
27. HAG: *MR*. 185, fls. 17v-18.
28. Antonio Bocarro, *Livro das Plantas de todas as Fortalalezas Cidades e povocações do Estado da India Oriental*, p. 154.
29. HAG: Ms. 782 – *Cartas e Ordens*, fl. not numbered.
30. HAG: *MR*. 93 B, fl. 408.
31. Alfred Plattener, *Jesuits Go East*, Dublin, 1959, p. 54. (Henceforth Plattener)
32. HAG: *MR*. 102 A, fl. 131. In 1732 there was shortage of nurses and servants. (HAG: *MR*. 99, fl. 286.).
33. HAG: *MR*. 133 B, fl. 435.
34. HAG: *MR*. 114, fl. 284.
35. XCHR : Mss. *Mhamai House Papers*, Doc 4915 dated 5th February 1785.
36. HAG: *MR*. 164 B, fls. 297-603.
37. HAG: *MR*. 185. fl. 17v-18.
38. *Ibid.*, fls. 19-20.
39. *Ibid.*, fl. 30.
40. HAG: Ms. 91 – *Cartas, Ordens e Portarias* fl. 82.
41. HAG: *RDA* Ms. 974, fl. 17.
42. *Ibid.* fls.7 and 38.
43. HAG: *MR.*, 204 A, fl. 234.
44. HAG : Ms. 646 – Regulamento do Hospital Real Militar; HAG; Ms. 1836 – *Regulamento do Hospital Real Militar*, 1830.
45. HAG: *MR*. 209, fls. 297-297v.
46. HAG: Ms. 1836 – Regulamento do Hospital Real Militar de 1830, fl. 61; HAG: Ms.

646 – *Regulamento para Hospital Militar de Goa e Botica Anexa*, 1830 fl. 70.
47. HAG: Ms. 1836 – Regulamento do Hospital Real Militar de 1830, fl. 61; HAG: Ms. 646 – *Regulamento para Hospital Militar de Goa e Botica Anexa*, 1830 fl. 70.
48. Appendix 5-D.
49. HAG: *MR.* 207 B, fl. 306v.
50. HAG: *MR.* 209, fl. 235.
51. *Ibid.,* fl. 247.
52. HAG: RDA Ms. 951 – *Livro de apontamento de medicamentos vendidos ao publico no Hospital Militar,* 1831, fls. 67-84.
53. HAG: *MR.* 209, fl. 236.
54. HAG: *MR.* 212 A, fl. 208.
55. *Ibid.,* fl. 1131.
56. HAG: *MR,* 207B, fl. 306v.
57. J.P.C. Soares, *Bosquejo das Possessões Portuguezas no Oriente,* Tomo I, Lisboa, 1851, p. 292.
58. *Boletim do Governo do Estado da India,* no. 18, 1839, p. 82. (Henceforth B.G.)
59. HAG: Ms. 1836 – *Regulamento do Hospital Militar 1840,* fls. 5.
60. *Jornal de Pharmacia e Sciencias Medicas da India Portuguesa,* Nova Goa, 15 de Novembro 1862, p. 53.
61. *B.G.* 11th January 1845, p. 3; HAG : Ms. 1224, *Estrangeiros,,* fl. 12v-13: refers to the expenses incurred with an American sailor Howard Horsely during his stay at the Military Hospital.
62. *B.G.* no. 10, 8th March 1850, pp. 73-74.
63. *B.G.* no. 14, 3rd April 1847, p. 93.
64. *B.G.* no. 51, 19th December 1851, p. 365.
65. *B.G.* no. 9, 31st January 1865, p. 56.
66. A.C. Germano S. Correia, *India Portuguesa – Prostituição e Profilaxia Anti-Vemerea – Historia, Demografia, Etnografia, Higiene e Profilaxia,* Bastora, 1938, p. 266.
67. *Relatorio Annual do Chefe dos Serviços des aude relativo ao ano 1920-1921,* Nova Goa, 1925.
68. To meet the needs of growing population the out-patient department was reorganised and free service was provided for the poor and victims of accidents. (LREI, 1935, Nova Goa, 1938, pp. 67-69.).
69. Antonio Camacho donated the land.
70. HAG: Ms. 921 – *Cartas, Ordens, Portarias,* fl. 18; HAG: Ms. 7740 – *Senado de Goa – Accordões e Assentos,* fls. 58-58v : gives a list of patients in the hospital of St. Lazarus as well as the date of death of patients who died in the hospital between 1694-1709. Majority of the patients were slaves. Many of them stayed in the hospital for a long period of time.
71. *Documenta Indica,* vol. I, ed. Josef Wicki, Rome, p. 126. (Henceforth DI).
72. DI, vol. XVI, Rome 1988, p. 720; Caetano Francisco Souza, *Instituições Portuguezas de Educação e Instrução no Oriente,* vol. I, Bombay, 1890, p. 43.
73. Francisco Souza, *Oriente Conquistado a Jesus Christo,* II parte, p. 29; Josef Wicki, ed. *DI,* VIII, pp. 314-318; Caetano Francisco Sousa, op. cit., p. 43. The hospital was housed next to the Holy Spirit Church.
74. DI, IV, p. 747. Patients were treated for tumours, running sores, fractures, etc.
75. HAG: *MR.* 14, fl. 31.
76. Alfred, Plattener, op.cit., p. 50. Each patient had his own special attendant.
77. The regulation was prepared by *Santa Casa da Misericordia* and approved by the

local Government.
78. HAG: Ms. 10425 – *Regimento do Hospital da Santa Casa Miserecordia*, fl. 1.
79. *Ibid.*, fl. 8.
80. HAG: Ms. 10426 – *Regimento do Hospital da Santa Casa Miserecordia para gente da terra e outros 1630*, fl. 3.
81. *Ibid.*, fl. 3.
82. LREI, 1902, Nova Goa, 1903, p. 77. The regulation was introduced to improve the available facilities.
83. *Ibid.*, p. 77.
84. To improve the conditions of the Hospital, the *Santa Casa da Misericordia* presented the hospital in 1919 with one more regulation. The regulation contained 20 chapters, 196 clauses, 33 sample maps and four tables. (B.O. no. 46, 10th June 1919; LREI 1919, Nova Goa, 1920.
85. *Arquivos da Escola Medico Cirurgica de Nova Goa*, Bastora, 1942, p. 166.
86. Antonio Bocarro, *Livro das Plantas de todas as Fortalezas, Cidades e Povoações do Estado da India Oreintal*, in A.B. de Bragança Pereira (ed.), *Arquivo Portugues Oriental*, vol. II, Bastora, 1936-1940, p. 255. The hospital was started when the city of Goa was facing a terrible famine and epidemic.
87. Albuquerque, Viriato, A.C.B. de, *Senado de Goa* Nova Goa, 1908, p. 166.
88. HAG: Ms. 831 – *Livro da receita e despesa de medicamento do Hospital do Convento de S. João de Deus*, 1733-1737.
89. F.D. Drewitt, ed., *Bombay in the Days of George IV : Memoirs of Sir Edward West*, London, 1907, p. 165.
90. HAG: Ms. *MR* 177 A, fl. 35.
91. Achilles Meersman, *the Ancient Franciscan Provinces in India*, Bangalore, 1971, p. 139. In 1784 Dom Manoel de S. Catharina, Archbishop of Goa was of the opinion that the Friars of Goa should have a place where they could go in the hot months. Hence he recommended that the Hospice of Valverde should be repaired and used for this purpose.
92. C.C. Nazareth, *Clero de Goa seus serviços a Religião e a Nação*, Nova Goa, 1927, p. 139.
93. HAG: Ms. *MR*. 205 A, fl. 129.
94. The *Asilo* was started by three priests Frs. Sebastião Zeferino Gabriel Botelho, Antonio Reginaldo de Mendonça and Conego Tomas Nunes de Serra e Moura.
95. HAG: Ms. 10550 – *Administração Civil – Saude a Benificiencia*, fl. 48.
96. *Asilo de N. Sra. dos Milqagres: Relatorio e Contas 1921-1922, 1924-1925*.
97. *Anuario da India Portuguesa*, Nova Goa, 1930, p. 198.
98. *Anuario do Estado da India 1930*, p. 196.
99. *Ibid.*, p. 201.
100. Albuquerque, Manuel João Socrate, *Hospicio do Clero – A historia da sua fundação contas*, Nova Goa, 1929, p. V.
101. LREI 1949, Nova Goa, p. 721.
102. Silvia Noronha, "Economic scene in Goa 1926-1961" in *Goa Through the Ages II*, ed., T.R. de Souza, New Delhi, 1990, pp. 277-278.
103. HAG: Ms. 11668 – *Correspondencia diversa* fl. 207; HAG: Ms. 1224 – *Estrangeiros*, fl. 65: A Goan patient was admitted in a Mental Asylum in Dharwar.
104. HAG: Ms. 10552 – *Administração Civil – Saude e Beneficiencia*, fl. 26.
105. *Relatorio dos Serviços de Saude do Estado da India, Novembro 1917 a Junho 1919*, Nova Goa, 1920.
106. Boletim Oficial (Henceforth B.G.) no. 58, 22 de Julho 1930.

107. B.O. no. 58, 22nd July 1930.
108. B.O. no. 93, 21st November 1930.
109. The asylum was in 1934 granted permission to accommodate twelve extra patients (B.O. no. 11, 6th February 1934). This number was further increased to sixteen in 1935. The expansion was necessary as the Portuguese Government was paying high fees to the British Government for the maintenance of mentally ill patients of Goan origin in mental hospitals in British India, (LREI, 1935, Nova Goa, 1938, p. 360.).
110. LREI, 1935, pp. 357-358. One nurse was paid Rs. 45 and the assistant nurse was paid Rs. 30 a month. Two servants were also appointed who were paid Rs. 14 each a month.
111. LREI, 1948, p. 510.
112. B.O. 2 de Abril 1959. Silvia Noronha in "Economic Scene in Goa 1926-1961" *op. cit.*, states that a Mental Asylum was established in Goa as late as 1948.
113. *Gazetteer of India – Union Territory Goa, Daman and Diu, Part 1: Goa*, Bombay, 1979, p. 714, (Henceforth Gazetteer). The following year a Committee was appointed by the Government to administer the institution (LREI 1931, Nova Goa, 1932, pp. 146-53.).
114. HAG: Ms. 3027 – *Provisões, Alvaras e Regimentos;* fl. 33v. The *alvara* was implemented from January 1521.
115. B.G. 26th May 1838, p. 157.
116. B.O. no. 110, 20th September 1892. Similar facilities were granted even as late as 1927. (LREI, 1927, Nova Goa, 1928, p. 82.).
117. Gazetteer, *op. cit.*, p. 713.
118. An extensive legislation was passed in 1927 defining the jurisdiction and duties of *Delegados de Saude* and sub-Delegados de Saude of Goa, Daman and Diu. (B.O. no. 36, 6th May 1927; LREI 1927, Nova Goa, 1928, pp. 139-151.
119. B.O. no. 60, 5th May 1910.
120. The doctor was to be paid by the Communidades of Astragar and Collomba. These two communidades had to contribute with Rs. 120 and Rs. 60 respectively. (LREI, 1908, Nova Goa, 1909, pp. 163-64.)
121. LREI, 1917, Nova Goa, 1918, p. 89. This appointment was the outcome of a petition sent by the inhabitants of Priol, Cundaim, Marcaim, Velinga and nearby villages. The doctor was paid an annual salary of Rs. 360 by the Municipality of Ponda.
122. Gazetteer, *op. cit.*, p. 715.

Hospitals and Extension Services

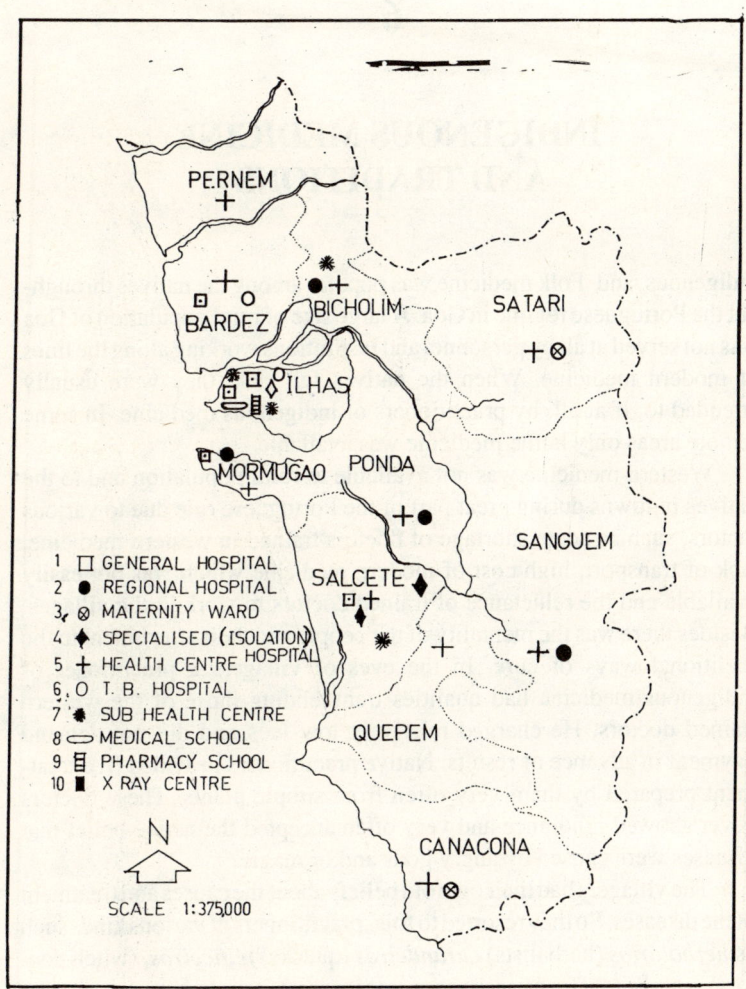

MAP 5.1: Health Facilities in Goa 1961

6

INDIGENOUS MEDICINE AND TRADITIONS

Indigenous and Folk medicine was popular among the natives throughout the Portuguese regime in Goa. A large size of rural population of Goa was not served at all by personnel and institutions working along the lines of modern medicine. When the natives fell sick, they were usually attended to, if at all, by practitioners of indigenous medicine. In some remote areas only home medicine was available.

Western medicine was not available to rural population and to the natives in towns during great part of the Portuguese rule due to various factors, such as acute shortage of doctors trained in western medicine, lack of transport, high cost of modern medicine which was not easily available and the reluctance of trained doctors to work in the villages. Besides there was the mentality of the people and their attachment to the traditional ways of cure. In the eyes of villagers a practitioner of indigenous medicine had qualities transcending those of the western trained doctors. He charged relatively low fees and did not demand payment in advance of results. Native practitioners provided free treatment prepared by them very often from simple plants. These doctors never showed ignorance and very often accepted the native belief that diseases were caused by angry gods and or magic.

The villagers had their own old beliefs about the causes and treatment of the diseases. So they resorted to folk practitioners of various kinds such as *herbolarios* (herbalists) *curandeiros* (quacks) *feiticeiros,* (witch doctors), *ghadis* (shaman) *sangradores* (bleeders), priests, astrologers, magicians, charm sellers, thorn pullers, wound experts, snake bite curers, *dais* (midwives), surgeons, bone setters and others. They have existed generation after generation and proved useful to the people. There were *hakims* (Muslim practitioners) and *vaidyas* (Hindu practitioners) who through centuries of practice became part of rural life. These practitioners received no formal training. Their therapeutic knowledge was handed over to them by their ancestors. Their remedies prepared from bark, herbs and other local products were of considerable value in the treatment of cholera, asthma and other diseases.

Vaidyas practiced ayurvedic medicine based on the threefold elements - wind, fire and water. Good health depended on balancing these elements, while disease was a result of imbalance. The treatment consisted in determining which kinds of humours were in excess or were insufficient. The causes of humoral imbalance were manifold : Errors in diet and excess of everyday life such as too much sexual intercourse, anger or exertion. The *materia medica* of Ayurvedic practitioners included vegetable drugs derived from indigenous plants. The therapeutics of *Unani* medicine is less well-recorded than for Ayurveda, but many ideas were the same. Unani system of medicine was of Greco-Arab origin. In Goa the system was introduced by the Arabs. Another category of indigenous medicine widely practised in Goa was homeopathy.

Indigenous Elite Medical Practitioners

Vaidyas : among the several types of practitioners of the indigenous medicine were *vaidyas* also known as panditos. *Vaidyas* were practitioners of ayurvedic medicine. These *vaidyas* learnt by trial and error. When a *vaidya* died, he usually left behind a note-book of prescriptions and practices to his son or a close relative who secretly studied the matter and learnt to practise the same.

Side by side with ayurvedic medicine practised by *panditos* we had in Goa some practitioners of *Unani* medicine. The practitioners were known as *hakims*.

Vaidyas played an important role, in the early Goan society, at a time when there was a dearth of efficient trained doctors in western medicine. They were in great demand both among the natives and the Portuguese. These *vaidyas* were well versed in tropical diseases and had good knowledge of many basic subjects, including medicine and therapeutics.

Garcia d' Orta the well known Portuguese naturalist, who came to Goa in 1534 was surprised to find that *vaidyas* were well versed in medicinal plants and several peculiar diseases.

Many of the European travellers who visited the city of Goa in the first two centuries of the Portuguese regime were unanimous in praising the native physicians. The Dutchman Linschoten who spent five years in

Goa (1583-1589) found them much respected and enjoying special privileges such as going about like the Portuguese whites under *sombreiros* (big umbrellas), an honour no other natives enjoyed, except ambassadors, and rich merchants.[1] Native physicians also enjoyed another privilege of going about for their professional visits on horse-back, palanquins and biers. This privilege aroused much jealousy among those Portuguese who enjoyed no such privilege.

Vaidyas had their own treatment for various diseases. External swelling was cured by applying the end of hot knife and then hot brass cup with long tube to suck the blood. In case of a colic the most efficient medicine was the hot iron applied to the umbilical region. It caused sudden convulsion and stopped colic. Leeches were used to lower the high blood pressure. In all cases rigorous diet was followed.

A seventeenth-century traveller François Bernier, paying tribute to the native physicians writes: "Although their art of curing differed much from European one, the principle which guided it might serve as a lesson to western physicians any time." He continues:" You must not give much food to the patient suffering from fever, the best remedy is abstinence nothing is more harmful to an ailing body, than meat broth as the later decomposes in the stomach. The patient should be bled only in extreme cases, for instance, when there are well founded fears of cerebral fever or inflammation in chest, liver or kidneys.[2] These methods according to him left the patient completely cured and were widely followed by the Arab, Hindu and Moghul physicians.

Native physicians cured the natives as well as the Portuguese, including the viceroys, archbishops, high government officials and friars. Native physicians had wider practice than the Portuguese ones. The latter charged fees for the treatment contrary to royal *alvara* (charter) of 1519.[3] Besides the Portuguese physicians could not communicate with natives due to language barrier and they had poor knowledge of tropical diseases. One friar from the Augustinian order, who had practised medicine for sixteen years in Portugal, found all his patients dying in Goa despite his best efforts. He called a *vaidya* to find out his secret of curing people. The *vaidya* told him that it was necessary not only to know the remedies but also the background and humour of the patient.

The *vaidyas* knew very well how to heal wounds, fractures, and cure fevers. However, they had no knowledge of the circulatory system. This could be one of the reasons they made no attempt to bleed their patients, but instead applied leeches. The *vaidyas* were ignorant about internal organs of the body as they performed no autopsy. The cause of the disease was not diagnosed. If a patient did not respond to the usual treatment, they often ascribed the cause to some supernatural forces, such as *Xetam* (devil) and advised the patient to consult their *bhat* and gods.

Native physicians received no encouragement from the Portuguese rulers. Their position deteriorated during Portuguese regime. Several restrictions were imposed on the practice of the native physicians. In 1563 Hindus were prohibited by a royal order from practising medicine and Hindu physicians in Goa were ordered to leave the place within a month.[4] This was the first order banning the practice of the native physicians. The order was finally not implemented. However, soon after some restrictive measures were imposed on them in the sixteenth and the seventeenth centuries by the Church Provincial Councils, Government and the Municipal Council (*Senado*).

The first Church Provincial Council held in 1567, imposed restrictions on native physicians probably as it did not wish the non-Christian physicians to treat Christian people on account of many evils resulting both to faith and to morality.[5] The same Council prevented Christian women from seeking help of Hindu *dais* at the time of child birth, because they used pagan rituals and witchcraft. It asked the Viceroy to tax the native physicians. Similar orders were issued by the Regent of Portugal Dom Henriques to the Viceroy Conde de Redondo, emphasizing the great harm caused by the Hindu physicians who treated the Portuguese and the native people.

The Third Church Provincial Council advised the native physicians to send for priests and advise the sick to confess before providing them with medical care. Those physicians who failed to advise the sick were fined 10 *pardaos* which they had to pay to the poor patients. If they repeated the same they could be sent away from Goa.[6] They were advised not to prescribe meat diet without the prior permission of religious authorities.

Restrictive measures were not imposed only by ecclesiastical authorities. In 1574 the Governor Antonio Moniz Barreto issued a notification banning native physicians from going about on horseback, biers and palanquins.[7] There was one exception. The native physicians of the viceroy continued to enjoy the privilege.[8] This was probably due to the fact that the viceroy depended on the native physicians in the absence of the efficient Portuguese physicians. The ban was a real blow to the native physicians, for whom it was impossible to walk around the city of Goa in order to reach the sick. Many *vaidyas* migrated to neighbouring courts. This move raised the mortality rate. Sick people preferred to die rather than seek help of the Portuguese physicians. Despite the ban it was not possible to get rid of all *vaidyas* due to paucity of western physicians.

The reason for these restrictions it appears were not exactly the incompetence on the part of the native physicians but the jealousy among the Portuguese physicians. They felt slighted for by not being called by patients of their own race including the viceroy. The Portuguese physicians used their influence with the Government and other agencies to damage the practice of native physicians and they succeeded in this to a large extent.

The Portuguese doctors often behaved in a high-handed manner and were hostile towards native practitioners. Once an Augustinian friar was sick with pain and swelling in certain part of his body. The Portuguese physician could not relieve the pain. He sought the help of an old woman living nearby who offered to cure him. She did so with the help of stewed leaves, which she applied to the painful area. The medicine relieved the pain but the woman had to pay the price. The Chief Physician got her arrested and she was forced to sell all her belongings to win freedom.[9]

On another occasion, the Chief Physician got a Hindu practitioner imprisoned for having refused to disclose the secret for curing scrofula. The practitioner was informed that he would win his freedom only if he disclosed the formula. The practitioner preferred to die rather than disclose it.

D. Ana Espanholim, the wife of the Governor Manuel Souza Coutinho (1588-91), who consulted native physicians, was condemned for doing it and was convicted by the Holy Inquisition to pay one thousand *pardaos*.[10]

In the early seventeenth century another attempt was made to regulate the practice of the Hindu physicians as may be inferred from a *postura* (regulation) of the Municipal Council in 1618. It directed that no one of any state or nationality is allowed to exercise the profession of physicians, surgeons, blood-letting or barber without first being examined and obtaining license. Any one who practised without a license was to be fined twenty *pardaos*.[11]

Native physicians were forbidden to move out of the city when the condition of the patient was serious. In case they really needed to go out they had to seek the permission of the Municipal Council. A physician violating the order would be struck from the Municipal roll never to be readmitted and would also pay a fine of 10 *xerafins*.[12] The same *postura* directed bleeders to have a signboard with a picture of a man being bled. This picture was to be placed above the door. Any bleeder violating this

Indigenous Medicine and Traditions

regulation would pay a fine of two *pardaos*.[13]

Thirty non Christians physicians, over forty surgeons and a number of bleeders were allowed to practise in the city of Goa with license of the Municipal Council, provided they possessed a certificate issued by the Chief Physician. License was issued to them by the Municipality for a fee of 10 *xerafins* on condition that they should not induce their Christian patients to make offerings to Hindu deities.[14] It is noticed that in the seventeenth century physicians were non-Christians while surgeons and bleeders were all Christians. Hindus probably did not take up the profession of surgeon or bleeder because of their belief in Ahimsa (non-violence). They had a distaste for cutting of flesh and to bleed. All *vaidyas* were men. Women were not taught medicine.

Folk Healers

While restrictive measures were adopted against indigenous elite practitioners, a vast majority of people continued to seek native medicine. Seeking the help of quacks, such as *curandeiros,* (quacks), *herbolarios,* (herbalists) feiticeiros (witch-doctors), snake bite curers and others was common not only in the villages but even in urban areas. These quacks had no real political power or legal sanction but had great influence on the people. These practitioners did not isolate their patients in the hospital far from relatives and friends.

Feiticeiros (witch doctors) had remedies for all kind of diseases. Each village had its own witch-doctor. Hindu witch-doctors were considered superior to Christian ones. The former performed rituals to cure diseases. Christian witch-doctors made use of holy water, prayers, relics, amulets, piece of cloth used to cover the saints, ribbon of the size of saints, rose of Jericho (a small shrub from Arabia brought by the missionaries). This rose, when immersed in water helped women to have easy deliveries.[15] Witch-doctor Simão da Cunha from Goa Velha made use of a cross which was placed over a rock in the river.[16] Some Christian witch-doctors also used non-Christian rituals to cure diseases. The Goa Inquisition tried several times to curb their activities. In 1786 Rodrigo Vieira and Francisco Vieyra both from Murmugão were condemned by the Inquisition for performing non-Christian rituals in order to cure the sick. The last one was exiled to *Casa de Polvora* for five years.[17] Again in 1794 Simão da Cunha of Goa Velha was sentenced by the Inquisition for same reason.[18]

Witches were bizarre people, who were believed to have some supernatural powers. They dressed in outlandish clothes, including a blue colour jacket with gold colour buttons. They wore usually silver bangles, ear-rings and a scarf around their neck. They carried a wand in their hand. Normally witches practised their craft in the forest or a cave, on a floor covered with cow-dung with burning fire and water nearby. The ritual would begin with an animal sacrifice. The witch then screamed and went into hysterical trance, and was then believed to be possessed by some force that inspired the witch in finding a cure or solution. Simão Faraz from Goa Velha performed his craft at night in an isolated place.[19]

Bardez taluka in the north and Salcete taluka in the south were full of *curandeiros* and charlatans.[20] In 1853 an attempt was made by the Government to control the activities of quacks. Taluka administrators and Government physicians were asked to report to the Health Board the activities of the quacks so that appropriate action could be taken against them as per the *alvara* of 22nd January 1810.[21] The authorities were unable to keep a check on them due to insufficient trained doctors. For instance, in Raia (Salcete), the professional skills of Remedio Piedade Soares were certified by the parish priest and local authorities. This practitioner guaranteed cure for dysentery, diarrhoea and skin disorders.[22]

In 1687 there was only one doctor trained in western medicine.[23] The Government was forced in the eighteenth and nineteenth centuries to issue diplomas to several individuals to practise as doctors. From 1782-1801 Goa did not have a physician trained in western medicine. Health care was left in the hands of native medicine men.[24] As mentioned earlier the practice of issuing diplomas had been stopped by the Government in 1838.[25] In 1860 another attempt was made to control the activities of the quacks. The guilty were to be punished.[26]

During this period there was acute shortage of doctors in Portugal and Goa. This acute shortage of doctors was responsible for the establishment of a Medical School in Goa in the year 1842. However, doctors trained in this school satisfied only the needs of the urban population.

In 1865 several individuals from Mapuça (a taluka town in Bardez) sent a petition to the Government requesting permission for one Tholentino Gabriel Fernandes to practise as a doctor. Similar petition was sent by the inhabitants of Siolim. Daniel Conçeição Luiz, a diploma holder in medicine was allowed to issue medical certificates to various individuals to practise.[27] New Conquests had no trained doctors in the first half of the nineteenth century with exception of military surgeons at Ponda, Bicholim and Pernem.

The medical scene at the beginning of the present century did not change much in rural areas. Therefore, it is not surprising that the majority

Indigenous Medicine and Traditions

of people in New Conquests resorted to indigenous medicine. The Census of 1910 indicates that Goa had 18 *curandeiros* of which four practised in Panjim, five in Salcete, three in Sanquelim and three in Sanguem.[28]

Women in rural and urban areas depended on a *dai* (midwife) at the time of delivery. There were no maternity homes for a long time. Even when these were established, women were reluctant to avail of the facilities. *Dais* had no formal training, but learnt their trade from their mother or an elderly woman in the family. She was illiterate usually middle aged or old and her only qualification was her experience. Unlike other male healers, she was of low caste, because among Hindus everything associated with confinement and to an extent with pregnancy was considered unclean. *Dais* had no knowledge of hygiene and were often responsible for the high infant mortality. *Dais* many times performed superstitious rituals at the time of deliveries.[29]

The Portuguese often resorted to *sangradores* (bleeders) who lived in the seventeenth century at Praça do Pelourinho Velho.[30] The Portuguese resorted to them even to cure slight fevers. In 1610 a bleeder was paid quarterly 5 *xerafins* at the Convent of Graça.[31] Bleeding a patient was not an easy task. It was necessary to find the correct vein. Barbers who were also bleeders were Christians. In year 1900 Goa had four *sangradores*, officially registered. Two bleeders lived in Ilhas and two in Bardez.

Dentists were few in Goa. Some had professional competence, but most were quacks. People lived without proper dental care. Caries was one major problem which the traditional extractionists tried to get rid by using oil mixed with garlic and mustard. The oil was allowed to cool and then poured with the help of a banana leaf (used as funnel) in the ear of the patient. On the side of injured tooth. After some time the patient was asked to empty the contents and the tooth puller would point out tiny threads as caries.

Every village or group of villages had curers against snake bite, the most respected among all medicine men. He learnt *mantras* to neutralize snake poison, perform many ceremonies and rituals. Snake curer was a man completely dedicated to his work. From the moment he was called he would refuse food and drinks until he found the cure for the snake bite. There were several curers against snake bite. They claimed that their ability to cure was an inherited one. For instance, a family of Mandrekars in Pernem claimed they could cure snake bite with water drawn by them from a particular well or spring which they splashed on the patient. This power was inherited by both male and female members of the family, but girls would loose their powers once they married. They could not charge fee for the treatment. It was believed that the privilege to cure snake bites was granted to the Mandrekar family by St. Thoma, the Apostle, who came to India.[32]

Snake bite curers performed a complicated ritual to cure persons bitten by a snake. The ritual started with *zaddo* or *zaddnim*. This involved beating the head of the patient with a branch of a tree known as *usky* (*Calycopteris Floribunda*). Next, the curer gave the patient a root to chew. The identity of the root was a closely guarded secret only known to the curer. Juice extracted from similar root was applied to the head and little juice was rubbed into the scalp. *Zaddnim* was performed several times on the first day. On subsequent days it was performed for half an hour in the morning and half an hour in the evening during seven days. On the seventh day, the patient was massaged with hot coconut oil and given a bath. The patient was kept on a diet of canjee made of *orio* (a kind of food grain).[33] This cereal was consumed by Hindu women as a substitute for rice during certain ceremonial days.

During the period of the above mentioned treatment the curer had to observe certain rituals: If he was eating his dinner, should his lamp blow off, he had to stop eating his food. He could have his next meal only on the following night. In case there was a solar or lunar eclipse he had to immerse half of his body in water until the eclipse was over. A woman who was menstruating could not speak to the curer during a meal. If this happened he had to live only on fruits for four days or until the said woman completed her menstrual cycle and she had her bath.

Snake bite was also cured in those days and even today by indigenous practitioners as well as by practitioners of western medicine with help of chickens. Small chickens were used to get rid of the venom. The anus of the chicken was applied to the area bitten by the snake. The chicken sucked the venom until it dropped dead. Several chickens were used in this manner until all venom was sucked out.

In the nineteenth century, *Diapana* was used for snake bite. This Brasilian plant was sent by Brown and Diner from Mauritius to Goa. The plant was a powerful antidote for snake bite and other injuries. The leaves or juice extracted from them could be used as an anti-venom.[34]

There was another person who practiced the art of healing in the villages. It was the *Bhat* who suggested "preventive medicine" by advising the people to perform rituals as a means of obtaining good health, prosperity and children. He prescribed similar rituals as cures for illnesses that were believed to be caused by religious laxity. Due to this belief he would advise pilgrimages to holy places such as Pandarpur, pouring water at the roots of sacred trees and conducting of sacrifices.

Deities, Rituals, Fetishes and Miracles

Superstitions were used to cure people of various ailments. Many believed in the effect of evil eye. It was believed that some individuals have faculty to cast spell on others by looking at them. As result of the evil eye things could perish and diseases could take place leading even to death. Children were believed to be susceptible to the effect of the evil eye. For this reason many would get upset if someone admired their children's beauty or strength, because they feared that such an expression of admiration was prompted by ill will.

A barren woman was not supposed to gaze at a child as her gaze was considered to be full of desire. It was believed that evil eye made the child cry too much and suffer from various diseases. Animals, plants and fields were also considered susceptible to the effect of evil eyes.

In order to escape from the influence of evil eye people made use of incantations and charms on Sunday, Wednesday or Tuesday. Salt and chilies were often used to get rid of the evil eye. These substances were waived around the head of the patient. Salt, dry chilies and alum were placed over hot charcoal and waived around the person. A piece of alum placed in the fire was believed to change into the form of a man or a woman. From this conjectures were made as to the sex of the person by whose evil eye the patient was affected. After the rituals the contents were placed on the roadside to repel evil eye. Chilies were probably used as they are pungent and red in colour. The red colour was said to attract the evil spirit.

The most popular charm against evil eye was soot which was smeared around the eyes or any part of child's face. Soot was prepared by filling a small earthen pot with oil, a wick of cotton lighted in it and a brass plate held over the flame. This soot is smeared around the eyes of the child to distract the eyes of the evil person from the child. In some communities a face is painted on the egg shell. The egg shell is waived over the person and placed at the junction of three roads to repel evil eye.

Coconuts were waived round the child and thrown at the boundary of the village and at places supposed to be haunted. To ward off or repel evil eye various charms and amulets were used.

An amulet is a material object, worn carried on the person or preserved in some other way. Amulets were used to cure diseases or to bring luck. Majority of children among the lower class wore amulets around their waist or neck. Some wore many amulets around their waist or neck. Some wore many amulets for a particular purpose. Adults also wore them in various forms. Amulets such as shoes and beads were attached to houses, fields, vegetable farms to protect from evil eye. It was looked upon as a weapon which protected the wearer against diseases and misfortune. Some of the material used were vegetables, roots, leaves, seeds, horns, animals, teeth, hair, claws, nails, relics, bones, strings, threads, beads of rudraksa and medals.

To protect against evil eye it was a practice to wear rings with elephant hair, tiger nails and bangles made of tortoise shell. Ladies often wore miniature band as a pendant. The same was worn by men on their waist. To protect children from diseases it was a practice to wear *doro* (black thread) or *taita* (effigy of Maruti).

Amulets were also used to cure and prevent various diseases. To cure dog bites a silver coin was applied to the wound. After 12 hours the coin was washed and applied to the wound on the other side. This procedure was carried on until the wound was healed. It was a traditional belief that silver had power to heal.

Women without children resorted to superstitious rites to conceive.[35] Offerings were made to *Bhut* (devil) to cure or prevent diseases.[36] The Goa Inquisition found several people guilty of making offerings to *Bhut*. Among them was Petornila Leitão of Chinchinim (Salcete) who made offerings for the good health of her son. In 1787 João Menezes of Dramapur, Salcete, was accused of keeping certain articles in his house meant for *Bhut* from which he was seeking good health.[37] Further he was accused of contributing towards the purchase of coconuts and roosters which were to be offered to the temple.[38]

The rural people believed that many diseases were caused by the wrath of gods and goddesses. It was believed that when a goddess was not given due recognition and reverence it would get angry and its wrath caused diseases and death. Propitiation of gods and goddesses was done through religious prayers, incantations and offering of animal sacrifices. Epidemic diseases such as cholera and smallpox are supposed to come from deities. People of all communities sought the help of goddess *Mhamai* in times of need. In 1785 João Benedito de Noronha was accused by Goa Inquisition of making offerings to goddess *Mhamai* in order to obtain cure of his sick child.[39] The following year Pedro also known as *Bombo* from Mandur, Ilhas was condemned for having sought the help of non-Christian gods and for taking other people along with him. As a punishment he had to spend six months at the Convent of *S. Cruz dos*

*Milagres.*⁴⁰ Luis Souza Ennum, a fifty years old farmer from Bastora (Bardez) was reprimanded by the same Inquisition for offering coconuts and promising to give cash to god Santipurso of a Nanora temple, in order to relieve him of a sickness.⁴¹

During the outbreak of smallpox Hindus appealed with special devotion to goddess Sitala Devi. People began to worship her after Puranic and Tantrika texts recommended her worship to avert fatal diseases and disasters. Sitala Devi was one of the minor goddesses but considered as goddess par excellence — a living medicine. It is stated that Sitala is so called because she soothes and cures the victims from the characteristic of extreme inflammation of pox. To appease this goddess animals of different types were sacrificed and many ceremonies were performed.

In one of the rituals the goddess was placed on a vessel of earthenware or metal with flowers and a lamp filled with coconut oil. No food was fried in the house of the patient because it was believed that the blisters would take a turn for the worse.

Tender coconuts, bananas and sugar were offered to the goddess Devi. If the disease erupted in a epidemic form the villagers performed a ceremony known as *Utar* to which all *Bagats* from the village were invited. A goat or seven to eight roosters were sacrificed in honour of the goddess. Following the ritual a procession was taken by the villagers to the outskirts of the village. They carried an earthenware pot containing coconuts, arecanut, betel, incense, flowers and fruits. The vessel was handed over to the inhabitants of the next village and passed from village to village. Finally the vessel was deposited on the border of Goa usually on the southern side or thrown in the sea. This symbolized the end of the disease in this territory.

It was a practice to burn incense and *agarbatis* daily when there was a case of smallpox in the house. The practice was probably followed to purify the air. The floor of the house was smeared with cow-dung. Visitors disinfected themselves by splashing water mixed with cow-dung. To propitiate the goddess they drank this water. The same procedure was followed during an outbreak of cholera.

Another ceremony performed at the end of a smallpox epidemic was the farewell ceremony. The inhabitants in a small basket of bamboo placed a new handkerchief, a coconut and flowers. This container was carried to the end of the village in a procession, where it was left under a tree. This ritual was performed to placate Sitala.

Just as smallpox was believed to be caused by an enraged goddess so was the case of cholera. Cholera was believed to be caused by goddess Durga. To appease her several ceremonies were performed.

Christians also believed that their saints have powers to cure disease. Goans have great faith in St. Francis Xavier and other saints. It is reported that soon after the arrival of Francis Xavier to Goa he visited the college of St. Paul in the City of Goa. On inquiring about the health of its inmates he was informed about a person who was critically ill with no hopes of recovery. Francis Xavier read the Gospel and blessed the patient. The patient recovered and lived for many years.[42]

Another miracle that is reported took place after the death of Francis Xavier. His body was brought in a casket and kept in the city of Goa. At this time a lady D. Joana Pereira wife of Christovam Pereira, was seriously ill for three months. She prayed to the saint and within a short time she was well again. Yet one more reported miracle was of Antonio Rodrigues a clerk in an orphanage. He was blind for seven years. He could recognize people only by their voice. One day he visited the college of St. Paul and touched to his eyes the relic of St. Francis Xavier and is reported to have recovered his sight.[43]

Miracles have also been reported to have taken place during the exposition of the body of Francis Xavier. For instance during the exposition of December 1859 at least six persons had miraculous cures. These cures were witnessed by people, certified by doctors and the church authorities. All these diseases were incurable. Bernadina Rodrigues a widow of 34 years suffered from paralysis of right arm for 12 years. She could not lift her hand to her mouth. On 14th December 1859 she went to Old Goa to pay homage to the saint and returned cured. Maria Isabel de Sousa wife of Pedro Noronha from Tivim had suffered from a uterine infection and other ailments which caused complete paralysis of her one side from neck downwards. The doctors had given her up as a hopeless case. She was preparing to resign to her fate when her mother carried her to the Basilica of Bom Jesus where she kissed the feet of the saint. Agonising pain followed — but soon after all pain disappeared and the woman could walk again without any help.

Another case was of João Thomas Fernandes of Panjim. He was cured at the age of nine of clubfoot. His condition was considered incurable until he visited Old Goa. He kissed the feet of the saint. He felt acute pain. His mother presumed it was the result of the long journey by foot. However, the next day the child could walk perfectly without any defect. Maria Antonia da Costa Campos, 13 years old daughter of an army official was paralysed on right side from waist downwards. She could not

Indigenous Medicine and Traditions

walk nor touch her foot to the ground. She kissed the feet of Francis Xavier. No change took place. On hearing the cure of João Thomas she decided to try again. She visited Old Goa for the second time and kissed the feet of the saint. She fell back with acute pain and loss of senses. She was helped by those around. Maria Antonia soon came to senses and began to walk. The right leg had resumed its normal shape and moved naturally. This cure was certified by the doctors one year later when Maria Antonia was 14 years old. As a thanksgiving she added the name of the saint to her name and came to be known as Maria Antonia Francisca Xavier da Costa Campos.

Fifty years old Antonio Jose da Cunha from Candolim was victim of tetanus in December 1855. As result he could not wear shoes. His knee was rigid for four years and he could not kneel. In 1859 he went to old Goa to kiss the feet of the saint. He was cured and in position to wear shoes and kneel down again.[44]

Popular Medicine and Practices during Child Bearing

Among the masses a *prima gravida* was bled in sixth or seventh month of her pregnancy. This was done probably to avoid high blood pressure. This practice of bleeding weakened the pregnant woman.

From the time the pregnancy was confirmed the pregnant woman was exempted from all laborious work. She was permitted only light work. Great care was taken to keep her segregated from all influences likely to distress her feelings. The duration of the eclipse was for her a period of inactivity. This was meant to prevent any disfigurement or deformities to the child. A pregnant woman was not allowed to visit or see a dead body as it was believed it would bring her bad luck.

Prayers and offerings were made for the safe delivery by close members of the family, usually by husband, mother or mother-in-law. Christians besides seeking help of their saints resorted also to *ritos gentilicos* (non-Christian rituals).[45]

The room used for the delivery was not the best in the house. They chose a dark room without proper ventilation and away from the family quarters. Child birth among Hindus was looked upon as unclean and the woman was treated as an outcast. She was kept confined to the corner of the house without any contacts with rest of the society. Close relatives could visit her and after that they had to change their clothes.

Cleanliness in the room was considered out of place. Windows and door were locked to prevent fresh air. Any openings on the walks were blocked up with papers or rags. Dirty old clothes were used during the delivery. They were good enough to pack around the woman to absorb the discharge.

Deliveries were performed either on a chamber pot or on two chairs placed in such a manner that they resembled a chamber pot. This practice was followed even fifty years ago. The child was received in a *sup* (winnowing fan). The umbilical cord was covered with pepper and bandaged with cloth. Through this bandage hot oil was poured daily on the navel. Many times instead of pepper they used ashes of banana leaf or *limbrå (Azadirachta Indica)* leaf. No bath was given to the child until the umbilical wound healed. However, the child was massaged with oil.

To bring the uterus to its original position, the mother was placed on a mat or bed. The *dai* would press the mother's stomach with the sole of her foot. At the same time she would try to raise the mother with her hands.

It was customary to place a container with live coal in the delivery room, in order to provide warmth to the mother and the child. To stop post delivery colics a hot smooth heated stone was applied to mother's stomach. A tampon of pepper was inserted in the vagina to prevent infection. This tampon was changed daily. Sometimes after the delivery the new mother was kept standing and the *dai* massaged her stomach to clear the bad blood from the uterus.

The penknife which was used to cut the umbilical cord was kept under the pillow of the child till the sixth day of the birth. Similar iron material was placed under the mother's pillow to prevent misfortune to the mother and child.

During the first six days a woman who gave birth to a child was not allowed to have a complete bath. She could have bath from the neck downwards. Some kinds of leaves were boiled in the water. She was allowed a complete bath only on the 21st day.[46] It was believed that head-bath before this period led to convulsions, tetanus and other problems. However, in some communities bath was allowed on the third day of the delivery.

The woman was regarded impure during the first eleven days of the delivery and during menstruation. If such woman participated in a religious ceremony it was believed that she transferred her impurities to the family or community, leading to misfortune or disease. She could not participate in any religious ceremony. Such women were quarantined and treated as outcasts.

A tradition was followed even among cultured people to decorate the door of the house of the newly born child with *marvel(Andropogan*

Annulatus). It was meant to drive away evil spirits. Possibly it was an antiseptic.

During the first three days a woman who had a baby was fed with a kind of cake made of flour and jaggery. After the third day jaggery was no longer used. Milk and *canjee* was not advised for the mother as it was considered harmful to health. Both the items had cooling effect which was considered harmful for a woman who had just delivered a child.

On the sixth day after the birth of the child a number of traditions and superstitions were followed: Seven types of vegetables cooked with coconut were distributed to seven houses. The clothes of the mother and child were changed. Flakes of garlic were tied around the wrist of the child. The family did not consume water from their house well. The whole family kept a vigil on the night of the fifth and sixth day. They spent the night singing and playing while they waited the visit of Dame Luck and Dame Fortune. It was believed that they visited the new child on this night. For this reason, the room of the child was rearranged. Close to the mother a mound of rice was arranged, and a vessel with cereal placed over it. The vessel was closed with coconut and flowers of a shrub known as *potcoli (Ixora Coccimia)*. The vessel represented goddess *Sotvi* and to her fruits and sacrifices were offered. These gifts were taken away by the *dai*. *Sotvi* was a custom followed even by Christians, despite repeated decrees both from the state and church against the custom.[47]

As the family waited for the Dame Luck/Fortune, the area from mother's bed to the front door was sprinkled with garlic flakes, mustard seeds and grains. The natives believed that both Luck and Fortune competed with each other on this night to be the first to enter the room where condiments were sprinkled to keep one of them busy collecting the grains while the other, usually Dame Luck, gave luck to the child and disappeared.

A mother was forbidden to nurse another boy whilst nursing her son. However, she could breast feed a baby girl. Boys were desired among the Hindus to carry on the family traditions. A mother could nurse a girl besides her son, probably because girls were not desired and they could do with less nutrition than boys.

Special ceremony was performed on the 20th day after the delivery. A sweet made of rice, coconut and milk was prepared. The *dai* took seven spoons one at a time, and waived it over the head of the mother and the child. At the end of the ceremony the sweet was placed in the bathroom where the mother had her bath during the first seven days.

Among the rural masses it was a practice to apply *lep* (paste) to the head and body of the mother. The *lep* made of leaves of *valicodul* and palm *fenny* (local drink) was applied on the 21st day after the delivery and the mother was given a bath.

After child birth a woman could move out of the house only after 40 days. On the 40th day she was given a bath and allowed to go out. Inspite of a episcopal decree of 1784 Christians women continued to follow this practice.[48]

It was also a practice for women to bath near the well for a period of two months after delivery. Many times betel and areca nut was mixed in the water. A decree issued in 1736 forbade Christian women from following this practice.[49]

Some Traditional Treatments and Medicines

Indigenous medicine was the only medicine available to vast majority of people. Indigenous medicine was looked down by educated people and doctors trained in western medicine dominated the scene.

Today it is regaining recognition all over India as a valid system after it was brushed aside as unscientific. The vogue for "soft medicine" and natural products in the western industrial world is assisting in this revival. Modern medicine grew out of traditional medicine with ingredients derived from plants.

Traditional medicine is not confined to extracts of plants. It includes bone setting and physical manipulation. Modern medicine has undesirable side effects. Indigenous medicine is generally free from side effects. However, home or folk medicine cannot be a substitute for scientific diagnosis and sophisticated modern therapies provided by modern medicine for certain specified diseases.

Abscess was opened with a paste of *nivol kanti (euphoria nerifolia)* fresh turmeric and cashewnut.[50] A leaf of *mavlinguini (citrus medica)* was applied to remove pus coconut oil mixed with melted wax was applied to heal the wound.

For anemia a patient was prescribed a decoction made from the bark of a tree known as *Santanacho ruk (Alstonia scholaries)*. About 1 oz. of the bark was boiled in 20 ozs. of water. The patient had to drink 2 ozs. at a time, two to four times a day. Another remedy prescribed for anemia was a decoction of bark of a tree *Davo Kudo (Halarrhena antidysenterica)*. It was lightly warmed and the juice extracted. The extract used as ear drop was considered beneficial for ear infection and pain.

An asthma patient were given to drink milk of wild boar mixed with water. Dr. Baronio Monteiro had a treatment for bed-sores. patient's spit was applied over the bed-sores with successful results.

Bleeding was stopped by placing thread in the form of a cross over the wound or cut. Sprained legs and other sprained areas of the body were cured by rubbing seven times a key or a sickle in the morning, evening and following day. It was also a practice to call a person who was born with his legs first. This person was asked to massage the sprained area.

Patients suffering from body-aches were advised by Dr. Baronio Monteiro to sun bath. This exposure to the sun relieved pain. Elements of nature were used by him to cure various illnesses. Water heated in the sun was considered good for health. He prescribed tamarind juice mixed with jaggery as a purgative. Typhoid fevers were cured with baths given every three hours.

Cataract in the eyes was reported to be cured by applying to the big toe the leaves of *Boram (Zizyphus Jujuba)* tree chewed by a *montri* (magician) for period of seven days. If the cataract was in the right eye, the paste was applied to the left foot, and vice versa.

In cases of cholera the native medicine men prescribed paste of *Teffolans (Xanthoxylum rhetesu)*, mustard seeds and garlic ground with vinegar. In Bicholim the people used a paste of mustard, drumstick, pepper and ginger ground with fenny.

Convulsions in children were cured by fumigating the head of the child with tobacco imported from Deccan. At the same time a packet of *sapus rintho* (camphor) and *hing (asafetida)* was hung around the neck and given to smell. The sick person was beaten on the head with a small branch of jackfruit tree or a plant known as *Usky*. Among the Christians it was a practice to make the child smell kerosene and burnt cloth. Many children having convulsions were treated with hot metal applied to the arm or leg. Another practice was to give cold water bath to the child.

Coagulated milk in the stomach was known as *gonxes* which the indigenous believed caused convulsion gastro-enteritis and dysentery. The child was given a concoction of a creeper known as *Gonsvel* and mint leaves to prevent convulsions.

Oddulso (Adathode Vasica) a common herb around the compound walls provided relief for coughs and fevers. Pieces of coconuts, bananas and some fruits were given to the monkey to chew. They were removed from monkey's mouth and given to chew to the person suffering whooping cough.

Diabetes patients were given the skin of a root known as *quivani (helicters ixora)*, wine of *jambulão (Eugenia Jambolana)*, juice of ripe figs *(Ficus Glomerata)*, decoction of the bark of *vodel (Ficus Indica)* or boiled flowers of banana tree. It was prepared by mixing 1 oz. of the bark with 1 oz. of water. Many people drank a decoction of *padvali roots (Cissampelos Pareira)* which was prepared with 1 oz. of roots and 20 ozs. of water.

Dysentery was controlled with decoction of the roots of *cuddo (holarrhena antide - senterica)* or *pitmari (marengamiaalata)*. Ear ache was relieved with garlic *(Allium Sativium)* in oil. Some people used the juicy stem of a wild cactus.

Eclampsy was prevented with a paste of mustard and garlic applied to the base of the feet and head of the expectant mother.

White onion, (roasted and ground) was applied to the forehead to get rid of headache and reduce fever.

There were many cases of leprosy in Goa during the Portuguese regime. It was an incurable disease in those days. However, it is reported that in the early stages some traditional remedies proved effective. About 50 gms. of sap of *Neem (Melia azadirachta)* was prescribed to the patient daily. The body was massaged daily with the sap. In case the sap was not available the patient was prescribed 5 gms of pepper and 10 gms. of neem leaves ground into a paste. This paste had to be swallowed for 40 days.

Mouth trash, popularly known as *Movem* or *Moem* was treated with a paste of dry lobster (head only) and honey applied to the affected area.

Nephralgia was cured with a leaf of jackfruit inserted in the nose in cone shape and the patient was beaten on the base of his head until he bled.

Rheumatism was cured by applying a solution made of 1 gm. of opium extract, 4 gms. belladone extract and 60 gms. glycerin with the help of cotton or cloth.[51]

A victim of smallpox was given a concoction made of *Poripat (Oldenlandia Corimvosa)*. The patient was fed on canjee without salt. The patient was made to sleep on a plain mat without a mattress. On the seventh day the body was massaged with wild flowers previously dipped in luke warm water. The patient was given a bath only on 21st day. No fish or any food stuff was fried in the house. It was believed that frying prevented eruption from taking proper course. The blisters were covered with dry cowdung.

Teeth problems: To remove caries the tooth puller boiled coconuts oil with garlic and mustard. The oil after cooling was poured with the help of funnel (made of banana leaf) in the ear, on the side of the injured tooth. After a few minutes the patient was asked to empty the contents and the tooth puller would show some tiny threads as caries. This treatment was

Indigenous Medicine and Traditions

not efficacious. Toothache was stopped by mixing pepper and fenny. The paste was applied to the side of the face. Pepper could be replaced by saffron or salt.

Tuberculosis had no cure in the early days. The sick sought the help of *herbolarios* and *curandeiros. The* victims and their families tried to conceal the disease due to stigma attached to it. Native medicine consisted of giving the patient everyday 2 gms. of powered skull of a small deer. The patient was fed on soup of boiled frogs and bandicoot. Garlic was considered a wonderful remedy for T.B. About 2 gms. of garlic with one kilo of sugar was boiled in 250 gms. of milk, till the quantity was reduced to one fourth. This decoction was prescribed to the patient three times a day.

There are a few home remedies for mumps. A thick paste of *dutro* is applied over the swelling. Some people covered the swollen portion with a paste of dry ginger. This was done to subside the pain and decrease swelling.

For wounds, inflammation and fevers the medicine men used *Taiquilo (Cassia)* plant.

Vomiting was stopped with the help of an egg. This egg was tied around the waist with the help of a cloth. The well known medicine man Madeva Oido of Querim, (Ponda) prescribed a simple method to stop hiccups by inserting in the nostril a toothpick and moving it to make the person sneeze. This was repeated if the hiccups did not stop.

Herbal and other Medicines

Goa abounds in myriad herbs, plants, spices which have great therapeutic value and have played an important role in the accumulation of medical knowledge. By observation and trial, the natives came to possess intimate knowledge of the medicinal properties of the vegetable kingdom. These remedies were the basis of health care in rural area. In fact remedies of elderly female in the family was often all that was available by way of medical help. Measurements were not precise. As the ingredients used were harmless, a little more or a little less did not matter.

Herbal medicine consisted of roots, bark, leaves, flowers, fruits, seeds, juices and gums of plants. The effect of medicine varied with the time or season, when the medicine was collected.

Medicine could not be used from a place covered with water, neither from dry sandy ground nor from one that had holes. Places destroyed by insects or where white ants had their nests, where bodies were burnt or buried. Sacred places were not proper places for raising medicinal plants. Soil in which there was much salt was unfavourable for the growth of medicine. The most favourable soil for medicine was situated near water. This soil helped the growth of trees.

The day and the time of the collection was also important to ensure cure of the disease. Medicines administered internally were taken for the first time on Mondays, Thursdays and Fridays. The medicine was collected when the auspicious stars were in ascendant. Before medicinal plants were gathered in the morning a prayer was said with face turned towards the north. Most medicines were taken on empty stomach for better effect.[52]

Allopathic physicians made use of herbal medicine. Some herbal medicines were used in the Royal Hospital and later in the Military Hospital probably because they were efficacious or no other drugs were available to cure particular diseases. Indigenous medicine was sent from Goa to various Portuguese *Feitorias*. There is reference in the Mhamai House records to drugs sent from Goa to Portugal such as opium, *xarope de brindão*, leaves of *malva*, eyes of crabs and others.[53]

Thermal Baths and Springs

The inhabitants of Goa visited periodically some of its beaches usually in the hot months of the year to find cure for many of their ailments. The sea water baths provided relief to health problems such as arthritis and skin disorders. Baga, Calangute, Colva, Benaulim, Miramar, Vagator beaches are well known for its medicinal value in folk medicine. However, it was believed that the sea water did not give relief to those staying near the sea all year around. Therefore, the inhabitants of coastal areas had spring bath to cure some of their health problems. Goa has about 40 well known fresh water springs.[54] Most of them are situated in Old Conquests. The spring at Ambora (Salcete) was mainly used by those having cutaneous eruptions. The one at Beloy (Margão) was supposed to help those suffering from nervous problems and patients suffering from hemorrhoids. Many visited the spring at Tollem (Assagão-Bardez) to get relief from lung diseases. The fresh water of Maina-Batim in Ilhas was considered to be a good blood purifier. The St. Peter's spring at Ponda was used by those having problems with their eyes.

REFERENCES

1. *The voyage of John van Linschoten to the East Indies,* ed., A.C. Burnell and P.A. Tiele, vol. II, London, 1885, p. 230.
2. *François Bernier's Travels in the Moghul Empire,* New Delhi, 1927, p. 338.
3. HAG: Ms 3027: *Provisôes, Alvaras e Regimentos 1518-1526,* fl. 33v. *APO,* Fasc. 5º, Part I, pp. 44-45.
4. *A.P.O.,* Fasc. 5º, Part II, Goa, 1886, pp. 543-545. This was the first order banning the practice of the native physicians. Since the newly converted Christians were at large extent influenced by native physicians who would perhaps be in a position to reconvert them the order banned the practise.
5. *Bullarium Patronatus in ecclesiis Africae, Asiae atque Oceaniae,* Tomo I, ed., V. de Paiva Manso, Lisboa, 1889, p. 69; A.P.O., Fasc. IV, 1857, p. 25. Any non-Christian physician found treating a Christian patient was to be sent away from the city.
6. *Ibid.,* p. 86.
7. HAG: *Ms.* 9529: *Provisões a favor de Christandade,* fl. I; HAG: *MR.* 93, fl. 363.
8. HAG: *Ms.* 9529 – *Provisões a favor de Cristandade,* fl. 83.
9. Nicolau Manucci *Storia do Mogor,* ed., W. Irwine, III, Calcutta, 1966, p. 128.
10. Antonio Baião, *A Inquisição de Goa,* Coimbra, 1930, p. 317.
11. HAG: Ms. 7795 *Livro das Posturas,* fl. 25.
12. *Ibid.,* fls. 25-27.
13. *Ibid.,* fls. 25-27.
14. HAG: *Ms.* 7795., fl. 25v; HAG: *Ms.* 7696: *Registos Gerais do Senado,* fl. 118. Madav Bhot was given a licence to fill the 30th place among the native physicians.
15. Jacinto Caetano Barreto Miranda, *Quadros Historicos de Goa,* III, Margão, 1865, p. 63.
16. Arquivo National da Torre do Tombo – Lisboa (henceforth Torre do Tombo): *Conselho Geral do Santo Oficio,* Maço 38, no. 7.
17. Torre do Tombo: *Conselho Geral do Santo Oficio - Maço 33, no. 20.*
18. Torre do Tombo: *Conselho Geral do Santo Oficio,* Maço 38, *no. 7.*
19. Torre do Tombo: *Conselho Geral do Santo Oficio,* Maço 38, *no. 7.*
20. Jose Antonio Oliveria, "Relatorio 11 de Junho 1853" *Jornal de Pharmacia e Sciencias Medicas da India Portuguesa,* Nova Goa, 1862, p. 56.
21. Boletim do Governo do Estado da India, no.19, 13 de Maio 1853.
22. *Jornal de Pharmacia e Sciencias Medicas,* ed., Gomes Roberto, March 1863, p. 56.
23. HAG: Ms. MR. 52, fl. 192. This native doctor was given informal training at the Royal Hospital.
24. HAG: Ms. *Monções do Reino,* 177 A, fls. 211-212 : Ignacio Afonso a native worked as a doctor in the Royal Hospital.
25. *Boletim do Governo do Estado da India,* 26 de Maio 1838, p. 157.
26. B.O., no. 38, 23rd March 1860.
27. HAG: Ms. 11668 – *CD,* fl. 142.
28. *Census 1910,* pp. 19-31.
29. Torre do Tombo : *Conselho Geral do Santo Oficio,* Maço 33, Appendix-1. no. 19, In 1785 Margarida Borges from S. Bartholomeo (Chorão) was found guilty of practising superstitious rituals during deliveries. As punishment she was exiled to *Casa de Polvorat.* Another woman by name of Catharina (Boteli) was reprimanded in 1790 by the Inquisição for same reasons. *(Conselho Geral do Santo Oficio* Maço 33, no. 24).

30. Pyrard, *Viagem de Francisco Pyrard de Laval*, ed., A. de Basto Magalhães, II, Porto, 1944, p. 54.
31. HAG: Ms. 2785 – *Despezas do convento da Graça*, fl. 96.
32. Barreto Miranda, *op. cit.*, p. 67.
33. A.B. Bragança Pereira, *Etnografia da India Portuguesa*, II, Bastora, 1940, p. 202. (Henceforth Bragança Pereira).
34. XCHR : *French Mhamai House Papers*, Vol. 6, fl. 25v (papers in French) and MMS. 14, 986.
35. Torre do Tombo: *Conselho Geral do Santo Oficio*, Maço 33, no. 19.
36. Torre do Tombo : *Conselho Geral do Santo Oficio*, Maço 33, no. 17.
37. Torre do Tombo : *Conselho Geral do Santo Oficio*, Maço 33, no. 21. He was also accused of contributing towards the purchase of coconuts and fowls meant to be offered to the temple.
38. *Ibid*. See Appendix 6-A.
39. Torre do Tombo : *Conselho Geral do Santo Oficio*, Maço 33, no. 19.
40. Torre do Tombo: *Conselho Geral do Santo Oficio*, Maço 33, no. 20. In the seventeenth century several people were punished for resorting to non-Christian rituals in order to seek cure. (Maço 38, no. 7; Maço 33, no. 27; Livro 369.).
41. *Conselho Geral do Santo Oficio*, Maço 33, no. 27, Appendices 6-B, 6-C.
42. Sebastiaao Gonçalves, *Primeira Parte da Historia dos Religiosos da Companhia de Jesus*, I, Coimbra, 1957, p. 380.
43. *Ibid.*, p. 421.
44. A contemporary manuscript copy in the private collection of Dr. Teotonio de Souza, Porvorim, Goa.
45. Torre do Tombo: *Conselho Geral do Santo Oficio*, Maço 33, nos. 18, 21 and 22.
46. *Boletim Geral de Medicina e Farmacia* 1934, Bastora, p. 77.
47. A. Lopes Mendes, *A India Portugusa – Breve descripção das posessões portuguesas na Asia*, II, New Delhi, 1989, (reprint), p. 42.
48. Brangana Pereira, *op. cit.*, p. 270; *Summario Chronologico de Decretos Diocesanos desde 1775-1899 – Decretos do* Arcebispo D. Francisco d'Assumpção e Brito, ed., Manuel Joço Socrates d'Albu querque, Bastora, 1900, p. 25.
49. Torre do Tombo: *Conselho Geral do Santo Oficio*, Mao 36, no. 23.
50. Filipe Nery Correia, *Medicina Indigena*, Margão, 1929, p. 1.
51. *Archivo de Pharmacia Sciences accessories da India Portuguesa*, ed., Antonio Gomes Roberto, 1863, Nova Goa.
52. Appendix – 6 D, Provides a list of some commonly used plants and minerals in Goa.
53. XCHR : *Mhamai House Papers*, Doc. 3314, fl. not numbered.
54. Esteves, *op. cit.*, p. 74.

7

WESTERN MEDICINE: TRAINING FACILITIES AND TRAINED DOCTORS
Goa Medical School
(Escola Medico-Cirurgica de Goa)

The Portuguese in Goa were probably the first to teach medicine and surgery of western kind in a systematic way in India. The first medical school of western medicine in Asia was opened in 1842 at the Military Hospital in Nova Goa. Earlier the informal education of medicine was carried out at the Royal Hospital in the city of Goa.

Jesuit missionaries taught philosophy, astronomy, theology, mathematics at St. Paul College and medicine at the Hospital for the Poor (*Hospital da Gente Pobre da Terra*) run by the Jesuits in the city of Goa. It appears that the Jesuits were convinced that knowledge of medicine was essential for their work among the poor. Medical care was generally at this time in the hands of non-Christians. Moreover, they knew medicine was a highly prized profession through which they could enter the courts of native rulers and receive favours on behalf of Portuguese kings. Furthermore, the Jesuits had missions in China and other parts of Asia where they needed personnel with medical knowledge.

The Portuguese rulers believed also that the teaching of medical science was important for gaining confidence of the people which later they could exploit to their own advantage. In addition there are other factors that contributed to the teaching of medicine, such as an acute paucity of trained doctors. Goa was dependent on Portugal for medical personnel. Portuguese medical doctors were reluctant to come to India on account of poor incentives, tropical climate and prevailing diseases. By the last quarter of the sixteenth century, the city of Goa was an unhealthy place. The city suffered from constant epidemics that reduced its population. Several viceroys and large number of soldiers died of dysentery, typhoid and other infectious diseases.

This chapter is divided into two sections. The first section is about medical training on western lines imparted at the Royal Hospital in the city of Goa and Goa Medical School at Nova Goa. Section II deals with contribution of doctors to Health and Hygiene in Goa, and of Goan doctors outside Goa.

I. MEDICAL TRAINING FACILITIES.

Royal Hospital (*Hospital Real*)

The prevailing unhealthy conditions in Goa forced viceroy D. Cristovam Souza Coutinho to initiate some measures. The viceroy requested the Home Government to send doctors who could teach medicine to the natives. It appears that the first steps to teach medicine at the Royal Hospital were started in the late seventeenth century. A reference is found in a Royal letter dated 23rd March 1691. In this letter the Portuguese king informed the local authorities about the appointment of two doctors to teach medicine in Goa.[1] Feleciano Gonsalves did not leave Portugal and the second doctor Manuel Rodrigues de Souza could not teach medicine as he fell ill on his arrival. Portuguese doctors were reluctant to take up appointments in India.[2] Finally after several appeals rudimentary teaching of medicine was started in 1702 with Cipriano Valadares as the master. During the first quarter of the eighteenth century students were taught only two subjects — *Cadeira Prima* and *Cadeira de Vespera*, besides practicals. The course was incomplete. During this period medical students in Portugal were taught five disciplines.

In March 1713 Manuel Rosa Pinto was appointed to teach *Cadeira de Vespera* with a salary of 500 *xerafins* paid quarterly.[3] It seems that in the next three years Dr. Rosa Pinto trained students to cure the sick. Dr. Pinto was followed by Dr. Jose da Silva Azevedo[4] and Dr. Francisco de Brito Vidigal in 1721.[5]

The earliest native doctor trained at the Royal Hospital is perhaps Gregorio Pereira Ribeiro. In 1732 he was considered the oldest trained doctor in Goa, probably at the time of Cipriano Valadares or Rosa Pinto.[6] Doctors trained at the Royal Hospital were absorbed in the hospital or had private practice. In 1735 King Jose instructed the Viceroy of India to grant permission to Manuel Caetano Alvares to practice as a physician in Portugal and all its colonies. He was the first and only Goan to be given *capelo gratuito* of Faculty of Medicine by an order issued by King Jose of Portugal.[7] Earlier his father Vincente Alvares was issued letter to practice by the Chief physician of Goa. Many others were given letters to practice. Among these were Pedro Roiz da Costa and Luis Alvares who worked as assistant physicians at the Royal Hospital. Antonio Xavier de Lima practised at S.Mathias and Antonio Tome dos Milagres practised at Panjim.

Teaching of medicine was not carried out on regular basis due to non-availability of teachers or because some of the Chief Physicians refused to carry out the teaching work as they were already overburdened with work in the hospital, as in the case of Dr. Costa Portugal who refused to teach on the grounds that the hospital lacked necessary equipment and books.[8]

In 1799 viceroy Souza Coutinho informed the Home Government of the need to have a Chief Physician and a good surgeon as the surgeon in the hospital was sick for the last one year and was unable to work.[9] The Royal Hospital had no trained doctor in western medicine between 1779-1801 after Dr. Costa Portugal left Goa.[10] Teaching of medicine was not carried out in Goa from 1775 to 1800. During this period the governors of Goa requested several times to the Home Government to send doctors who could teach medicine. It was felt that Goan youth would do well and would be useful in the field of medicine.[11] After the death of the native doctor Ignacio Afonso, the hospital had no doctor capable of running the institution.[12]

In 1800 the Portuguese Government appointed Dr.Antonio Jose Miranda e Almeida, a professor trained at Coimbra University to teach medicine in Goa.[13] He was also well versed in pharmacology and botany and a good administrator.[14] Dr. *Miranda Almeida* started a three years course in medicine and surgery at the Royal Hospital, Panelim, in 1801. Students seeking entry to the course required knowledge of Latin and French as most of the books used were written in these languages.

In the first year the students were provided with knowledge of anatomy. Pathology was taught in the second year together with botany and chemistry. In the third year the students learnt all about diseases. A total of eight disciplines were taught in the 3 years course.[15] There is no doubt that this course was an improvement upon the earlier one. A detailed list of books prescribed for this course is available.[16] The course had several limitations. The teaching of medicine was more theoretical than practical. Dr. Bernardo Peres da Silva was appointed to help Dr. Miranda Almeida and later when Dr. Almeida fell ill, Dr.Peres da

Silva a native, taught medicine in the hospital.[17] Many Goans joined the course.[18]

Dr. Almeida was followed by Dr. Antonio Jose de Lima Leitão.[19] He started a new course of four years.[20] The academic year was from June to March. Theory classes were held on alternate days and practicals were held daily. The students daily accompanied the teacher on his visits to the wards. Any student missing ten theory classes was not allowed to appear for his final examinations. A student failing twice had to leave the course. A dissertation had to be submitted at the end of the year. This dissertation had to be written in a closed classroom without the help of any book. Examinations were to be held at the end of every academic year. At the end of the four years the student was to be given a certificate of proficiency either in medicine or surgery, depending on the branch selected by the student. The *Curso Medico-Cirurgião* of 1821 consisted of following disciplines: Anatomy, physiology, *materia medica*, internal pathology and *nosografia medica e cirurgica*. In the fourth year the students were required to study internal organs and treatment. This course paved the way for the formal teaching of western medicine as early as 1842.

Goa Medical School

The Goa Medical School was established on 5th November 1842. It was set up along the lines of similar schools in France and Portugal. However, the facilities provided were limited as the best teachers did not find incentives to teach and the standard of teaching remained low. The staff at first consisted of four teachers who belonged to the health cadre, including the Director who was the Chief Physician of the State. These four teachers were entrusted with several disciplines of medicine. The school lacked proper equipment for class room work and research. Books prescribed for the course were either not available in Goa or were outdated. Some of them were published in the earlier century.

The school required entrants to be over 16 years of age and to have a good knowledge of Latin, grammar, philosophy and drawing. In addition the student was required to pass the first year of Mathematics School. The medical course was spread over four years, with the following subjects: Anatomy, physiology, *materia medica*, pharmacology, hygiene, pathology, surgery, history of medicine, internal pathology, medical clinics and forensic medicine. The school had a course of three years in pharmacy. The school was legalized on 26th March 1847 and provided with proper rules. It was known as *Escola Medico-Cirurgica de Nova Goa*. The first batch of students who graduated in 1846 consisted of Agostinho Vicente Lourenço, Felizardo Quadros, Gonzaga de Melo, Joaquim Lourenço de Araujo, Francisco Xavier Lourenço, Fremiot da Conceição, Luis Moreira and Bernardo Wolfango da Silva. Among the pharmacy course students Cosme Damião Pires received his diploma in 1846.

In 1856 the school council submitted a plan to the Home Government, requesting to improve the standard of teaching and to restrict admissions to the school. Students were to be admitted on alternate years. This was essential as qualified teachers were not available. Besides many graduates from the school remained without practice due to scarcity of jobs. Jobs in Government services were few and not easily accessible to the natives. Fifteen posts of military surgeons were occupied by the Portuguese doctors. Old Conquests with 2,47,846 inhabitants had 128 trained physicians. Hence, one doctor for 1,936 inhabitants. Margão, a small town in south Goa had 16 doctors. Moreover, non Christians rarely consulted doctors trained in western medicine. They resorted to *vaidyas* and other native medicine men. Graduates from Goa Medical School refused to work in rural areas because of poor amenities.

A plan was proposed to raise the number of subjects to nine, including general and topographic anatomy. The descriptive anatomy introduced earlier was of no help to the students. They could not learn many details because of scarcity of dead bodies and bones. The course was to be extended to five years. A report enclosed along with the plan of 1856 explained the difficulties faced by the school. The school had no buildings of its own. It was run in the Military Hospital with inadequate facilities. One lecture room was used for three classes. A building started five years earlier for the school was incomplete due to lack of funds. Anatomy was imperfectly taught from pictures and models. The scarcity of bodies prevented the school from having regular practicals in anatomy. Students had no proper training in obstetrics. It was also taught with pictures since female patients were not admitted in the hospital attached to the school. Therefore, the school had placed orders in Paris for a doll and parts of female organs made of synthetic material. The existing equipment was limited. The plan of 1856 was approved only in 1865 with minor changes. The Director of Health Services was appointed the Director of Medical School.[21] In 1859 the school received books from Lisbon.[22]

During this period an unsuccessful attempt was made to merge the Military Hospital with *Hospital da Misericordia*. This merger would have solved some of the problems of the school in the field of gynecology and pediatrics.

Another plan was submitted in 1871 by the Director of the school Dr.Fonseca Torrie. This plan stressed the need for further improvements in the school. The existing course failed to meet the needs of the native population. For example, there was no midwifery course in the school. This course was judged essential because of high incidence of maternity and infant mortality. Women at the time of their deliveries sought the help of untrained *dais*. The report recommended establishment of wards for women and children. This need was not satisfied until the early twentieth century. The report also recommended laboratories for research and a botanical garden.

The school library had a collection of 205 books. Between 1870-1880 it acquired 3,711 books. The school received also some plants and some material needed for anatomy practicals. This was possible due to loans granted by Visconde de S. Januario to the tune of 3,880 *xerafins*. In addition the Archbishop had ordered for some instruments through the *Banco Ultramarino*.

Contemporary sources indicate that the school authorities constantly pressed for the improvement of facilities in the school. Their demands were motivated probably by their professional ethos and concern for the institution.

Several plans were submitted to the Government between 1871-1896. Every plan demanded changes in the curriculum, better service conditions for the staff and a properly equipped course for midwives. None of these plans were approved by the Government.

A complete apathy on the part of the Government was noticed. In 1888 one more report was sent to Portugal emphasizing the need to have well organized medical care, which was regarded necessary to perpetuate colonial rule and economic exploitation. A course of six years with 21 subjects and a pharmacy course of three years were proposed.[23] The report recommended that the school should have at least ten teachers and four substitute teachers. It was also proposed to rename the school as *Escola de Medicina Naval e Colonial*. The plan further suggested that the school should be sponsored by the Ministry of Overseas Colonies. Consequently, the graduates of Goa Medical School could be appointed to the overseas health services.

Most of the plans submitted to the local Government were not processed due to dearth of funds and deficiencies noticed in the plans. In 1894 further changes were demanded asking the Government to set up a laboratory for anatomy, pathology and bacteriology. The study of these subjects was to be made compulsory for the students after finishing their medical course. The plan also proposed the introduction of new subjects. The new curriculum would consist of general and descriptive anatomy in the first year. The same subject was to be repeated in the second year together with general biology and human physiology. In the third year the students would learn all about *matèria medica*, pharmacology, general pathology, dermatology and clinical surgery. In the fourth year again the students would be taught pathology (internal and tropical), surgery, hygiene, practical medicine and surgery. Finally in the last year they would learn obstetrics, legal medicine, clinical surgery and medicine.

The school decided to start courses for nurses and midwives. Two new departments were attached to the school to cover experimental physiology and diagnosis.[24] It also asked for more teaching staff.

By the end of the nineteenth century the Military and Mathematics school was closed down. As a result students joining the medical course no longer required the first year of Mathematics School. Instead the knowledge of English, Geography and Science was made compulsory. Incidentally science taught in Goa was outdated.

Despite severe limitations, the achievements of the school were quite commendable. Eight to ten doctors graduated annually as general practitioners. These doctors practiced in Portuguese India and Portuguese colonies of Africa, Macau and Timor. In 1881 about 43 graduates of Goa Medical School worked outside Goa in the Portuguese colonies. The Goa Medical School was the only medical school in Portuguese colonies. Portuguese doctors were still reluctant to work in India because of poor incentives and ban on private practice. The scales of Higher Secondary School (*Liceu*) teachers were higher than the scales of the teachers in the Medical School. Besides the latter had additional duties in the hospital and outside in times of epidemics.

The Goa Medical School faced several problems in the early twentieth century mainly due to lack of proper equipment, teaching staff and complete apathy from the Home Government.

In January 1905 the school council sent one more appeal to the Ministry of Overseas Colonies demanding changes in the existing medical course.[25] It proposed a curriculum with twelve disciplines spread over a course of five year, increase in number of teaching staff and improvement in their service conditions. Establishment of a course for midwives was also proposed. Primary school certificate and 21 years of age were suggested as minimum qualifications for those seeking admission for the course of midwives. But there was no response from the Home Government. However, it approved the establishment of an Institute of Bacteriology. The purpose was to investigate the causes of various epidemics that occurred regularly in Goa. The Institute was established in 1907. The school was still being governed by decrees issued in the nineteenth century.

An apparent lack of interest from the Government prompted some members of the school council to discuss its future. They suggested that the Government should close down the school. However, the Director Dr. Miguel Caetano Dias and some others opposed the move. The Director submitted fresh proposals to the Government. He stressed the pioneering work done by the school in training young doctors and expressed regret about the attitude of the Government. Many young Goans preferred to join medical schools in Bombay. After the British had made themselves the undisputed masters of the Indian sub-continent Goa had lost its importance. Besides medical schools, Bombay offered better facilities for training. The Director of Goa Medical School warned the authorities that this exodus would encourage decolonization. Further, it was suggested that Goa was the right place for the teaching of tropical medicine.[26]

The issue was discussed in the Portuguese Parliament. It was suggested that the school be closed down if it did not meet the required standards. In lieu of the school some deputies recommended granting of scholarships to Goans to pursue their medical studies in Portugal. The Portuguese press also expressed its opinion. It stressed the need to train doctors in their own environment. Teaching of tropical disease could be imparted better in tropical countries.[27]

The discussions and appeals resulted in three orders being issued by the Government between 1913-1919. They allowed *adhoc* changes in the school curriculum. The medical course included 18 disciplines to be taught during five years with seven teachers, one substitute teacher and two assistant teachers. Descriptive anatomy, physiology and histology was to be taught in the first year. In the second year the students would learn all about topographic anatomy, human physiology and microbiology. During the third year the students learnt pathological anatomy and dermatology, *materia medica*, external pathology, general pathology and pharmacology — both theory and practicals. Internal pathology, exotic pathology, surgery and hygiene was to be taught in the fourth year. Finally, in the fifth year the student learnt all about clinical medicine, clinical surgery, obstetrics, gynecology and general medicine.[28]

The school was still experimenting with various disciplines of

Western Medicine

medicine and as a result many new disciplines were included from time to time while some existing ones were dropped.

In 1922 the School Council proposed certain changes in the existing decree of 11th October 1865, probably because it found some deficiencies and revision was necessary to meet the needs of the time. The changes gave extra powers to the School Council, such as to approve the teaching plan prepared by the teaching staff for each academic year. This plan had to be published 15 days before the new academic year. The Council was empowered to issue passing certificates to those who completed their studies in medicine and pharmacy as well to award prizes to the students. In the beginning of each academic year the teaching staff was to be given a time table. Each teacher was to be given a maximum of nine teaching hours. Teachers who failed to enter a class room within 15 minutes after the bell were to be marked absent. Any teacher who was absent 20 times without any explanation would lose one third of their teaching allowance. The teaching staff was asked to sign the muster daily and to write down the work discussed in the class. The amount to be collected from the students for issuing a decree was fixed by the legislation. It also revised the fees to be paid by the students. Admission fees for the medical course was 34:04:07 each year. The degree of *medico cirurgião* was granted for 85:11:05. (Rs. tgs. rs.).

The library was put in charge of a substitute teacher who was responsible to the School Council. Newspapers and journals were not to be issued to the staff. Any staff member who wished to take a book home from the library had to apply for the same in writing. Reference books could be issued to the teachers only during summer holidays. Other books could be issued for 15 days and reissued if there was no claim from others.

In case all the students stayed away from a class the teacher could consider the matter as done. This step was taken so that the curriculum was not affected due to the absence of the students. Each lecture was of ninety minutes. The first thirty minutes were for revision of the matter discussed in the previous lecture. In each subject there were three lectures per week. However, the practicals were to be held daily. Students missing 10 lectures in each subject of three weekly lectures or 20 in subjects with six weekly lectures without proper reason would not be allowed to appear for examination in the subject. The Council and the teachers were warned not to help the students in this matter.

There were written and practical examinations. All final examinations had to begin in March. Each student had to submit a dissertation. A committee was appointed to go through the matter. The guide of the student could not be a member of this committee.[29]

The medical course now consisted of eighteen disciplines. In the first year the students were taught descriptive anatomy, general physiology and histology. In the second year students learnt all about topographic anatomy, human physiology, and microbiology. Pathologic anatomy, dermatology, *materia medica*, external pathology and *propedeutica cirurgica* was done in the third year together with general pathology, theoretical pharmacology and practicals. In the fourth year internal pathology, *propedeutica medica*, exotic pathology, surgery, general hygiene and demographic sanitation, climatology and intertropical hygiene and practicals was taught. Finally, in the last year they learnt about medicine, clinical surgery, obstetrics, gynecology and general medicine. This course was to be conducted by eight full-time teachers, one substitute teachers and three assistant teachers.

A new curriculum for the school was proposed in 1927 by Dr. Froilano de Mello, the Director of the School.[30] In this curriculum the medical course would be spread over six years with 21 subjects including physics, zoology, biology and bio-chemistry. Dr. de Mello suggested the introduction of specialized courses in ophthalmology, E.N.T., physiotherapy, pediatrics, venereal diseases and the study of Ayurvedic medicine. These courses were thought necessary because otherwise in their absence the sick had to avail themselves of facilities in far away places in British India.

The teaching staff of the medical school was burdened with the work in the school, hospital and the health services. In 1946 the teaching staff of the school succeeded in their attempts to separate the school from the Health Services. The Goa Medical School was made an autonomous body with Dr. Germano Correia as its director. A new plan of reform was approved by the Ministry of Overseas Colonies. The new course was spread over five years. The school was granted permission to engage assistant professors and substitute professors in addition to full-time professors. Nevertheless, the teaching staff continued to be overburdened with work in the hospital.

In 1946 the Goa Medical School was provided with a new curriculum. In a five-year course the students were taught anatomy, histology, embryology, physiology, bacteriology, medical zoology, pharmacology, surgery, medicine, climatology, hygiene, endemology, legal medicine, obstetrics-gynecology and orthopedics. The Pharmacy course was also reorganized. The school still lacked proper facilities. Some of the existing laboratories remained with the Health Services. The grants from the

Government were too small to meet the needs of the time.

The planned transfer of laboratories from Health Services to the Medical School did not materialize. Attempts were made in 1952 to transfer them to one centrally located building so that both the institutions could use them. This attempt also failed. Finally in 1958 the Ministry of the Overseas Colonies determined the following:

The laboratory for clinical analysis and bacteriology, the laboratory of chemical analysis, bramatology, toxicology as well the X-rays and physiotherapy units were to be attached to Goa Medical School.[30] As soon as these laboratories started funtioning, the laboratory of analysis established in 1952 was to be closed down. The staff working in this unit as well in the X-rays unit (started in 1944) were to be transferred to the new laboratories with the same designation. The laboratory of clinical analysis would have a director, assistant doctor, two laboratory assistants, one clerk and two peons. The laboratory of chemical analysis would be in charge of a Director with one assistant doctor, one mechanic cum photographer, one male nurse, one female nurse and two peons. The posts of assistant doctors were to be filled with graduates from Portugal or Goa Medical School. The selection was to be done through interviews. The post was on contract basis. The post of the pharmacist was also to be filled in the same manner. Technical qualifications were required for the post of a technician. In case qualified candidates were not available the post was to be filled with candidates having 5th year of Lyceum.

In 1949 the school received large grants from the government for, equipment diets and medicine. Between 1949-1959 several decrees were issued to introduce changes in the curriculum. Due to a fire in 1957 several laboratories were destroyed. At the end of the Portuguese regime there were plans to put up a new building for the school but could not be implemented due to a change of regime.

II. EMINENT DOCTORS

Goans have made a distinct contribution in the sphere of medicine since the early eighteenth century and they have continued it till today. They have contributed as general practitioners and as specialists in various branches of medicine. They have worked to eradicate contagious diseases and have devoted themselves to valuable research in the field of medicine, not only in Goa but outside the territory. Joaquim Francisco Colaço, Caetano Florencio Colaço, Caetano Francisco Xavier, Bossuet da Piedade Rebelo, Joaquim Bernadino de Santana Pinto, Antonio Micael de Azaredo and others worked in Portuguese colonies of Africa to eradicate several epidemics. Doctors in medicine enjoyed great prestige in early days. Some doctors who graduated from the medical school did not practise as doctors. They involved themselves in non-medical work, probably because it was potentially lucrative or it appealed to them. These doctors became famous in administrative field, politics, anthropology, economic and cultural life. Thus for instance, Francisco Luis Gomes, Gerson da Cunha, Nicolau Fonseca, Blasio Paes, Constancio Mascarenhas and Mariano Saldanha. Many of them might have joined the medical profession, not because they were inclined towards the profession, but due to the fact that higher academic courses were very limited or to keep up the tradition in the family. Besides, the title of doctor was considered prestigious. Such doctors have not been included in this study. As in Portugal, Goa also has a tradition of "doutores" without a degree from a medical school or any college for that matter.

This chapter only includes medical doctors who became known for the their work in the medical field. It has not been possible also to include all eminent doctors due to lack of reliable information. Majority of doctors were Christians. There were very few Hindus in the profession. It could be due to the restrictions imposed by the *varna* and the belief that touching a dead body was "polluting".

a) **Trained in Goa — working in or outside Goa**

Goans not only earned fame at home but also in the international field. The first Goan doctors trained in the Royal Hospital who crossed the seas were Vicente Dias Ataide from Taleigão, Antonio Fernandes from Ribandar, Mateus Pereira and Manuel de Conceição, both from Panjim.

Agostinho Vicente Lourenço (1822-1896) from Margão was one of the first students of Goa Medical School. After completing his medical studies he joined Goa Medical School. His great desire was to go for further studies in Portugal but he could not afford it. A scholarship of *Camaras Agrarias* enabled him to go to Portugal and another scholarship helped him to study in Paris. Agostinho Vicente Lourenço worked under renowned scientists Wurtz and Bunsen. In 1855 he made important discoveries on the derivatives of glycol and glycerin and polyhydric alcohols. He took a degree in engineering and returned to Portugal to teach there. He organized the chemistry department of the University of Lisbon. He undertook a series of chemical analyses of the mineral waters of Chaves, Vizela and Vidago (Portugal). His research was presented at a scientific session at the University exhibition in Paris. The Portuguese Government gave him an award for his work.[32]

Augusto Carlos de Lemos was the precursor of preventive quininism. This prophylactic which he used in Goa in 1869 was put into practice on a wider scale half a century later by the French during the First World War in the course of the Macedonian campaign.

Jose Antonio Valeriano Coutinho from Aldona completed his studies in 1876. He worked in the island of Cabo Verde and organized an excellent plan to eradicate smallpox in the colony. At this time graduates from Goa Medical School were not allowed to practise in Portugal, neither they were promoted to grade I in the colonies. Valeriano fought against this discrimination. Portuguese whites in the colonial armies were promoted without having any studies, while the doctors graduated from Goa Medical School were not promoted to more than a lieutenant in the army.[33]

Jose Pedro Ismael Sertorio Caridade Moniz was the first to use with successful results an arsenic compound in tripanosomiasis human, revealing thereby a rare clinical knowledge of a sickness, the etiology of which was unknown. Moniz was also the first to combine arsenic with iodine just as Moore and others had combined it with atotoxil.[34]

Luis Caetano Santana Alvares was in the health cadre of Guine and Mozambique. He was born in Margão. In 1888 he graduated from Goa Medical School with brilliant academic record. He did equivalent medical studies in the city of Oporto (Portugal). He worked to eradicate plague. He also rendered his services during the military operation at Geba and Bissau. The Portuguese Government honoured him with awards of *Torre e Espada*, medals of *Christo e Avis* and a gold medal for his outstanding work in the Overseas colonies. He retired in 1910 as medical captain in the army.[35]

João Vicente Santana Barreto died in 1913 at Lisbon. He studied medicine at Goa Medical School and later studied in Portugal. He was appointed to lead the committee to inquire about sleeping sickness at Guine for which he was honoured. His important works are: *A tripanossomiase humana na Guine Portuguesa O beriberi na Guine Portuguesa, Historia de Guine, Insectos Henatofogos de Goa, Encefalite Tuberculosa e Menigite celebral para meningocica, Plague in Portuguese India, Estudos Epidemiologico sobre a peste na India Portuguesa, Os Indios e as Farpas.*[36]

Francisco Antonio Wolfango da Silva (1864-1947) was the Director of Health Services of Portuguese India between 1915- 1926. He studied at Goa Medical School, later he repeated his medical studies in Lisbon.[37] Wolfango da Silva acquired an additional degree in pharmacy. Before joining the Goa Medical School as a professor he worked in the health cadre of Angola. He was the first surgeon to perform operations for strangulated hernia and laparastomy in Goa. Francisco Wolfango da Silva took an active part in the campaign against plague that broke out at Ribandar (Ilhas) in the early twentieth century. A good orator and writer, he was born at Nova Goa.[38] He was given several awards by the Portuguese Government for his work to end the epidemics of smallpox in the island of S. Tiago, cholera in Salcete (Goa) and Daman.

Pedro Joaquim Peregrino da Costa (1890-1960) born in Navelim, Goa, completed his medical studies in 1912 and equivalent studies in Lisbon. He studied also at the Institute of Histology of the Faculty of Medicine Lisbon. Peregrino Costa specialized in problems of digestion and heart at a well known hospital of Paris. In 1916 he joined the health cadre of Macau and worked to eradicate meningitis and cholera from the area. He organized also units for leprosy, tuberculosis and pediatrics at Macau. He attended the Congress of Far Eastern Association of Tropical Medicine at Tokyo in 1925, at Calcutta in 1927 and at Hong Kong in 1938. The Portuguese Government awarded him *Ordem de Avis* and *Benemerencia*. He started *Boletim Sanitario de Macau* and has a number of works to his credit. [39]

Jose Camilo Aires da Conceição Sa (1882-1956) from Nova Goa hailed from a family of doctors. He obtained a degree from Goa Medical School in 1907. He specialized in equivalent medical studies with distinction at the University of Oporto. His thesis entitled "Hygiene de Panjim" was published in Goa. He acquired a diploma in Tropical Medicine from Lisbon. This diploma was a requirement to all desiring to join health services. After a brief stint in Portuguese colonies of Macau and Timor he was transferred to Goa Medical School as a professor. During the First World War he took active part in the plague campaign in Margão where he was posted as special doctor in the Health Board. The precautionary measures taken by him helped to control plague and improve the health and hygiene of the town. Since it was war time it was not possible to easily import machines. The small sulfur disinfection. Clayton type of machine owned by the Health Department was required at the outpost of Colem. This led Aires de Sa to improvise a machine which could be manufactured locally. This machine was named Airiston. The same was later imitated by Dr. Ed. Bonjean of Paris who named it

Western Medicine

Notial. Aires de Sa modified Willets pincers used in obstetrics and was responsible for starting the department of radiology and electrotherapy at the Goa Medical School.[40]

Antonio Augusto T.R. do Rego (1887-1972) son of João Filipe do Rego was born at Nova Goa. He was professor at Goa Medical School and took an active part in campaign against plague that broke out in Margão during the First World War.

Froilano de Mello (1887-1955) born at Benaulim (Goa) concluded his medical studies in Goa, and later repeated the course at Oporto (Portugal). In 1910 he returned to Goa with an additional diploma in Tropical Medicine of the University of Lisbon. He joined the Goa Medical School and also took charge of the Bacteriological Institute — a small shed in Campal (Goa) which became the center of his great activities as scientist.[41] In his research with a microscope Froilano de Mello discovered thousand of protozoa, parasites and microbes which today bear the Latin names given by him, followed by his own surname de Mello, as the discoverer. He published more than 200 research papers on bacteriology in Portuguese, French and English journals. He was colonel in the army and was later appointed Director of Health Services of Portuguese India from 1927-1947. He was the Dean of Goa Medical School. In 1945 he was elected member of the Portuguese Parliament.[42]

Froilano de Mello worked to eradicate tuberculosis in Goa and malaria from Old Goa. Due to his efforts two important institutions were established namely the Leprosarium at Macasana (Salcete) today known as *Leprosaria Froilano de Mello* and *Dispensario Virgem Peregrina* at St. Inez (Panjim). He succeded in opening a ward for lepers in Daman. He headed a Portuguese delegation to the World Leprosy Conference in Cuba and attended at least 37 World conferences. The President of Cuba honoured him with the *Grau de San Martin*. Pope Paul IV and Queen Juliana of Netherlands awarded him medals of honour. Froilano de Mello was a great orator and always in demand to raise toasts for Goan weddings

His work in French entitled *A la veille du Centenaire* describes in a nutshell the contribution of Goa Medical School during the first hundred years of its establishment.[43] Froilano de Mello was responsible for introducing measures to improve urban sanitation including the establishment of Sanitary Police in the capital town.[44]

Alberto Carlos Germano da Silva Correa doctor of the military corps, professor and Director of Goa Medical School was born in Nova Goa in 1888. He studied in Goa and Oporto and acquired additional diploma in Tropical Medicine before joining the teaching staff of Goa Medical

School in 1912. In 1946 when the Health Services where separated from Medical School he was appointed the Dean of Goa Medical School. He attended various medical conferences in Lisbon, London and Cairo. He was interested in anthropology, history, ethnography and climatology. He has written more than twenty papers and several books on health and hygiene of Goa and Angola. He was awarded many medals by the Portuguese Government and the Pope. He reached the rank of colonel in the Portuguese army.[45]

João Manuel Pacheco de Figueiredo (1901-1990), the last Dean of Goa Medical School and the first Dean of Goa Medical College was born in Margão. Pacheco de Figueiredo studied medicine in Goa and Coimbra. He obtained also a diploma in Tropical Medicine in Lisbon. After a brief stint in Mozambique, he joined the Goa Medical School as professor. In late 1940's Pacheco Figueiredo was appointed the Director of Goa Medical School. He occupied several honorary posts and attended many conferences and congresses. He represented Goa Medical School in 1952 at the Luso-Spanish Congress held at Coimbra, International Congress of Tropical Medicine at Lisbon in 1953, VI Medical Conference in Pakistan. He represented the Portuguese Government at the following conferences: At the second, third, fourth and fifth South East Regional Conferences of W.H.O. held in different parts of Asia in 1949, 1950, 1951 and 1952, at the first National Congress of Tropical Medicine Lisbon 1952, third Medical Conference of Pakistan in 1953, the first World Conference of Medical Education in 1953 at London, IV Congress of International Society of Hematology Boston 1956; VI International Congress of Blood Transfusion and the IX Annual Meeting of American Association of Blood Bank in 1956. In 1953 he visited France, Spain and Switzerland as a scholar of W.H.O. Pacheco de Figueiredo was a member of many medical associations including *Academia das Ciencias e do Instituto de Coimbra*, *Sociedade das Ciencias Medicas de Lisboa* and *Instituto Brasileira de Historia da Medicina da Goa*. He has a number of papers to his credit. He was doctor of Medicine *Honoris Causa* from Coimbra University 1961.[46]

Escolastica Gracias e Amaral Peres (1904-1992) was Director of Hospicio de Sagrado Coração, Margão. She studied medicine at the University of Lisbon and obtained an additional diploma in Tropical Medicine from Lisbon. She was a professor of the midwifery course. Her thesis on leprosy was published in Lisbon.

Fernando Albuquerque was born in Panjim in 1910. He graduated from Goa Medical School in 1932 and from the Faculty of Medicine of Lisbon in 1936. Later he obtained a diploma in Tropical Medicine in

Lisbon. In 1948 he was appointed professor in Goa Medical School. In 1957 he represented this school at the third Congress of P.I.O.S.A of Indian Ocean held at Madagascar, where he read a paper entitled Human Ecology. Albuquerque has many works to his credit.[47]

Pondarinath S. Borcar from Ponda completed his studies at Goa Medical School in 1934. He practised for a while in a private nursing home at Gogol, Margão, before joining the Health Services of Portuguese India. In 1950 he was one of the two doctors selected by W.H.O to undergo training at the Malaria Institute at Delhi. He was in charge of Malaria campaign in Sanguem. In 1960s when the Malaria department was established in the Health Services he was put in charge of the department. In 1955 he attended the W.H.O. conference at New Delhi and Bandung. Pondarinath Borcar is still an active clinician. He has many published papers and he is the author of a Marathi book on some problems of health during the Portuguese rule in Goa.

Jose Filipe P. Fernandes Mesquita born in 1910 at Benaulim (Goa) was Deputy Director of the Health Services of Portuguese India. He graduated at Goa Medical School at the age of 22 with several prizes. He did his post graduate studies under W. H. O. fellowships. In 1952 he acquired a diploma in Public Health from Calcutta and received training in control of tuberculosis at Dacca in 1955. In 1961 he received training in Public Health Administration in Puerto Rico and Brasil. Jose Filipe Mesquita was put in charge of campaign against Filarasis. He was one of the two delegates who represented Portugal the at the W. H. O. conference at Bangkok and Kandy. He attended also the First Conference on Malariology in Bangkok (Thailand) held in 1953. He has published papers on medical subject in Goa and Portugal.

Francisco C. T. da Silva (1911-1992) was born in Benaulim, Goa. He completed his medical studies at the Goa Medical School in 1935 with a gold medal and several prizes in microbiology, physiology, obstetrics-gynecology and hygiene. He studied at the Institute of Tropical Medicine in Lisbon before joining the Health Services of Portuguese India. In 1950 he was sent by the Government on a W. H. O. scholarship to the Malaria Institute in New Delhi for a course in malaria. After further training in Bombay and Orissa he was posted at Canacona (Goa) to eradicate malaria which was done successfully. Few years later he was posted at Quepem for the same purpose. In 1953 he attended the first International Conference on Malaria organized by W. H. O at Bangkok and later together with Dr. Jose Filipe Mesquita attended the W.H.O. meeting held at Bangkok as a delegate of Portugal. He was in charge of campaign against smallpox in Goa and has contributed papers to the *Anais de Medicina Tropical*, Lisboa.

Emidio Afonso (1916-1990), son of Bossuet Afonso from Betalbatim, comes from a family which has given Goa several eminent doctors. After graduating from Goa Medical School in 1938, he was a Government analyst, the first Principal of the Pharmacy College, professor of Biochemistry, Director of Public Health Laboratory and Director of Health Services. A modest person, he was a good clinician. In 1959 the local Government sent him on a one year W.H.O. scholarship to study in New York. Emidio Afonso published no less then one and half dozen papers in renowned international journals such as *Nature*, the *Lancet, Immunochemistry* a journal of clinical Pathology and the *Clinica Chimica Acta*. He reconstructed a simpler version of J.C. Bose's crecograph, an instrument to find the sensitivity of plants. His major work *Cor In Vitro* contains experimental studies in embryology, histology, physiology and pathology of the heart. He wrote a number of papers for *Boletim do Instituto Vasco de Gama*.[48]

Skoda Afonso (1923-1992) was the brother of Emidio Afonso. After studying in Goa Medical School, he went for further studies to U.S.A. In 1965 he was awarded a doctorate in physiology by the University of Wisconsin. He became the Associate professor for cardiovascular physiology at the same University. Skoda Afonso developed a method for measurement of coronary blood flow.[49]

Goans from Goa Medical School have distinguished in the army right from Pedro Gonzaga de Melo, one of the first eight student of the school. Caetano Florencio Colaço, Albino Pascoal de Rocha, Jose Antonio Valeriano Coutinho, Luis Fernando Colaço, Feliciano Primo de Menezes, Antonio Maciel de Azaredo, Joaquim Francisco d a Silva, Afonso Aniceto de Souza, Graciano Andre Ribeiro de Santana, Cosme Valerio Dalgado, Domingos Joaquim Menezes, Caetano Francisco Xavier Bossuet da Piedade Rebelo, Miguel Dias, Aires de Sa, Victor Dias, Froilano de Mello, Germano Correia, Pedro Joaquim Peregrino da Costa are some of the many Goan doctors who were in the army.

Aristides da Costa, Jose Pedro Godinho, Demostenes Mascarenhas, Caetano Rosario Dantas, Joaquim Lourenço de Araujo, Luis Cabral, João Filipe de Souza, Octaviano Moniz, Arminio Ribeiro de Santana, Sacarama Gude, Honorato Sousa, Pestaninho de Veiga, Jose Inacio de Loiola, Pedro Joaquim Peregrino Costa, Elinio Colaço, Sales de Veiga Coutinho, Manuel da Veiga Coutinho, Atmarama Borcar were known clinicians. Antonio Colaço was another great clinician who became a member of the

Western Medicine

Indian Parliament. Many of the students were health officers throughout the Portuguese regime. Some where doctors of the hospitals, Municipalities and *partido* (Communidades).

b) Doctors who worked in Goa

Garcia d'Orta the renowned physician was born at Elvas in Portugal. He was given license to practice by the Chief Physician of Castelo de Vide after appearing for a test. He came to India in 1534 as the Chief Physician of the State. He carried detailed research in India, specially concerning the use of various medicinal plants. He is well known for his famous work *Os Colloquios dos Simples e Drogas*.[50]

Francisco Manuel Barroso e Silva arrived in Goa as the Chief Surgeon in 1786. He brought along with him from Portugal a number of instruments to be used in the Military Hospital and for the teaching of medicine to the natives.

Antonio Jose de Miranda Almeida studied at the University of Coimbra where he taught for a while before coming to India. He was responsible for starting a three years course in Medicine at the Royal Hospital at the city of Goa.[51]

Antonio Jose de Lima Leitão a graduate in medicine from the University of Paris occupied several posts in Portugal and Mozambique before coming to India as the Chief Surgeon of the State. He started the four year course in medicine at the Royal Hospital. Later he had to resign from his post as he got involved with political activities of the time which were directed against the Government. He has written a number of papers in medicine and translated some books.[52]

Mateus Cezario Rodrigues Moacho a graduate in medicine from the University of Lisbon, received his doctorate from the University of Lovama. He improved the conditions of the Military Hospital of Goa. It is on his advice that the local Government decided in 1840s not to issue licenses to individuals desiring to practise as doctors unless they appeared for a test.

Francisco Stuart da Fonseca Torrie arrived in India in 1862 and was appointed to the post of Director of Health Services in 1871. He has many works to his credit on maritime hygiene, environmental hygiene, military hygiene, cholera and prostitution in Portuguese India. He was given many awards by the Portuguese Government for his contribution to health.[53]

Rafael Antonio Pereira the first Goan to be given charge of the Health Services of Portuguese India, was born at Benaulim in 1847. A graduate in medicine from the University of Lisbon he worked in the Portuguese navy as doctor of grade II before he was transferred to Goa in 1875. He was appointed acting Director of Health Services in 1884 and he was confirmed in this post in 1885. In 1896 he was transferred to the Portuguese colonies of Cabo Verde and Guine as the Director of Health Services. The following year he was promoted in the army as colonel. He was awarded a silver medal for good behaviour and the award *Real Ordem de S. Bento de Aviz* in 1897.[54]

Caetano Antonio Claudio Julio Raimundo da Gama Pinto a famous ophthalmologist and professor of the University of Lisbon, was born in 1853 at Saligão (Goa). He did his secondary education in Goa and Portugal. He passed his medical course with distinction from the University of Oporto. Very keen in learning ophthalmology he visited Paris, Munich, Leipzig, Halle and Berlin. In Paris he worked under famous doctor Wecker. In Heidelberg he studied under Kuchne and Arnold and in Vienna he specialized with famous ophthalmologists Arit and Jacger. In 1880 he joined the Goa Medical School as a professor, but soon thereafter he was invited by professor Otto Becker to work with him in Germany, where he was appointed lecturer of ophthalmology and ocular surgery at the University of Heidelberg. After ten years he returned to Portugal and set in 1892 the Institute of ophthalmology, today named after him. He was member of various associations and contributed a number of papers to reputed medical journals of Portugal, Germany, France and United States.[55]

Roberto Belarmino do Rosario Frias (1853-1918) from Arpora was a well known surgeon born in 1853. He studied at Oporto and later he returned to Goa. He taught at Goa Medical School for some time. In 1887 he joined the medical school of Oporto and was promoted to the post of professor of clinical surgery. He wrote *Compendio de Quimica*. His other works were in the field of tuberculosis, filaria, peritonitis, influenza, etc. He died in 1918.[56]

Miguel Caetano Dias (1854-1936) was the Director of Health Services of Portuguese India and Goa Medical School. He was the last Goan General when he died in 1936. He studied medicine at the Faculty of Medicine of the University of Lisbon and joined the military medical cadre of Mozambique. The Portuguese Government bestowed on him several honours including the medal given by Queen Amelia. Miguel Dias was responsible for eradicating the bubonic plague from Panjim in 1908.[57] His son Antonio born in 1898 was a medical graduate from the University of Lisbon. He was well known as surgeon and Director of

Hospicio de Sagrado Coração, Margão. It is said that Antonio Dias found a new cure for polio. Miguel Caetano's other son Victor (1892-1949) studied medicine at the University of Lisbon. "The anti-social reaction of the alcoholics" was his theme for the doctoral thesis for which he was awarded the degree of *Doutor em Medicina e Cirurgica* by the University of Lisbon. He obtained an additional diploma in Tropical Medicine before joining the health cadre of Angola. In 1923 he was transferred to Goa Medical School as professor of surgery, physiology and histology. He was Director of the Health Services in late 1940s. Victor Dias was entrusted by the Portuguese Government with the Sanitation Scheme at Old Goa, which he successfully concluded before his death in 1949.[58]

Bossuet Afonso (1880-1957) son in law of Miguel Caetano Dias, became well known for his famous thesis entitled "The action of X-rays on the eye", for which he won the *Benemerenti* medal awarded by the University of Wuerzburg (Germany) and was granted the title of professor of the same university. This title was not granted to a foreigner until that time. He proved that lens of the eyes were subject to the damage of the X-rays. Another important work of this doctor was *The thyroid gland and Haemolisis of puerperal streptococci*. Bossuet Afonso studied at the Universities of Vienna, Berlin, Wuerzburg and Heidelberg. He has several contributions to his credit. During the First World War he rendered medical care to German soldiers in Goa.

Adelia Costa was the first woman neurologist in Portugal. Born in 1928 at Loutolim, Goa, she joined the Goa Medical School where she completed second year of medicine and proceeded to Lisbon to study medicine there. She joined the Faculty of Medicine of the University of Lisbon and graduated from there in 1952. In the same year she joined as an intern in *Hospitais Civis de Lisboa*. In 1953 she passed one year diploma course in Tropical Medicine at the Institute of Tropical Medicine of Lisbon and the following year she obtained licentiate in Public Health from *Instituto Superior de Hygiene Dr. Ricardo George*, Lisbon. At this time it was common for women doctors in Portugal to specialize either in pathology or gynaecology or pediatrics. However, Adelia Costa chose a different branch for her specialization which no women in Portugal had so far joined. She specialized in Neurology at *Hospital dos Capuchos* and appeared for a test from *Ordem dos Medicos*. She took a keen interest in clinical electroencefalography. She practised in *Hospital Julio Matos* (a hospital dealing with mental problems) before returning to Goa in 1958 to join the Health Services. She was appointed Director of Mental Hospital renamed soon after as *Hospital Abade Faria*. In 1962 she returned to Lisbon to further specialize in psychiatry from *Ordem dos Medicos*.[59]

During the last two decades of Portuguese rule some outstanding Portuguese surgeons visited Goa and worked in the Medical School Hospital and *Hospital da Misericordia*. Among these was Dr. Baptista Souza who introduced several changes to improve the conditions of the Goa Medical School Hospital in late 1940s.

c) Goan doctors outside Goa.

Jose Caetano Pereira — was born at Divar, Goa in 1821. He finished his medical studies in 1851 and joined the army as chief surgeon. He saved the life of Dom Afonso V at a time when his brothers were already dead due to an illness. He was rewarded by the Portuguese King with an appointment as honorary doctor of the Portuguese Court. He fought to end the epidemic of cholera and yellow fever that broke out in Lisbon in the years 1856-1857. The Portuguese king bestowed on him the award *Torre e Espada*. His career suffered a setback due to a crime committed by his wife. He was accused as an accomplice was later proved not guilty. He published his thesis entitled *There is no connection between the virus causing blenorragia and cancer*. He contributed to many medical journals.[60]

Jose Camilo Lisboa a renowned botanist hailed from Assagão, where he was born in 1823. After his elementary education in Goa he went to Bombay to study in Grant Medical College. He was appointed Assistant Surgeon at J. J. Hospital and professor of Anatomy in the Grant Medical College. Later he was appointed surgeon in the J.J. Hospital and lecturer on Anatomy in the College. He distinguished himself as surgeon in western India. He was in Europe for two years and on his return studied botany and leprosy. He contributed several papers to various journals. The Government of Bombay appointed him to study the Flora of the Presidency. He discovered several plants some of which have been named after him. He was a member of Bombay University Syndicate and President of Grant Medical College Society. He was a distinguished member of the Royal Asiatic Society and Bombay Natural History Society. He was a Fellow of the Geographical and Medical Society of Lisbon. The Royal Academy of Science elected him Fellow of the Linnaean Society of London. The *Academie Internationale de Geographie Botanique* of France elected him corresponding member and awarded him a medal "Merit Scientific".[61]

Andre Paulo de Andrade was born in Parra (Bardez) in 1834. He did his early studies in Goa and then joined a Medical College in Bombay. He completed his medical studies on the top of the list in 1834. He worked as assistant surgeon at J.J. Hospital in Bombay before he was appointed Assistant Medical Officer to a newly set up venereal hospital at Bandra. He was a Fellow of the Medical Society of Grant College. He distinguished in legal and religious field as well.[62]

Luis Caetano Santana Alvares belonged to the Guine and Mozambique Health Cadre. Born in Margão, he died in Lisbon in 1915. A brilliant student of Goa Medical School, he repeated his medical studies at Oporto (Portugal). He fought one of the most violent epidemics of his time in Mozambique, and to improve the sanitary conditions of the place. He joined the army and took part in the military operations as medical doctor. He was honoured by the Government with the cross of *Torre e Espada*, and awards of Cristo and Avis, besides gold medal for outstanding work in Portuguese colonies in Africa.

Jervis Pereira who played an important role in Africa was born in 1862. After a brilliant career at Grant Medical School he proceeded to England where he took a diploma of medicine at the Universities of Glasgow and Edinburgh. He specialized in gynaecology and obstetrics. He was appointed a life member of the Medical Society of Edinburgh. In 1888 he left England for Portugal to work as Medical Officer in Mozambique and took over the charge of the hospital of Lourenço Marques. He took active part in the Municipal life of the city and occupied several posts. He was appointed Italian consul in Lourenço Marques and Consul for Greece in 1900.

Alfredo Costa (1859-1910) was born at Margão (Goa). A graduate from the Medical School of Lisbon, he joined the school first as a demonstrator and promoted later to the post of a lecturer in obstetrics. Probably, he was the first surgeon to perform colostamy and Estlander operations in Portugal and to introduce Volkmann method in the cure of hydrocel. Alfredo Costa was one of the first surgeons in Portugal to make use of autoclave. His great dream of setting up a maternity home did not materialize in his life time. However, he was responsible in setting up a temporary maternity ward in the hospital where he was working. He published several scientific works. In 1932 a Maternity Home was established in Lisbon and named after him.[63]

Bernado Bruto da Costa was born in Goa in August 1878. After graduating in medicine from the University of Lisbon and obtaining a diploma in tropical medicine he joined the Portuguese overseas health cadre. He was appointed to lead a team to eradicate sleeping sickness in Portuguese colony of Principe from 1911 to 1915 and at Benguela from 1916 to 1918. He discovered that the tse-tse flies were responsible for the sleeping sickness in S.Tome and Principe. He was Director of the Hospital of S. Tome, President of the Municipality and Administrator of the same island. Besides contributing to end the sleeping sickness at S. Tome and Principe, he worked to improve the hygiene of the colony. The Portuguese Government honoured him with a gold medal for his services in Africa.[64]

Luis Cupertino Saldanha born in Goa in the year 1886, completed his primary education at Anjuna at a very early age of seven. He finished his secondary education in Bombay before proceeding to England to study medicine in the University of Edinburgh. He obtained his Master in Surgery and later studied at the faculty of Medicine and Surgery of Glasgow. He was appointed member of the Royal College of Doctors. He was nominated Fellow of the British Medical Association of the London and Scottish Geographical Society. Luis Saldanha worked in hospitals of London, Paris, Berlin, Aberdeen before returning to India. He occupied various posts in India and distinguished himself by his measures against the violence of plague that raged in India at the end of the 19th century. He died of plague in 1903.[65]

Agostinho de Souza was born in Calangute, Goa. He went to Oporto to take his degree of Medicine. As early as 1880 he made a name for himself by publishing his famous work *La theorie de l'Atomicite et la loi perodique de M. Mendlejeff*. In 1888 his theory of cardiac rhythm made him popular not only among the Portuguese but even among the French physiologists. He enjoyed vast practice as an expert of Dermatology and Venereal Diseases. He died at a comparatively young age in 1919 at Oporto.[66]

Ramkrishna Vital Lad commonly known as Bhau Daji, was born in Mandrem (Pernem) in 1822 and settled in Bombay. He was one of the makers of modern Bombay. He was one of the first student of Grant Medical College.[67] He was well-known as a physician and surgeon. In surgery he distinguished himself by operating on tumors and eye cataracts and by doing obstetrical operations. As a physician, he enjoyed the reputation of having cured a Goan suffering from leprosy.[68] Bhau Daji was a man of varied interests in life. He took interest in chemistry, mineralogy, botany and numismatics. He earned the honour of being one of the first Indians to be appointed as a member of the Royal Asiatic Society and later was appointed the Vice-President of the same Society.

Acacio Gabriel Viegas from Arpora earned reputation for his

brilliant diagnosis of bubonic plague that raged in Bombay at the end of the nineteenth century. His diagnosis helped the Bombay Government to take timely action in successfully combating plague in Bombay. He had the unique distinction of being the first Indian Christian to be elected to the Bombay Municipal Corporation in 1888. In 1906 he became its first Catholic President.

Francisco Xavier da Silva Teles (1860-1930) was born at Nova Goa . He graduated in medicine from the University of Lisbon. He joined the overseas health cadre and later joined the navy. In 1905 he represented the naval doctors in the National Congress of T.B. held at Coimbra. Earlier he attended the International Congress of Medicine in Paris. He taught Tropical medicine and joined the University of Lisbon as its Rector. Teles da Silva was the Secretary General of Geographical Society of Lisbon, and in this capacity he attended several meetings. He published several works in the medical and non-medical fields among these was his thesis *A tuberculose e o problema.*[69]

Luis Manuel Julio Frederico Gonsalves was born in Nova Goa in the year 1881. He graduated from the University of Lisbon with the highest marks and joined the naval medical services. He participated in many military expeditions in Africa and was bestowed several awards. He designed a special type of stretcher for the Portuguese navy. He was Director of *Gabinete de Estudos da Armada*, Naval Arsenal Health Services and Naval Hospital. He attended several congresses and has many papers to his credit.[70]

Francisco Xavier da Costa who specialized in London was the first Goan and second Indian to be a Fellow of the Royal College of Surgeons of London. He was the director of the well known St. Marta Hospital of Bangalore.

Aires de Souza was born in Goa in October 1905. In 1929 he graduated in medicine from the University of Lisbon and specialized in Tropical Medicine. In 1932 he joined the Civil Hospitals of Lisbon as radiologist. Few years later he was promoted as the head of the department of radiology and posted at Hospital de Desterro. Aires de Sousa specialized in France, England and Italy. He attended the II Congresso Luso-Espanhol of Dermatology, IV Hispano- Portuguese Congress of Urology, II Hispano-Portuguese Congress of Radiology, and II Medical Congress of electro-radiologists. He was the president of various medical associations of Lisbon. His works were published in well-known journals such as *Lisboa Medica, Imprensa Medica, Boletim Clinico e de Estatistica dos H.C.L* and many others from France.[71]

Alfredo Araujo was in charge of the psychology department of the Julio Matos Hospital and Director do Instituto da Orientação Professional.

Jeronimo Acacio Gama who was born in 1845 at Verna (Salcete) was one of the first ophthalmologists from Bombay. He founded the Bombay Charitable Eyes and Ear Infirmary. He presented several papers to British Medical journal of London and *Annales d'Oculistique of Paris*. He was awarded with order of Christ by the Portuguese Government.[72]

Herculano de Sa (1881-1958) from Piedade (Ilhas) started his medical career as tutor at the Grant Medical College and in 1926 he was appointed professor of Midwifery and Gynaecology at G.S.Medical College. He set up a maternity home at Chowpatty. His daughter Juliet de Sa–Sousa (1912-1986) became in 1939 the first Goan woman surgeon of Bombay. Later she was put in charge of Midwifery department of Grant Medical College. On her father's death she took over his nursing home. His son Joseph (Joe) Vincent de Sa after advanced training in U.S.A. and Great Britain joined the K.E.M. Hospital as the head of the E.N.T. department. He became a member of International College of Surgeons, Fellow of the American College of Surgeons and some other associations.[73]

Socrates Noronha specialized in London, Paris and Vienna. He was a professor of dermatology in the National Medical College, Nair Hospital, St. George Hospital, Polish Red Cross Hospital. He worked to combat venereal diseases in Bombay and set up a league for the purpose. He established the V.D. Department at St. George's Hospital and the Military Hospital at Colaba. He was awarded the Order of British Empire, Kaiser-i-Hind Medal and some others for his outstanding services. Socrates Noronha was the founder member of the Catholic Medical Guild of St. Luke, Bombay.[74]

Jose Luis Pinto do Rosario was the deputy Director of the Health Services of Bombay Presidency and Director of Vaccine Institute of Belgaum. He was the Director of Health Service of Gujarat. Pinto do Rosario represented Bombay Presidency at the Congress of Tropical Medicine in Calcutta and Congress of Social Hygiene in London.

Ernest Borges is remembered for his great human qualities and solicitude for his cancer patients. He studied medicine in Bombay and went to England for his F.R.C.S. later he specialized in cancer. He joined the Tata Memorial Hospital in 1939 and made Tata Hospital one of the best cancer centers of India. Honoured both by the Church and the State, in 1961 he was knighted in the order of St. Gregory the Great and in 1964

Western Medicine

the Pope appointed him Privy Chamberlain with cape and sword. In 1965 the Government of India awarded him the Padma Shri. He died in 1969 at the age of 59 years.[75]

In 1950's Charles Pinto received advanced training in plastic surgery in the U.S.A on his return he started a department of plastic surgery in the K.E.M. Hospital. Ten years later he was appointed President of the Association of Plastic Surgeons in India and a member of the British Association of Plastic surgeons. Charles Pinto became famous for developing a technique to correct cleft-palate.[76]

Ivan Pinto was probably the youngest Indian to be a member of American College of Cardiologists. He specialized in the U.S.A and England. He was appointed the Head of the Department of Cardiology of K.E.M and G.S. Hospitals in Bombay. He was a member of the Executive Committee and the Research Committee of the International Society of Cardiology Council in Arteriosclerosis. In 1977 he was elected President of Cardiological Society of India and presided over the first National Conference on Pacemakers. He was a honorary cardiovascular consultant to the W.H.O. He helped to set up the first pacemakers bank in the K.E.M. Hospital.[77]

The first department of neurology in India was set up at Grant Medical College by Menino de Souza. He specialized abroad and in 1957 represented India at the World Neurological Conference at Brussels. In 1951 he was elected Dean of the Faculty of Medicine of Bombay University.[78]

V.N. Shirodkar was a gynecologist of great repute. He was born at Shiroda a village in Ponda (Goa). After obtaining M.D degree from Bombay University he proceeded to England for further studies. He obtained a fellowship of the Royal College of Obstetrics and Gynaecologist and a Fellowship of the American College of Surgeons. He designed half a dozen techniques in gynaecological surgery: a technique to prevent abortions commonly known as Shirodkar stitch ; a technique for cure of the descent of the womb; the Shirodkar technique for opening blocked fallopian tubes and the cervical hood and a technique for creating an artificial vagina. He was an authority in Tuboplasty. He attended several congresses abroad where he was asked to demonstrate his technique.

REFERENCES

1. HAG: *Monções do Reino*, 56, fl. 75.
2. HAG: *MR.* 59, fl. 305, Majority of doctors in Portugal at this time were Jews.

3. HAG : Ms. 23 – *Livro das Merces Gerais*, fl. 204.
4. HAG: Ms. 7 – *Livro das Merces Gerais*, fl. 205v.
5. HAG : Ms. 25 – *Livro das Merces Gerais*, fl. 134.
6. HAG: *MR.* 99, fl. 286.
7. Torre do Tombo : *Chancelaria de D. Jose – Livro 66*, fls. 357-357v.
8. HAG: *MR.* 161 D, fl. 2149.
9. HAG: *MR.* 180 A, fl. 272.
10. HAG: *MR.* 159 C, fl. 712: Costa Portugal was accused of several irregularities and bad temper.
11. HAG: *MR.* 159 C, fls. 712-713; HAG: *MR.* 164 C, fl. 1057.
12. HAG: *MR.* 178 A, fl. 272. Ignacio Afonso was accused of over drinking and causing problems in the Hospital.
13. HAG: *MR.* 180 A, fl. 90; HAG: *MR.* 185, fl. 6.
14. HAG: *MR.* 180 A, fl. 465.
15. HAG: *MR.* 185, fls. 26v-29v.
16. HAG: *MR.* 180 A, fl. 48.
17. HAG: *MR.* 196 A, fl. 321; HAG: Ms. 91 – *Cartas, Ordens e Portarias*, fls. 58v-59, says that Bernardo Peres da Silva together with Gonzaga Vincente da Fonseca and Antonio de Noronha were dismissed from the Royal Hospital in 1820.
18. HAG: *MR.* 198 A, fls. 144-144v.
19. HAG: *MR.* 198 B, fl. 420.
20. HAG: Ms. 91 – *Cartas, Ordens e Portarias*, fl. 98v.
21. *B.G.* no. 54, 7th July 1922.
22. HAG: Ms. 125 – *Cartas, Ordens e Portarias*, fl. 99.
23. J.M. Pacheco de Figueiredo, "Escola Medico-Cirurgica Esboço Historico", offprint of *Arquivos da Escola Medico-Cirurgica de Goa*, Bastora, 1960, p. 20.
24. Germano Correia, *Historia do Ensino Medico na India Portuguesa*, Nova Goa, 1917, p. 25.
25. Pacheco de Figueiredo, *op. cit.*, pp. 156-158.
26. *Ibid.*, pp. 159-164.
27. *Ibid.*, pp. 179-180.
28. *LREI* 1913, Nova Goa, 1914, pp. 277-281.
29. *B.O.* no 54, 7th July 1922, The presiding member was to be paid Rs. 10 and other members received Rs. 5 each.
30. Pacheco de Figueiredo, *op. cit.*, pp. 171-172.
31. LREI, 1958, Nova Goa, 1958, pp. 1-5.
32. Abreu, Miguel Vincente de, *Noção de Alguns Filhos Distinctos da India Portuguesa*, Nova Goa, 1874, p. 13.
33. *Escola Medico-Cirurgica de Goa*, 1842-1957, Bastora, 1957, p. 58.
34. *Ibid.*, p. 160.
35. Aleixo Manuel da Costa, *Literatura Goesa – Apontamentos bibliograficos para sua historia*, Lisboa, 1967, pp. 69-70. (Henceforth *Literatura Goesa*); P.J. Peregrino da Costa, *A Escola Medica de Goa e a sua projecao na India Portuguesa e no Ultramar*, p. 31.
36. *Ibid.*, p. 133.
37. The degree of Goa Medical School was not recognised in Portugal and in order to practice there one had to study medicine all over again.
38. *Anuario da Escola Medico-Cirurgica de Nova Goa*, 1916-1917, Nova Goa, 1917. (Henceforth *Anuario da Escola*).
39. *Literatura Goesa*, op. cit., pp. 369-371.

40. Aires de Sa, *Hygiene de Panjim,* 1908; Navhind Times 29th August 1982.
41. *Anuario da Escola Medico-Cirurgico de Nova Goa 1925,* Nova Goa, 1925, pp. 56-60.
42. *GEPB,* vol. XVI, Lisboa, p. 806.
43. Alfredo Froilano Bachmann de Mello, "Froilano de Mello (A centenary tribute)", *Boletim do Instituto Menezes Bragança* no. 153, Bastora, 1987, pp. 1-13.
44. *Escola Medico-Cirrugica de Goa – Monografia,* Goa, 1959, pp. 100-103.
45. *GEPB,* vol. XXVIII, Lisboa, pp. 856-857; *Anuario da Escola* p. 61.
46. Offprint *"O Medico"* no. 511, 1961.
47. *Literature Goesa,* op. cit., p. 54.
48. Information compiled from various published works of Dr. E. Afonso.
49. *World Who's Who in Science from Antiquity to Present – A Biographical Dictionary of Notable Scientists from Antiquity to Present,* ed. Allen G. Dubes, Chicago, 1968.
50. Anuario *da Escola Medico-Cirurgica de Nova Goa 1916-1917,* Nova Goa, 1917, p. 15; More details about *Colloquios* are given in Bibliographical Essay.
51. *Ibid.,* pp. 18-19.
52. *Ibid.,* pp. 19-20.
53. *Ibid.,* pp. 29-30.
54. *Ibid.,* pp. 38-39.
55. *GEPB,* vol. XII, pp. 118-119.
56. *GEPB,* vol. XI, Lisboa, pp. 880-81.
57. *Dr. Miguel Caetano Dias,* Nova Goa, 1937.
58. Victor Dias, *Velha-Goa – Seu Saneamento,* Fasc. I, Cidade de Goa, 1949.
59. Carlos Garcia *A primeira mulher neurologista Portuguesa"* in *Neuronoticias – Boletim da Sociedade Portuguesa de Neurologia* no. 1, Lisboa, 1990.
60. *GEPB,* vol. XX, Lisboa, p. 153.
61. P.J. Peregrino da Costa, *A Expansão do Goes pelo Mundo,* Goa, 1956, p. 128; *Indo-Portuguese Review,* vol. 4, Calcutta, 1921, p. 35. (Henceforth Peregrino da Costa).
62. *Ibid.,* p. 130.
63. João Filipe de Rego, *Mestre Alfredo da Costa – Medico e Apostolo,* Bastora, 1959; *GEPB,* vol. VII, Lisboa, p. 857.
64. *GEPB,* vol. VII, Lisboa, p. 865.
65. *The Indo-portuguese Review,* vol. 3, Calcutta, 1921, p. 29.
66. *The Indo-Portuguese Review,* 1923-1924, vol. VI, Calcutta, 1924, p. 92.
67. Peregrino da Costa., *op. cit.,* p. 129.
68. Antonio Cruz, *Goa – Men and Matters,* Vasco da Gama, 1974, pp. 205-214.
69. Dr. F.X. da Silva Teles – *Homenagem da Escola Medica de Goa* offprint of *Boletim Geral de Medicina e Farmacia* Bastora, 1934; *GEPB,* vol. XXVIII, Lisboa, p. 897.
70. *GEPB,* vol. XVI, p. 559.
71. *GEPB,* vol. XXIX, pp. 755-756.
72. Peregrino da Costa, *op. cit.,* p. 130.
73. Teresa Albuquerque, *To Love is to Serve,* Bombay, 1986, p. 40.
74. *Ibid.,* p. 39.
75. *Ibid.,* pp. 40-41.
76. *Ibid.,* p. 42.
77. *Ibid.,* p. 44.
78. *Ibid.,* p. 42.

8

AN OVERVIEW

Every individual regards health as an important element of his well-being and of the well-being of those close to himself. Indeed, the enjoyment of health has come to take a place among the "human rights".[1] The preamble to the constitution of W.H.O. states that "the enjoyment of the highest attainable standard of human health is one of the fundamental rights in every human being without distinction of race, religion, political beliefs, economic and social conditions".[2] Improvement of health conditions of people as a whole, rather than of better-off individuals or groups, is being stressed in the context of the Third World health standards. This marks a development in the holistic understanding of health. It is a language of "rights of the people" rather than the traditional western capitalist discourse of *individual* "human rights" that makes more sense in the context of the colonial-imperialist exploitation of natural resources by the western countries for the benefit of the western countries, but resulting into a global threat to the whole planet and to all life on it.[3]

Western and eastern systems of medicine originated from man's view of himself in continuity with the nature around him. The doctrine of humors was common to both systems of medicine. Consequently, knowledge of astrology was regarded as essential in the medical world. Hence the classic Spanish saying of Judaeo-Arabic medieval writings: *Ciego es el medico que no sabe astrologia* (= Blind is the physician who is weak in astrology).[4] However, in the course of time western man's concern seems to have become more self-centered and individualistic to the detriment of an awareness of man as part of the community and as a part of the whole cosmos.

At the risk of being simplistic the image comes to my mind of the hunters and gatherers of old. The west with its hunting instincts more active explored ever new avenues of economic gain and political

An Overview

dominance. They arrived in the east. They met a people in this country whose ways of life might conform to the image of the gatherers and whose philosophy of life had made them more receptive to gather the best of the thought and life of the new-comers. The colonial powers tried to ride over a culture that they considered primitive from their ethnocentric viewpoint, without caring to realize that it was a more evolved culture and in some ways superseded their own.

Apparently, when the Portuguese first came to India they were not concerned with the health conditions of the native population. The first Hospital in Goa was established in the city of Goa to cater to the needs of the Portuguese soldiers in need to recover from long sea-journeys, from wars of conquest and sea-monopoly they sought to enforce, and from the infectious diseases which they imported or acquired locally. Hospitals and other facilities were designed with the interests of the Portuguese as their priority. Similar situation also prevailed in British India in the nineteenth century.[5] It was the missionaries and the Holy House of Mercy that tried first to introduce western medicine among the masses, including natives, in the city of Goa, but it was still restricted to the areas where the Portuguese lived. The majority of the native population continued to have recourse to their traditional medicine. Their indigenous practitioners were cheaper, more easily available and the natives had faith in them.

Initially it appears that the western system of medicine and the eastern one could co-exist peacefully. Some Portuguese physicians, including Garcia d'Orta took keen interest in indigenous ways of healing.[6] Many viceroys, high government officials and nobles sought the help of the native *panditos*. Probably because so few western doctors were available, and also because they believed that the local diseases could be best treated by the native practitioners. This happy situation ended when the Inquisition intervened and imposed restrictions on the practice of the native medicine men, probably because of their moral influence upon their clients. Also the Portuguese doctors in Goa were openly hostile to the native practitioners, and they used their influence in the ruling quarters to check the practice of the native doctors.

The efficacy of indigenous medicine is difficult to assess at this point as new diseases were brought in by the colonial powers. The indigenous systems were unable to cope with new diseases. While one can say that Goa's high mortality rates mean that indigenous treatments were not effective, no other treatment could have done better, since mortality rates were closely linked with poverty, famines and environmental problems intensified with the creation of western-type urbanisation in Goa. Goa had never before seen a degree of urbanisation and eco-disturbance as the one introduced by the Portuguese in the sixteenth century.

As elsewhere in South Asia health conditions were correlated with the income and levels of living in Goa. These levels depended on Portuguese imperial fortunes. The upper strata with better standards of living were probably able to avoid deficiency diseases, but not the transmittable diseases.

Level of living was low for the masses. This condition was responsible for their level of nutrition. Majority of our people during colonial time lived on subsistence agriculture and on remittances from across the borders. Since most lived in conditions of chronic economic stress, they could not afford to spend much on their food. Malnutrition and undernourishment were responsible for many diseases and for morbidity in Goa at least till the beginning of this century. Malnutrition was one of the chief causes of infant mortality. It also caused a chronic debility that impaired people's labour input and reduced their resistance to disease.

Environmental problems may not have been as serious and extensive as we face them today, but they were there. Over-urbanisation of the capital city had grown beyond the capacity of the existing methods of sanitation. Poverty, ignorance, non-cooperative attitude of the natives, lack of sufficient potable water and poor drainage were also responsible for the environmental problems. Goa was blessed with a large network of rivers, but there was scarcity of potable water, chiefly in the summer months of April and May. Colonial politics did not give priority to solving this problem. Wells and rivers were also polluted and responsible for many water-borne diseases.

Contrary to the general view-point in the West today that many infectious diseases are a heritage of the Third World, we know that the European colonial scum was responsible for bringing many of the infectious diseases to the rest of the world, including Asia. As Europe succeeded in freeing itself from such diseases, it has also forgotten that it was the cause of spreading them elsewhere where they have been left as a part of the legacy of poverty inherited by the Third World. Syphilis known in Goa as *baili pidda* is attributed to the Portuguese and other whites. Diseases like tuberculosis were brought to Goa in the later period by emigrants returning home for holidays. Improvement in means of transport, pilgrimages and trade were also responsible for diseases which often assumed epidemic proportions.

Only in the last decades of their rule the Portuguese tried to extend western medicine to the masses as a result of growing realisation that the health of the Portuguese whites could not be secured through measures directed at their health alone. The reduced difference between the urban and rural life-styles after mid eighteenth century and a greater shift of the Portuguese and administrative personnel into the countryside also explains the extension of the health policies beyond the urban centres.

The introduction of the western medicine and health legislation are considered by many as some of the benefits of the Portuguese rule in Goa. However, western medicine benefited only a small section of the population, mainly in the Old Conquests. The New Conquest territories were neglected. The living conditions of most inhabitants remained appalling with high morbidity and mortality rates till the last few decades of the Portuguese rule. It was only towards the fag end of the Portuguese rule that more health services reached the masses, and that too largely through private initiative. Apologists for the colonial rule believe that its limitations in the field of health were mainly on account of the poverty and ignorance of the people, and not due to inadequate colonial policies. Although this may have been true to some extent, colonial rulers were responsible for the depressing socio-economic conditions in Goa. Elsewhere in India the fall in mortality rates from 1920's onwards is related to grace of gods of weather, resulting into improved levels of nutrition and resistance to infections.[7] The impact of the same factors in Goa cannot be ruled out, though the other regional political and socio-economic characteristics studied in this dissertation need to be taken into account.

Daniel R. Headrick lists medicine among several "tools of empire" that enabled or facilitated western penetration and domination of the non-European world.[8] It was not the political rulers only that saw in medicine a wider utility. The missionaries too appreciated the opportunity it offered them to establish contact with the native souls.

In order to control diseases a series of measures were introduced from the nineteenth century onwards. There was emphasis on epidemic rather than endemic diseases, and upon curative rather then preventive medicine. The preventive aspects were confined to areas inhabited by the ruling class to begin with. Later epidemic measures were spread to the masses. But they were not fully implemented because of the attitude of the inhabitants. The people were reluctant to cooperate on account of religious taboos, superstitions and other beliefs. They were resisting vaccination on such grounds.

The colonial government was also reluctant to make financial commitments and to enforce measures that might provoke resistance and revolt. A fear of the consequences of compulsion was thus an important check on the State. It was from the second decade of the twentieth century that the State powers were used to enforce sanitary and medical measures. This, together with absence of famines, introduction of new medical technology, improvement in the standards of living and education, helped to eradicate epidemic diseases in the last two decades of the Portuguese regime in Goa.

Religion played a dominant role in western as well as native medicine in Goa. It was a tool used to implement some measures and an excuse for non-implementation of others. Some medicinal practices were made a part of religious rituals, specially among the Hindus. Belief in *ahimsa*, caste and socio-religious factors prevented non-Christians from taking up to western medicine for long. Dead bodies were considered a source of pollution, and this discouraged the non-Christians from practising medicine or joining medical studies.

Colonial rulers made Goa dependent on them for health services. Colonial health services were not always popular with the Portuguese whites themselves. The best Portuguese medical talent did not seek employment in the colonies and punitive measures had to be taken to force many doctors to practise in the colonies, including Goa. To supplement its own limited man-power the Portuguese looked for native recruits.

Political forces played a dominant role in the shaping of the health services. Colonial policy was greatly responsible for the state of affairs in the *Estado da India*. The colonial rulers had their politics of health. Lack of enforcement and lethargic attitudes were also responsible for poor health conditions. Having stated that the western medicine did not reach all sections of the population during the Portuguese rule in Goa, it must be admitted that the Portuguese did establish what is considered as the first medical school in Asia, one of the first hospitals of western medicine, and many far-sighted health measures. Besides, the graduates of the Goa medical school made significant contribution despite the limitations of their training and technical facilities.

Medicine in the world today has made great strides in the preventive and curative fields. Unfortunately the world has experienced negative impact too of the toxic effects of the so-called "scientific medicine".[9] Violence has also been done to human mind, body and environment. Today one begins to see a tendency in the west to investigate and practise traditional remedies and medicinal practices, including Indian yoga and vegetarianism. The eastern systems of medicine and health-care are seen as having less harmful side-effects. It looks as if man has come full circle in seeing himself as a part of the larger cosmos, nothing more and nothing less.

Le Roy Ladurie writes about the "unification of the globe by disease in the period after 1300".[10] It appears to me even more true today that any polarisation of the world into the first world and the third world, or developed and under-developed world is not really helpful for the well-being of the humankind. We are growing into the awareness of the inter-relatedness of all things in the Universe and the mutual impact of societies. Maintenance of harmony between man and nature is of paramount importance and everyone has to cooperate in the task. Those who have contributed to greater exploitation and ecological destruction in the past may need to feel the obligation of contributing with larger investments for the eco-restoration, rather than using the environmental issues to add insult to injury and prevent the poorer nations from gaining the benefits of development and to retain their own monopolistic domination.[11]

Through an accident of history we have encountered in Goa attempts at combining eastern and western approaches to medicine. Somewhat symbolic of this was the practice in the famous Royal Hospital of Goa of prescribing a glass of cow urine three times a day for recovering their colour, after the patients were bled several times to cure their illnesses.[12] The Portuguese succeeded to quite an extent in introducing the western medicine in Goa, but its overall colonial failure[13] made the Portuguese empire much less deleterious and some traditional approaches to health care have continued to be popular in Goa. A follow-up in the direction of bringing about a healthy balance of the western and eastern systems of medicine could lead to a better quality of life for all.

REFERENCES

1. Gunnar Myrdal, *Asian Drama*, III, Middlesex, Penguin Books, 1968, p. 1537.
2. *Ibid.*, p. 1536.
3. K.R. Nayar, "Changing International Gaze on Environment and Health Issues", *Social Action*, vol. 41, No. 1, Jan.-Mar. 1991, pp. 54-63; Andre Beteille, "Distributive Justice and Institutional Well-Being", *Economic and Political Weekly*, XXVI, Nos 11 & 12 (Annual Number 1991), pp. 591-600.
4. G.V. Scammell, "The New World and Europe in the Sixteenth Century", *The Historical Journal*, XII, 3 (1989), pp 389-412.
5. Roger Jeffery, *The Politics of Health in India*, Berkeley, 1988, p. 19.
6. Garcia d, Orta, *Colloquios dos simples e drogas e cousas medicinaes da India e assim de algumas fructas achadas nella*, Lisboa, 1877.
7. Sumit Guha, "Mortality decline in early twentieth century India: A preliminary

inquiry", *The Indian Economic and Social History Review*, XXVIII, No. 4 (Oct.-Dec. 1991), pp. 371-391.
8. Quoted by David Arnold, "Disease, Medicine and Empire", *Imperial medicine and indigenous societies*, ed. D. Arnold, New Delhi, 1989, pp. 1-26.
9. Manu L. Kothari and Lopa A. Mehta, "Violence in Modern Medicine", *Science, Hegemony and Violence*, ed. Ashis Nandy, Delhi, Oxford University Press, 1990, pp. 167-210. Carries a very useful list of reference material on the subject. Cf. also Eugene Linden, "Lost Tribes, Lost Knowledge", *TIME*, Vol. 138, No. 2 (September 23, 1991), pp. 38-46.
10. David Arnold, *op. cit.*
11. Nurul Islam, "External Environment for Development in Third World", *Economic and Political Weekly*, Sept. 7, 1991, pp. 2107-2112; Anil Agarwal and Sunita Narain, "Technology Control, Global Warming and Environmental Colonialism: The WRI Report", *Social Action*, Vol. 41, No. 1 (1991), pp. 3-28.
12. *Jean-Baptiste Tavernier's Travels in India*, Vol. 1, ed. William Crooke, London, 1925, p. 160.
13. M.N. Pearson, *The Cambridge History of India : The Portuguese in India*, Cambridge, Cambridge University Press, 1987, p. 2.

BIBLIOGRAPHICAL ESSAY

This essay deals with important relevant primary and secondary sources used in writing of this dissertation. All other sources not discussed in this essay have been listed in the Bibliography.

Primary sources have been divided into archival sources and published primary sources. Archival sources in Goa have been divided under three headings: I.(a) Archival Sources at the Directorate of Archives, Archaeology and Museum. I.(b) Manuscripts at the Xavier Centre of Historical Research. I.(c) Church Records at the Patriarchal Palace (*Paço Patriarcal*). II. Archival Sources at *Arquivo Nacional da Torre do Tombo*-Lisbon (Portugal). The published primary sources are covered under four headings: Missionary reports; Travellers; State Papers; Medical Journals.

Secondary sources have been grouped and discussed under five headings: Hygiene; Diseases and Epidemics; Medicinal plants; Institutional care and training; Miscellaneous.

A. ARCHIVAL SOURCES

I.(a) Sources at the Directorate of Archives, Archaeology and Museum (Historical Archives of Goa) Panjim, Goa.

The Historical Archives of Goa has a large number of documents which form valuable primary sources for the history of the former *Estado da India Portuguesa*. Some of these sources have been used for the first time in this work. The bulk of the documents in Goa Archives are in Portuguese. Many of these documents are inadequately catalogued. Even a brief description with some comments on their value could be of help for someone desirous of undertaking further research in this theme. That is what is attempted here.

1. *Monções do Reino*

Monções do Reino is one of the largest collection at the Goa Archives, with over 450 manuscript volumes covering a period from 1560 to 1914. These volumes contain instructions, letters and other official matters sent by the Home Government in Portugal, some replies sent from Goa and extracts of many original documents. It includes information regarding administration, health, salaries, legislation, population statistics and other matters. Salaries paid to various officials in the seventeenth century are given in *Ms.* 203 B. *Mss.* 84 B, 86 A, 125 B, 159 A, 159 D, 169 A, 170 B 173, 177 A, 187 B, 190 C provide population statistics for the pre-census period, Mss 14, 85, 121 B, 131 B, 143 A, 161, 173, 196 C and 197 give information on health conditions. Prices of commodities are found in codex 168 C. They contain also information concerning the Royal hospital (*Mss* 185, 102 A, 133 B, 114, 164 B, 185, 209, 207 B, 212 A), various epidemic diseases, diseases suffered by soldiers during the journey to India and medical training facilities (*Mss* 56, 59, 161 D, 180 A, 178 A, 196 A, 198 A, 198 B). On an average each volume has about 300 folios. Many of these volumes have been published in the series entitled *Documentos Remetidos da India.* Some documents concerning the sixteenth and seventeenth century were published in J.H.Cunha Rivara's *Archivo Portuguez-Oriental.*

2. *Provisões a favor de Cristandade*

These are two codices (9529, 7693) with laws and decrees for promoting Christianity in India. Several restrictions imposed against the practice of native physicians are mentioned in these volumes. Ban imposed on non-Christians concerning slaves is also given. These documents have been published in *Livro do Pai dos Cristãos*. Codex 9529 — *Provisões a favor de Cristandade* has 206 folios and covers a period 1513-1840. It contains instructions issued in 1595 by Fr. Alexander Valignano (in Goa) to *Pai dos Cristãos*. It contains also additional instructions issued later. Majority of these documents are dated around 1670. These documents have been indexed in Panduronga Pissurlencar's *Roteiro dos Arquivos da India Portuguesa*, Bastora, 1955, pp. 63-95. A list of the documents of this codex are found also in the *Boletim da Filmoteca Ultramarina*. Codex 7693 — *Leis a favor da Cristandade* consists of 93 folios. The list of documents belonging to this codex were published in *Documenta Indica*, (vol. III), in above mentioned *Roteiro* and in the *Boletim da Filmoteca Ultramarina*, vol. I.

3. ***Provisões, alvaras e régimentos*** (1515-1598).

These two volumes are copies of regulations issued in the sixteenth century. They include many original documents. *Mss* 3027 and 3028 contain regulations issued for the Royal Hospital in the first two decades of Portuguese regime in Goa. Some of these documents have been published in *Archivo Portuguez-Oriental*. These codices have about 250 folios each.

4. *Vencimentos Civis e Eclesiasticos* (1626-1804).

Vencimentos civis provide information about salaries paid to various Government servants. MS.3068 lists the salaries paid to Government servants right from the Governor to the peon in 1626. Codex 2317 with 492 folios is concerned with salaries of Government servants in 1771-1772. Codex 1832 has a list of salaries paid to government servants between 1775-1804. In addition there is another codex 1598 with salaries paid to the clergy. These MSS. help us to judge standards of living of various classes in Goa.

5. *Records of the Goa Municipal Council (Senado de Goa)*

It is a very extensive series of MSS at the Goa Archives. They cover a period from 1535 to 1879. They are records on judgments passed by the Senate, charters, provisions, edicts, letters, patents, general registers, sale of stamped papers and other matters. Among these the *Registos Gerais* consist of codices with texts of licenses issued to various native Christians as well as non-Christians to practise as physicians, surgeons and bleeders in the city of Goa, besides licenses issued to artisans and merchants from 1570 to 1875. Ms. 1795 is an early nineteenth century copy of regulations issued in 1618 to improve the hygiene and other matters in the city of Goa. Some of these measures were in force until the nineteenth century.

6. *Livro da receita e despesa de Medicamentos do Hospital do Convento de S. João de Deus*

The manuscript is in good conditions and contains the daily prescriptions to the patients of the hospital and the expenses incurred by the hospital during 1733-1737.

7. Regulamento do Hospital da Misericordia de Goa

These are MSS 10425 and 10426. They contain regulations issued for the *Hospital da Misericordia* in the seventeenth century. These two MSS are small and not in a good condition. However, the writing is clear. Both the codices consist of about 12 folios each.

8. Regulamentos (1830-1839)

These deal with regulations issued to the Military Hospital in 1830 and 1840. Ms 646 consists of two parts. The first part deals with *Regulamento do Hospital Real Militar de Goa 1830*, and consists of 103 folios. The second part concerns the *Casa das Moedas* (Mint House), *Regimento provisiorio de Typografia de Goa* (Provisional regulation for the Printing Press of Goa), and *Trem Geral de Exercito de India Portuguesa*. The second part has 194 folios. The manuscript is not in good conditions. Ms.1836 — *Regulamento para bom Governo do Real Hospital Militar de Goa e Botica annexa: coprehendendo os diversos ramos da sua administração, economia e politica* is a rewritten copy of the regulation issued by the local Government on 31st December 1830 for the Military Hospital. This copy was made in 1883. There is yet another copy (Ms. 1829) of the same regulation of 1830. This copy is wrongly dated on the cover as 1835. The second part of this manuscript has a new regulation issued for the same hospital in 1840.

9. *Directorate of Accounts : collection of income and expenses of the Military Hospital.*

It is part of a very large series covering many areas of administration of Estado da India. There are more than 150 manuscripts volumes on income and expenditure of the Military Hospital from 1811 to 1887. Many of these manuscripts contain lists of medicine bought and sold at the hospital's pharmacy, inventory of clothing, utensils, furniture, list of employees and other matters. Some volumes include prescriptions given by the doctors and the methods to prepare them. They have also the lists of patients treated in the institution. Several of these volumes are in bad conditions. They are moth eaten and have fungus marks. They are valuable sources of information concerning the hospital in the nineteenth century. Most of them have not been used until now.

10. *Papers of suppressed Convents (Papeis dos Conventos Extintos)*

Another large collection at Goa Archives belonged to the suppressed Convents in 1835. Some of these MSS are wrongly labeled. They provide information of income and expenses of the convents, the wages paid to the labourers and prices of various commodities. Fees paid for medical care are also mentioned. These Mss are good sources for information on the cost of living of various sections of the society in the city of Goa during the period they cover, namely from 1612-1835.

11. *Correspondencia Diversa*

This series consists of orders and circulars issued by the local Government to its various departments. They include orders concerning health and hygiene issued between 1888-1927.

I.(b) **Manuscripts at Xavier Centre of Historical Research.**

(i) *Fonseca's Collection*

Fonseca's Customs and Manners/ Question and Responses gives us a fairly good idea about the standards of living in Goa during the later half of the nineteenth century. They are sources of information about the prices of different market commodities, wages paid to different categories of labour, household expenses of various classes and many customs followed by the people around 1880s. It contains also information on the architecture and cost of building a house. Questions and Responses contain the replies sent by Parish Priests, Village Magistrate (*Regedores*) and Taluka administrators to the queries sent by Jose Nicolau de Fonseca while preparing his work entitled *An Historical and Archaeological Sketch of city of Goa*,(Bombay, 1878.)

(ii) *Mhamai House Papers*

Mhamai House Papers consist of nearly 200, 000 loose papers and 250 codices from the last quarter of the eighteenth to the first quarter of the nineteenth century. They deal with trade that Mhamai family had with west coast of India, as well as with Portugal, Africa, Brasil and some Eastern countries.

The family was also involved in slave and opium trade. Some of the documents refer to medicinal plants and medicine imported to Goa from Brazil, Macau and the French Colony of Mahe. They mention also the cash transactions between the Mhamai family and the Military Hospital of Goa. The Mhamai brothers also supplied local medicine to their personal clients and kept records of the treatment. These papers are written in Portuguese, French, Old Kannada script, Persian, Modi script and Gujarati.

I. (c) **Church Records** (*Paço Patriarcal*).

Church records for socio-demographic studies have not been much used. Some of them contain important information on historical demography. The Archives of the Patriarchal Palace in Panjim (Goa) has a large collection of Church Rolls, Pastoral Visits and Parish Registers from the seventeenth century onwards. Some of these parishes no longer exist.

(i) *Rois das Igrejas* (Church Rolls)

They contain yearly statistics issued by Parish Priests from 1773-1941 indicating the number of Christian inhabitants and information concerning their age, health, sex, occupation and reception of sacraments. *Rois das Igrejas* were not always accurately maintained and were often filled without accurate field work. But these micro statistics can be an useful source for historical demography and for information concerning emigration among the Catholics in Goa. Latter rolls also include Hindus in their statistics.

(ii) *Visitas Pastorais*

They cover Pastoral visits from 1747-1927 to various Parishes in Goa, Belgaum, Khanapur, Malwan, Ratnagiri, Beed, Azra, Vingurla, Pune, Karwar and Sadhashivgad. They contain statements signed by sworn witnesses and taken down by the notary assisting the Archbishop during his visits to the parishes. In the eighteenth century the Pope had determined that the Archbishop should visit the parishes at least once every four years. The purpose of these visits was to check the state of faith and morality of the parishioners and to advise them to improve. The non-Christians in Goa living in predominantly Christian areas were also subject to these checks through secular authorities. The Christians were checked through the parish priest or his assistant. The Christians were often involved in abuses such drunkenness, usury, prostitution, slavery, adultery, exploitation of labour and non-observance of religious practices. These documents also deal with matter concerning *confrarias*, churches, chapels, cemeteries and financial problems. They provide lists of children confirmed by the Archbishop. These records consist of 19 volumes. Each volume is made up of two original separate books with independent numbering of folios.

(iii) *Parish Registers*

The registers pertaining to existing parishes are well maintained and upto date. They are copies of registers maintained by parishes in Goa, Daman and Diu. All births, marriages and deaths among the Christians were registered at the parishes. They give us indication of causes of death, the age of the concerned individuals and professions. They are a rare source of information on infant mortality and its causes among the Christians population.

II. Archival Sources at the Arquivo Nacional da Torre do Tombo

Arquivo Nacional da Torre do Tombo, Lisboa, has a rich collection of material. Many of these series are now well indexed with separate index books. Relevant material from *Conselho Geral do Santo Oficio* has been included in this work. This material was not included in the original thesis. It has been subsequently collected by the author during her April-May 1993 trip to Portugal.

Conselho Geral do Santo Oficio is a very large collection containing material about the Inquisition. This material is available in *Livros* (books) and *Maços* (loose bundles). Material concerning the Goa Inquisition is mostly in *Maços*. There are also about seven *Livros* on Goa in this series. The documents on *Inquisição de Goa,* contains list of *Actos de Fe,* decrees, accounts and correspondence between the Governemnt and *Inquisidor Geral de Goa* and others. Some of these documents provide information regarding various rites and superstitious practices used to cure diseases.

B. PRIMARY PUBLISHED SOURCES

1. Church and Missionary Reports

These have been included among primary sources, because unlike the other passing travellers the Church had become a local institution and the missionaries had more stable and permanent contact with local population. As such they were more involved in the living conditions of the people for whom they worked.

Missionaries have written many reports on Goa and other parts in the East where they had their missions. Some of them are good sources of information on the conditions of health in the sixteenth and the seventeenth centuries

Documenta Indica

Documenta Indica edited by Josef Wicki are published in 18 volumes so far. Volumes XIV, XV, and XVI are edited by Wicki jointly with John Gomes. They contain documents and letters written by Jesuits to their superiors in Rome and Portugal, and to their counterparts and friends in Europe. The letters were a kind of progress reports written to keep the Superiors in touch with their Missions. Some letters were given wide publicity in the sixteenth century. They were meant for the enlightenment of the members of the Order and its friends. These letters had profound influence on the Catholic world. As a result many joined the Society of Jesus. They cover a period from 1540 to 1597. Missionaries sent interesting news about their activities, customs, religions, conditions of life, health, hygiene and study of races.

Documentação para a Historia das Missões do Padroado Portugues do Oriente: India

This series edited by Antonio da Silva Rego consists of 12 volumes covering 1499 to 1582. Many of these documents provide details about the expenditure and income of the Royal Hospital and other health matters of the time. Several of the Jesuit documents included in these volumes have also been published in *Documenta Indica*. However, it includes documents concerning the Franciscans, Augustinians and Dominicans as well.

Bullarium Patronatus

Bullarium Patronatus in ecclesiis Africae, Asiae atque Oceaniae, Tomo I, edited by V. de Paiva Manso contains the proceedings and decrees issued by Church Provincial Councils held in 1567, 1575, 1583, 1592, 1602, as well as those of the Synod of Diamper. The Church Councils were held in Goa to implement the directives of the Council of Trent held between

Bibliographical Essay 219

1545-1563. The proceedings of these Councils discussed various issues concerning local society including certain local customs which were seen as problems for the practice of the new faith. Among such problems mentioned are: People seeking help of Hindu *dais* and native Hindu medicine men who were accused of inducing their patients into making votive offerings to the Hindu deities and temples. The minutes of these Councils were also published by J. H. da Cunha Rivara in vol. IV of *Archivo Portuguez-Oriental*.

2. Travellers Accounts

These could be regarded as quasi-primary sources for being contemporary witnesses of events. However, all that they reported was not always necessarily from their personal observation. Some travellers drew information from earlier travellers when they published their travelogues years after their visit to Goa. Many also included heresay information which can be accepted if corroborated by other accounts of the period or by official records.

Many European travellers have visited Goa in the past. Some like Bernier, Careri, Freyer and Manucci were medical practitioners who left accounts on the state of health in Goa. The accounts of the travellers also contain abundant references to topics connected with life in the city of Goa.

One of the first travellers to whom detailed reference has been made in this work is the Dutchman John Huygen van Linschoten who visited Goa at the close of the sixteenth century when the Portuguese empire was still displaying its glory. He has described in detail the conditions of health, certain habits in personal care that he noticed in Goa, the uses of many medicinal plants and superstitions followed in Folk medicine. Accounts about the life in the city of Goa are also found in the works of Ralph Fitch and James Forbes.

A similar account to the one given by Linschoten and very interesting is of Pyrard de Laval, a Frenchman who was a patient at the Royal Hospital in the early seventeenth century. Pyrard gives a vivid description of the Royal Hospital and other aspects of city life. He was impressed with personal care of the people.

John Albert Mandelslo was a member of the embassy sent by the Duke of Holstein to Muscovy and Persia. He visited Goa around 1638. He provides a glimpse of life-style of the upper strata and describes a dinner party he attended in one of their homes.

The Italian Pietro della Valle noticed the declining conditions of the city of Goa around 1623. François Bernier one of the first French physician who came to Goa in 1656 paid tribute to native physicians and their art of treating the sick.

The deteriorating conditions of the Royal Hospital once described by Pyrard as the best in the world are found in the accounts of Thevenot Tavernier and Careri. Tavernier blamed the declining conditions in Goa to the effects of war with the Dutch. The system of constant bleeding, corruption and malpractice are considered as factors responsible for the decay of the Royal Hospital. Dr.John Fryer who arrived in Goa at the end of 1675 has left behind vast amount of small information which would escape more scientific minds and which is always interesting. He describes the habits of hygiene of the natives and unusual practices followed by them in the disposal of waste. Manucci refers to health conditions and many malpractice of Portuguese physicians in Goa. Manucci came twice to Goa. He visited Goa for the first time in 1667 and subsequently in 1681. His large professional practice in Goa aroused the jealousy of the Portuguese physicians. The declining standards of living are described by Kottineau de Klogen who visited Goa in early nineteenth century.

3. State Papers

Archivo Portuguez-Oriental

These 10 volumes edited by J.H. da Cunha Rivara (Nova Goa 1857-76). Most of the documents belong to the sixteenth century. Fascicles II, III, IV, V and VI have been much used in this work. They contain various regulations concerning hygiene and medical care as well as regulations issued for the Royal Hospital of Goa. Many of the regulations are no longer available in its original form at the Goa Archives. Fascicle IV contains the minutes of the ecclesiastical councils of Goa.

Census of Estado da India

The first census was carried out in 1881 as a result of the Anglo-Portuguese Treaty. Decennial censuses were carried out in Goa from 1900 onwards. These censuses took into account all population present and temporarily absent. They are of importance to a demographic historian. The censuses provide information about population density, sex ratio, literacy, occupation, marital status and fertility rate. Some of these censuses are in bad physical conditions specially the ones of the early twentieth century.

Bibliographical Essay 221

Earlier in many places the census enumeration was done by village *regedores* (village magistrate) without on the spot checks.

Legislação relativa ao Estado da India

This series covers all laws and decrees issued for *Estado da India* from 1901 to 1960 by the Government, Municipalities and other bodies. This series contains among other things measures approved by the Government to tackle epidemics and diseases, to provide health care and medical training during the last 60 years of the Portuguese regime.

Secretaria dos Serviços de Saude do Estado da India reports

These are annual reports submitted by the Directors of Health Services to the Governors of *Estado da India* in the present century. The reports were based on the information sent by various taluka Health officers and doctors in charge of medical institutions in Goa, Daman and Diu. They are useful sources for the twentieth century health conditions in the State and measures planned and implemented to improve the conditions of the inhabitants. The bulk of these reports in the possession of Health Services of Goa have been destroyed when the department was shifted after liberation of Goa from the old building to the present one. The Central Library Panjim and Bibloteca National (Lisbon) have some copies of these reports belonging to the late nineteenth century and first three decades of the twentieth century. A set from the Secretariat is now with the Goa Archives but is not made accessible to the readers.

Government Gazettes

Boletim do Governo was started in 1837 and *Boletim Oficial* in 1879. These weekly state papers contain orders issued by the Government among other matters concerning medical care, legislation, appointments of medical personnel, etc. They had two parts, namely oficial and unofficial. The Goa Archives and the Central Library (Panjim) have almost a complete collection of *Boletim do Governo do Estado da India*. However, some numbers are in bad conditions.

4. Medical Journals

Revista Medico-Militar da India Portuguesa

Revista Medico-Militar da India Portuguesa edited by Augusto Carlos de

Lemos, was published in early 1860s at Hospital Regimental. It was a monthly consisting of about 24 pages in the months of February, May, August and November, and 20 pages in the remaining months. Few issues of this journal are now available. It provides information about the climate and sanitary conditions during various seasons of the year.

Archivo de Pharmacia e Sciencia Accessorias da India Portuguesa

This monthly journal was edited by Antonio Gomes Roberto. It started in early 1860's and closed in December 1871 and contains information on conditions of health and hygiene. The uses of several medicinal plants and minerals are also mentioned in many of its issues.

Archivo Medico da India

Archivo Medico da India a monthly journal of medical and pharmacopic science, was edited by Pantaleao Ferrao, Bastora. The journal was started in July 1894 and closed down in May 1896. The issues contains among other things information about medicinal plants.

Boletim Geral de Medicina e Farmacia

Boletim Geral de Medicina e Farmacia was a six-monthly journal started by Dr. Froilano de Mello in 1911. It contains information concerning health conditions in Goa, Daman and Diu. Many of its issues give detailed information about folk medicine and traditions followed by people to cope with disease. This journal continued to be published as late as 1954.

Arquivos da Escola Medico Cirurgico de Nova Goa

Arquivos da Escola Medico-Cirurgica de Nova Goa was started by Dr. Froilano de Mello around 1927. It was published in two series. "Series A" contains exclusively scientific investigations carried out by the teaching staff and students of the Goa Medical School. "Series B" provides reports on the health conditions of Goa and academic matters of the Goa Medical School. These volumes are an important source of information about health of the inhabitants of Goa in the last six decades of the present century. It is a useful source of information also on infant mortality, epidemics and the work done to control them. It also provides statistics of the patients treated in hospitals in Goa and information about doctors graduated from the Goa Medical School.

Anuario da Escola Medico

Anuario da Escola Medico Cirurgica de Nova Goa was published by Goa Medical School and covers the activities of the School. It also contains lists of the staff in addition to short bibliographical sketches of some important staff members of the Goa Medical School including its Director. The first issue was published in 1909. Volume for 1909-1910, 1911, 1916-1917, 1922-1923, 1924 and 1925 are available at the Central Library, Panjim.

C. SECONDARY SOURCES

1. Hygiene

Although hygiene played a very important role in health very little has actually been written about hygiene in Goa during the colonial regime.

Germano Correia has touched on problems of hygiene in the city of Goa during the rise and decline of Portuguese empire in India in his work *La Vieille Goa* (Nova Goa, 1931). In early twentieth century Aires de Sa published his *Higiene de Panjim* (Nova Goa, 1908). It is a critical work on sanitary conditions of Panjim in the late nineteenth and early twentieth centuries. In this work he has made several suggestions to improve the sanitation of the capital town. There is practically nothing written about rural hygiene.

2. **Diseases and Epidemics**

Works on diseases and epidemics are mainly published in medical journals such as *Boletim de Medicina e Farmacia* and *Arquivos da Escola Medico -Cirurgica de Nova Goa* and in form of of small booklets. This topic has been discussed by doctors in charge of health services or by those directly involved with epidemics. F. Wolfango da Silva, Antonio A. de Rego, Froilano de Mello, Germano Correia, L.J. Bras de Sa and some others have discussed at length the epidemic and endemic diseases in Goa.

There are also few works published in book form: Garcia d'Orta's *Colloquios dos Simples e drogas e cousas medicinaes da India e assim de alguns fructas achadas nella* (Lisboa, 1877) discusses many diseases prevailing in the country in the sixteenth century and provides various methods to heal them.

Another work on this subject is Germano Correia's *A cholera-morbo na India Portuguesa, desde a sua conquista ate a actualidade —Estudo nosografico, epidemiologico e climato-sanitario*, (Nova Goa, 1919). A reliable and comprehensive account of cholera in Portuguese India from 1543-1919. Correia's other work entitled *As pestilencias na India Portuguesa*, (Nova Goa, 1922) is small book that describes many epidemics in Goa that broke out from early times.

Luis de Pina in his booklet entitled *Subsidios para historia da medicina Portuguesa Indiana do seculo XVII*, (Porto, 1931) gives a brief description of diseases and the methods of treatment used by the Portuguese to cure fevers and some other diseases in India . It also discusses medical facilities on the board of ships sailing between Portugal and India.

1a. Conferencia Sanitaria 1914 (vol.II)

Proceedings of the First Sanitary Conference 1914 (Nova Goa 1917) contains papers presented at the conference by many Goan doctors. Epidemics and causes of various infectious diseases are discussed in these papers. They provide also information on infant mortality in Goa in early twentieth century.

3. Medicinal Plants

A great deal of work has been done on this topic by Goan doctors and the Portuguese ones who have worked as physicians in Goa.

Garcia d' Orta, the first writer on tropical medicine has left a very interesting and useful work on plants and drugs available in Goa and some other parts of India. It describes the uses of these various plants in healing diseases. Many of these plants were cultivated by Garcia de Orta in the gardens attached to his residences in Goa and Bombay. Garcia d 'Orta who was in India for about 30 years travelled extensively and studied plants of Ghats, Central India and other places.

Another Portuguese physician who made a study of plants in India is Cristovão da Costa also known as Cristobal Acosta. He came to Goa in 1568. On his return to Europe he settled in Spain where he published *Tratados das Drogas e Medicina das Indias Orientais* (Lisboa, 1964). There are many things in common between this book and Garcia de Orta's *Colloquios*. Cristovam Costa used extensively the work of Garcia. Besides describing plants he explains how they were propagated.

D. G. Dalgado who worked as a medical officer for 22 years at Savantwadi has written two books on plants of Goa and Savantwadi. *Flora de Goa e Savantvadi,* (Lisboa, 1898) provides botanical names as well as English, French and Konkani names of the common plants. It lists more then 1,000 plants including 275 exotic plants brought to Goa by the Portuguese from Brasil and other parts of the East.

Dalgado's other work is entitled *Classificação botanica das plantas e das drogas descriptas nos Colloquios da India de Garcia d'Orta* (Bombay, 1894). It is a scientific classification of plants described by Garcia d' Orta in *Colloquios*. The book has an index of *colloquios*, name of the drugs and plants in Konkani and five pictures of useful and important plants.

Lencastre Pereira in his *Plantas Medicinais de Goa* provides a list of plants in Goa along with their botanical and vernacular names. It also mentions the places where these plants are found in abundance, their history, description, methods of propagation and their therapeutic uses.

Caetano F.X. Gracias describes plants with their mythology, classification, botanical names, medicinal and other uses of plants. His work entitled *Flora Sagrada da India* (Margão, 1912) studies also chemical composition of various plants and fruits.

Another book on medicinal plants is that of J.R. dos Remedios Barreto's *Plantas medicinais de Goa,* Bastora, 1959. In this work the author describes the use of many medicinal plants of Goa.

4. Medical Institutions and Training Facilities

The history of Goa Medical School has been written by João Manuel Pacheco de Figueiredo (senior) in various papers published in the *Arquivos da Escola Medico Cirurgico de Nova Goa* and other medical journals as well as in papers presented at various conferences abroad.

Germano Correia has two works on the subject. The first one entitled *O ensino de Medecina e Cirurgia em Goa nos seculos xvii,xviii, xix: Historia do ensino medico-cirurgico no Hospital Real de Goa antes da fundação da Escola Medica- Cirurgica de Nova Goa* (Bastora, 1941) narrates the type of medical training provided to the natives in the Royal Hospital before the establishment of Goa Medical School. His *Historia do ensino medico na India Portuguesa* (Nova Goa, 1919) describes the formal training provided at the Goa Medical School from 1842 to 1917.

The history of *Santa Casa Misericordia de Goa* is narrated by J.F. Ferreira Martins in 3 volumes entitled *Historia de Santa Casa*

Misericordia de Goa. It covers a period from 1520 to 1910. He produces several documents concerning *Santa Casa* in Goa. These volumes have several errors and is often confusing as well as disorganised. But it is a basic publication on the subject..

Enciclopaedia Portuguesa Brasileira (Lisboa) is a good source of information about some eminent doctors who worked in Goa and Goan doctors who worked in the Portuguese colonies in Africa. These volumes contain few errors concerning date of birth. Another source of information about eminent doctors is *Escola Medico-Cirurgica de Nova Goa 1842-1957* (Bastora, 1957) published by Goa Medical school and *Escola Medico-Cirurgica de Goa — Monografia* (Nova Goa ,1959). J. P. Peregrino da Costa in his *Expansão do Goes pelo Mundo* (Goa, 1956) gives information about the contribution of many Goan doctors in different parts of the world . His other work concerning Goan doctors *Medicos da Escola de Goa nos Quadros de Saude de Colonias*, (Bastora, 1944) is a detailed account of work done by some Goan doctors in the Portuguese colonies. In his *Escola Medica de Goa e a sua projecção na India Portuguesa e no Ultramar* (Bastora,1957) he describes briefly the contribution of some Goan doctors - graduates of Goa Medical School to Portuguese India and Portuguese overseas colonies.

The Indo-Portuguese Review (Calcutta, 1921-1925) is also a good source of information on some Goan doctors specially concerning those who worked in British India.

Miscellaneous

O Oriente Portugues-revista da Comissão Archeologica da India Portuguesa, Bastora, 1904-1920 and 1931-1941, contains useful information on diseases (vol. II), institutional care (vols. I, IV, VI) medical training facilities medical personnel (vols. IV, IX, X, XI) population statistics (vol. XIII) by various contributors.

CHRONOLOGICAL INDEX
OF SOME HEALTH LEGISLATION

A considerable volume of health and sanitary legislation was enacted in the colonial era. Health legislation particularly the legislation concerning sanitation was largely restricted to urban areas where the whites lived, and meant to safeguard the interests of the ruling class.

Most of the health legislation, excepting the measures in times of epidemics was not well enforced. Sanitary measures were not given top priority. Legislation was lacking in vital subjects. For instance, over a long period there was no legislation forbidding the quacks to practise medicine, probably because of shortage of trained doctors mainly in rural areas. In the same way no legislation was issued to control the sale of adulterated food and drugs.

The plague, cholera and smallpox epidemics of the late nineteenth century and early twentieth century provoked some of the most drastic legislative responses. The victims of various epidemics were isolated in the hospital set up for the purpose, their residences and shops were sealed, families were advised to leave their homes for certain period of time. Travellers were medically inspected. These measures were inadequately explained and few people accepted the rationality of it. Some resisted openly. Traders rejected bans on the movement of their goods. Cases of plague were not reported to the concerned authority due to fear of isolation. Many infected people and their families refused to leave their houses. Some victims would leave their homes and move to other areas. People influenced by superstitions refused vaccination. Vaccinators had to deal with frequent rumors of the dangers of the treatment.

In many instances, legislation was outdated. Legislation about the control of epidemics was issued after the outbreak of the epidemic. Often preventive measures issued from the nineteenth century onwards were not always implemented, because of the general lack of stringent penalties for non-compliance and poor administration. The masses of the people in rural areas were hardly touched by preventive medical work undertaken in the colonial period, barring few edicts making smallpox vaccination compulsory and some measures to prevent epidemics.

All health laws were difficult to enforce due to popular ignorance and apathy in matter of hygiene. Government officials were also reluctant to enforce legislation on the people in order to avoid hurting the feelings of the people. Besides there was paucity of personnel to enforce measures. The work had to be paid for with revenues raised in *Estado da India*. During the later period of the Portuguese regime the *Estado* could not spend on health as funds were required for other urgent needs.

Legislation pertaining to health and hygiene was issued by the Home Government (Portugal), by the local government in Goa and by other agencies, such as *Senado de Goa* (Municipal Council), *Santa Casa da Misericordia de Goa* (Holy House of Mercy) and the Church. The legislation issued by *Santa Casa da Misericordia de Goa* and the Church were subject to the approval of the local Government. Legislation issued by the Home Government was earlier issued separately for each colony but from the nineteenth century onwards it was issued jointly for health services of all overseas Portuguese colonies.

Among the institutions which were characteristic of Portuguese empire were the Municipal Council (*Senado de Camara*) and Holy House of Mercy (*Santa Casa da Misericordia*). They were the twin pillars of Portuguese society from Brazil to Macau. In Goa it was said that " whoever wanted to live high, wide and handsomely should try to become an alderman of the Municipal Council or brother of the Misericordia or preferably both.(Source: C. R. Boxer, *The Portuguese Seaborne Empire 1415- 1825,* Middlesex, 1969, p. 288.)

The Municipal council consisted of aldermen or councillors, justices of peace and a Municipal attorney. They were collectively known as *Oficiais de Camara* (Council officers). The officials had to be old Christians and not of Jewish descent. To be elected as alderman a candidate had to serve earlier as market inspector, justice of peace or city attorney.

These members were elected through a complicated system of balloting. General elections were conducted every three years in the sixteenth century. The *oficiais da Camara* enjoyed certain judicial rights. They could not be arrested arbitrarily nor subjected to judicial torture, nor imprisoned in chains, save in cases of high treason which involved death penalty. They were exempted from military service and they were paid allowances to attend certain functions like the feast of *Corpus Christi*. There were instances of nepotism, corruption, and embezzlement of municipal funds.(Source: *Ibid., p.278.)*

The decision of the *Camara* in Municipal matters could not be revoked by any authority save only if they involved unauthorized innovations. The *Camara* acted as a court in summary cases. It supervised leasing of Municipal lands, fixed sale prices of the commodities, licensed street vendors, checked quality of wares, public work and was responsible for policy of towns and public health and sanitation. (Source: *Ibid.*, p. 275.) The Municipal council issued a number of *posturas* (laws) concerning health and hygiene of the city of Goa.

In the middle ages *posturas* were issued only by the king, but from the eighteenth century onwards laws issued by other administrative bodies came to be known as *posturas*. These posturas applied only to the area of the Municipality issuing the same. The Municipalities could issue *posturas* on matter within their jurisdiction and matters not involved in general laws. Village bodies were also permitted to issue *posturas*.

As regard the Holy House of Mercy (*Santa Casa Misericordia de Goa*) it is not possible to pinpoint the date of its establishment. However, there are references to it around 1519 or even earlier. The Holy House of Mercy was a lay confraternity closely patterned on the lines of the mother house in Lisbon which was founded under royal patronage in 1498. The members of this institution were known as brothers and belonged to the upper strata of the society. The Holy House of Mercy began with 100 brothers rising through 400 in 1595 to 600 in 1609 but thereafter the number declined rapidly with the economic decline of the city.(Source: *Ibid.*, p. 288.).

Wars and conquests had taken heavy toll of life leaving behind widows and orphans. Besides, the moral degradation of the sixteenth century had created problems. To remedy the situation the Holy House of Mercy set up in early seventeenth century homes for widows, orphans and women who had gone astray. The institution helped the orphans to find husbands by offering dowries and jobs to men prepared to marry them. The *provedor* or the president of the board of the guardians was the most important of the elected officials who served in the Misericordia. No brotherther could be elected *provedor* in the first year after he was received in the brotherhood. In Goa such posts were often filled up by Governors, Archbishops, Inquisitors, Captains, Judges and others. Many times these dignitaries had no time to look after affairs of *Misericordia* and the routine work of the institution was run by the *Escrivão*. The funds of the *Misericordia* were derived from private charity and legacies.

The Holy House of Mercy in many places maintained a hospital of its own and in Goa besides its own *Hospital de todos os Santos,* it also managed for sometime the Royal Hospital. To run these institutions the Holy House of Mercy issued regulations from time to time.

Finally, the Catholic Church in Goa gained importance only after Goa was made the headquarters of the Portuguese empire in the East. Until 1533 it was dependent of Funchal (Madeira island). In 1577 it was raised to the rank of a metropolitan archdiocese. The diocese of Goa embraced the whole of the East from the Cape of Good Hope till China. (Source: Teotonio R. de Souza, *The Afro-Asian Church in Estado da India*, in Ogbu U. Kalu (ed.) *African Church Historigraphy: An Ecumenical Perspective. Papers presented at a workshop on African Church History held at Nairobi, August 3-8, Berne, 1988.*

The Church of Goa was headed at first by Vicar General, followed by Apostolic Commissaries, Bishops, Archbishops and after 1866 by Patriarchs. They were appointed for life and many of them belonged to the religious orders, generally Franciscans, Augustinians and Dominicans.

The Catholic Church also issued decrees which affected the social and moral lives of the people. The Church was a powerful institution in the early centuries of the Portuguese regime. It was a State within the State. The Church in Goa was controlled both by the Church and the State represented by Viceroy and the Archbishop chosen by the crown. The appointment of the Archbishop was approved by the Pope. The Church provided funds to the State. The Archbishop and the Church Council issued decrees relating to the lives of their followers.

Women of ill fame

First Provincial Council held in 1567 forbade non-Christian women of ill fame from living with Christian women. It ordered that the former should live separately beyond the Hospital of S. Lazarus in the city of Goa. Source: *Bullarium Patronatus Portugallie Regum, Tomo I*, Olisipone, 1872, p. 25.

Sick slaves to be sheltered by Holy House of Mercy

The fifth Provincial Council(1602) determined that the incurable sick slaves thrown out by their masters should be given shelter by Holy House of Mercy in the city of Goa.

The same Council forbade the inhabitants from moving about in closed palanquins to prevent illicit affairs.
Source:*Bullarium Patronatus Portugallie Regum, Tomo I*, Olisipone,

1872, p. 142.

Wet nurses

Women engaging wet nurses were advised by the fifth Provincial Council to do so only after consulting their husbands.
Source: *Ibid.*, p. 138.

Postura to improve the sanitation of the city of Goa

The Municipality of Goa issued a detailed postura on 3rd November 1618 to improve the health conditions of the city inhabitants. The Postura remained valid upto mid nineteenth century.

By this postura the inhabitants were forbidden to dump filth in places other than fixed by the Municipality. A penalty of 100 reis was imposed on the defaulters. Slaves faced whipping for the same offense.

People throwing filth around Se Cathedral and other churches were fined 5 pardaos. Anyone staying in the vicinity of the outdoor pit had to get the pit's boundary cleaned before the monsoons. The inhabitants were prevented from throwing dirty water between Rua Direita and Fortaleza in the drains meant for rain water. Further the inhabitants were not allowed under penalty to carry excreta pots to the quays. They had to be emptied in the sea.

The inhabitants were instructed not to dump manure in the streets. The postura directed the owners of dead animals to bury them away from the suburbs. Rearing of pigs in the city and nearby places was forbidden.

The practice of frying fish in the streets was put an end to by this regulation as the smoke and smell polluted the area. The postura also put an end to the consumption of meat of dead horses. No meat could be sold in places other than fixed by the Municipality. It prohibited washing of clothes in the water springs of the fountains of S.Domingos and Bangeunim.

The postura of 3rd November 1618 imposed many restrictions on native physicians. Physicians were to be fined twenty pardaos for practising without license. The bleeders were asked to display at the door a poster showing a bleeding man. The postura compelled the Municipal officials to visit all pharmacies every six months. They were given permission to destroy adulterated medicine. It limited the number of Hindu physician to thirty. Christians were forbidden to employ non-Christian physicians for preparing medicine.

Bakers were asked to prepare clean bread. In case of violation he was to be fined 100 reis. If caught thrice his oven was to be destroyed and he would forfeit the right to pursue his profession. Badly baked bread was to be confiscated and given to the prisoners. A master expelling an ailing slave was liable to a fine of 10 pardaos for the first time and 20 pardaos for the second time.

Source: *HAG : Ms. 7795 — Livro de Postura*, fls. 72-73.

Measures issued by the Archbishop

The Church Councils were not the only ones to issue decrees. Very often the Archbishop issued decrees to control the activities of the faithful, to improve their moral and health conditions.

In addition to general decrees issued by the Church and the Archbishop, there were some measures passed at the time of pastoral visits to parishes in Goa. These measures were applied to specific villages. The sentences were executed by the Parish Priest or assistant Parish Priest. Non-Christians who lived in predominantly Christian areas were also subjected to checks imposed by the Archbishop but these checks were executed by secular authorities. Checks were imposed to curb prostitution, homosexuality, drunkenness, adultery and non-observance of religious practices.

Prostitution

Prostitution was common throughout the period specially in port area of Marmugoa, and areas near Military camps. During Pastoral Visit of 1748 several women of Marmugoa were accused of offering their services to Frenchmen and Portuguese soldiers. Portuguese officials were also accused of having bailadeiras in their residence.

Many people including parents of young girls were accused of keeping brothels. *Visitas Pastorais* refer also to instances when husbands encouraged their wives to go into prostitution. There are cases when prostitutes worked as cooks and maids in the houses of their masters. Penalties were imposed on those indulging in prostitution. They were fined, imprisoned, beaten up, their hair shaved off and sometimes sent away from their villages. Usually the ones from Bardez were sent to Salcete. Many times such women were sent to Portuguese possessions in Asia and Africa.

Source: PP: *Visitas Pastorais*, 1747-1750, vols. I and II, fl. 132. (henceforth VP); VP, 1750-1754, vols. V and VI, fl. 96; VP, 1766-1772, vols XI and XII, fl. not numbered; VP, vol. 16-17, fls. 149v-150; VP, 1785-1787, vols 18-20, fl. 40; VP, vol. 24-26, fl. 87v; VP, vol. 24-26, fl. 77.

Casual sex

Casual sex prevailed among the lower class people. Widows were often involved in such activities. Probably due to economic conditions and other reasons. One widow at Betalbatim was accused of killing her illegitimate child after birth. When she conceived again she left the village to avoid being reprehended by the Parish Priest. She returned after some months showing no signs of pregnancy.

There are cases of Kunbi women giving birth to children after the death of their husbands. One them was accused in 1771 of getting pregnant for the second time and throwing her foetus for the pigs to eat.

There are instances of men living with women with permission of their mothers. One Custodio from Margão whose wife was away was accused of keeping a woman in his house with the approval of his mother. Many women whose husbands were away were accused of adultery with other men including brothers of their husbands. Such women were ordered as punishment to attend church services on holy days with their heads uncovered.

During a pastoral visit of 1772 one Parish Priest was accused of having a woman in his residence. Another priest was accused of getting his widowed sister-in-law pregnant for the third time. He was also accused of helping her to get rt rid of her foetus.

A Hindu man of Nerul was ordered during a pastoral visit to throw out of his house a woman who worked as a cook but was presumed to be his mistress.

Source: PP: VP, 1779-1785, vols. 16-17, fl. 83v-84; PP: VP, 1747-1750, vols. I and II, fl. 119; VP, 1772-1785, vols 13-15, fls. 2-3, 49-51, 129v-130.

Homosexuality

Homosexuality was not uncommon in Goa. Young slaves were preferred for such activities. In 1779 two kunbi boys were accused during pastoral visit to Nerul of perversion and living with three Hindu men.
Source: PP: VP, 1747-1750, vols. I and II , fl. 65.

Ban on sixth day celebration

The episcopal decree dated 27th July 1784 put an end to various traditions and celebration on sixth day of the birth among the Christians. These were Hindu customs followed by the Catholics. It disapproved also women staying away from the Church in the first forty days after the delivery.
Source: *Summario Chronologico de Decretos Diocesanos desde 1775-1899 — Decretos do Arcebispo D. Francisco d'Assumpção e Brito*, ed. Manuel João Socrates d'Albuquerque, Bastora, 1900, p. 25.

Organization of overseas Health Services

The first steps to organize the Health Services of the overseas Portuguese colonies were taken by the decree of 14th September 1844. The decree fixed the number of doctors, their salaries and privileges. It proposed the establishment of four medical schools in the colonies to train doctors who could work as auxiliaries in the health cadre. Only one school was finally established in the Portuguese colonies.
Source: CLP: 9749 — *Ministerio dos Negocios da Marinha e Ultramar*, p. 531.).

Establishment of Goa Medical School

The establishment of *Escola Medico-Cirurgica de Nova Goa* was approved by the Portuguese King only on 11th January 1847, although it had started functioning from 1842.
Source: *Boletim do Governo do Estado da India*, no.13, 26th March 1847.

Incentives to Portuguese doctors working in the colonies

A decree issued on 11th December 1851 provided incentives to Portuguese doctors who were willing to work in the colonies. The same decree allowed medical graduates to work as surgeons in the Portuguese colonies of Moçambique, Solor and Timor.
Source: *Ministerio dos negocios da Marinha e Ultramar — Organização dos Serviços de Saude das Provincias Ultramarinas*.

Doctor candidates from colonies to be helped

Carta da Lei dated 11th August 1860 authorised the local Government to

Chronological Index of Some Health Legislation 235

sponsor a certain number of aspiring doctors of the overseas colonies to study in Portugal.
Source: *Anuario do Estado da India,* 1930, Nova Goa, 1930.

Cadre for Health Services Overseas

It appears that Portuguese doctors were still reluctant to work in the colonies due to absence of proper service conditions. Consequently, there was acute shortage of medical personnel in Portuguese colonies particularly in Africa. These conditions led the Portuguese Government to issue a decree on 23rd July 1862 to improve the service conditions of the doctors working in the overseas colonies and to encourage the new ones to join the services.

It decreed that the doctors working in the Naval and Overseas Health cadre would receive same salary as the members of Naval and Overseas Council who had worked in the army. Doctors in this cadre could retire with full salary after working for 16 years in Asia and 10 years in Africa. Doctors at the time of retirement were to be promoted to the next higher grade. All staff of the overseas health cadre were entitled to leave travel allowance when proceeding home. Doctors and pharmacists of the Overseas Health cadre working in India had also the duty of teaching in the medical school. Their salary was fixed at 20$000. In addition those who completed 16 years of teaching were entitled to additional one third of the salary as teaching allowances.

The decree of 23rd July 1862 had made provision for statutes to be drawn up for the Health Services of overseas colonies. The decree was approved on 28th October 1862. The following were the main provisions: The Health Services of the Overseas colonies were to be manned by doctors, pharmacists and nurses of the Naval and Overseas cadre. Doctors of class II and pharmacists of class II were to be appointed after selection by Naval and Overseas Health Council. In the absence of doctors trained in Portugal the same posts could be filled up with candidates qualified in Medical School of Goa and Funchal as per the rules framed in December 1851 and November 1855. The selected candidate before the appointment had to be examined by the Health Council for Naval and Overseas colonies or by the Health Board of Estado da India. Only doctors trained in Portugal and belonging to grade II could be promoted to grade I. The Chief physician of Estado da India, Moçambique, Angola and Cabo Verde and Chief Surgeons of S. Tome e Principe and Macau were also appointed as Health Directors of their respective colonies. The Director of Health

Services, the Chief Surgeon and the first pharmacist had to reside in the capital city. The teaching staff of Goa Medical School also had to live in the capital city.

In all capitals of the colonies, a Health Board was to be constituted with the Director of Health Services as its President, and two other senior doctors of the Health cadre, one among these would act as the Secretary of the Board. Health Board was responsible for the health matters of the colonies.

Source : *Legislação Novissima do Boletim do Conselho Ultramarino*, 1857-1862, II, pp. 757-765.

Further Priveliges to doctors working in the colonies

The decree of 23rd July 1867 was followed by Carta da Lei dated 3rd April 1867. This document granted further privileges to the staff of Health Cadre of the Overseas Colonies. The decree was issued to encourage young doctors to join the cadre.

The Overseas Health Services were further reorganized by a decree dated 2nd December 1869. It tried to improve the conditions of the Health Services and fixed rules for the recruitment, seniority, promotion and retirement of the employees of the Health Services. It made provisions to increase the medical personnel in the colonies. In the Health Cadre of Estado da India candidates with distinction were to be admitted to teach in the medical school.

Source: CLP: 9749 — *Ministerio dos Negocios da Marinha e Ultramar.*

The aim of the new decree was to reorganize the Health Services without additional expenses and at the same time to provide certain amount of autonomy to the Health Services. The Health Services were to be in charge of a doctor from Overseas cadre. The deputy Director was to be appointed for a term of two years and selected from among the doctors of grade I from Health Services of Overseas Colonies. The decree created the posts of doctors and pharmacists in grade III.

This staff was to be promoted to the next grade within a year after joining the services. The earlier decree permitted doctors of grade II to join the Overseas cadre. As a result young men who had just joined the army without much experience were placed in high positions. The decree of 1895 granted the Directors of Health Services powers to take action against the staff and also to implement various sanitary measures in urban and rural areas. The Directors of Health were responsible to the Governors of their respective colonies. They were given wide powers. Doctors working in the Health Services had to provide free medical care to the poor at health offices as well as at the homes of the patients. In addition they had to work in the hospitals and any other institution of charity in their areas which required their services. They would be renumerated for these services. These doctors had to submit accounts of the income and expenses of any hospital under their care. A Health Board was to be organized in every colony. They had a number of functions to perform. In Goa every taluka would have one member of the Board, these members were to be selected from among those who occupied a post in the Municipality or Communidades. The member of the Board had to live in the taluka headquarters.

The decree granted special concessions to the Europeans working in the cadre. These European doctors could enjoy six months leave in the mother country with full salary and travel expenses paid by the Government.
Source: *Reorganização Geral dos Serviços de Saude do Ultramar de 13 de Julho 1895.*

Colonial Hospital

In 1902 a colonial hospital was established in Lisbon to treat members of the armed forces when they returned from the colonies and to teach tropical medicine to doctors desiring to join the overseas Health Cadre.
Source: *LREI 1902,* Nova Goa, 1903, pp. 242-248.

Compulsory vaccination in colonies (1902)

The Ministry of Overseas Colonies ordered compulsory vaccination in all Portuguese colonies. This was necessary due to recurring smallpox epidemics in the colonies. Vaccination was to be carried out twice a week in all villages by Health Officers and missionaries trained for the purpose.
Source: *LREI 1902,* Nova Goa, 1903, pp. 216-217.

Sanitary measures in the colonies

The urgent need to organize sanitation in the colonies led the Home Government to pass a legislation on 30th November 1904. The aim was to preserve the health of the Europeans living in the colonies and to protect the natives from contagious diseases. The Governors of the colonies and the autonomous state of Timor were asked to find ways to improve water supply, sewage system, removal of garbage and the hospital system. Together with their report they had to submit statistics about births, deaths and important diseases prevailing in the colony as well as their causes.

Source : *LREI 1904*, Nova Goa, 1905, pp.147-148; Boletim Oficial, 24th November 1911.

Village Committees for cholera victims

To control incidence of cholera and to provide care to the victims, the Governor General of Estado da India approved a proposal put forward by the Director of Health Services. Among other things a committee was appointed in every village presided by Parish Priest to take care of sanitary problems of the village. The legislation came into force from 27th December 1907.

Source: *Boletim Oficial*, no. 103, 27th December 1907.

Measures against plague

Cases of plague and death of rats had appeared in the capital town of Goa in early twentieth century. The Governor General issued an edict on 9th August 1908 ordering: (1) Inspection of all houses in the capital town. The town was divided into zones and each zone was to be in charge of a physician appointed by the Health Board. (2) Houses having victims of plague were to be isolated for 10 days to control the spread of the disease. During this period all the neighbouring houses were to be inspected to find cases of plague. Houses and areas with dead rats were to be disinfected. Those failing to report cases of fever or dead rats were to be punished. (3) Houses considered to be the source of plague were to be destroyed.
Source: *Boletim Ofical*, no. 65, 21st August 1908.

Inspection of Passengers from Bombay

On 26th August 1908 the Governor General Jose M de S. Horta e Costa issued another edict to prevent any infectious disease from being carried to Goa by boats from Bombay.

All passengers were to be examined by a doctor before landing. Any passenger or crew member found with plague or suspected of the disease were to be sent directly to the isolation ward at Reis Magos. Dirty clothes

were to be carried to the isolation ward for disinfection. Passengers and crew staying in Goa had to report for a medical check during a period of 10 days. Sanitary measures at the Panjim jetty were to be carried out by a doctor from Health Services.
Source: *Boletim Oficial,* no. 67, 28th August 1908.

Measures to control plague in Salcete

Several cases of plague in Margão and rest of Salcete including Marmugoa led the Governor General of Estado da India to approve measures to control the disease. These measures became effective from 22nd December 1910.

Roads, drains, compounds and shed in Margão were to be cleaned and holes in the compound were to be filled up with mud. The garbage was to be destroyed in the dumping grounds. However, the garbage of the affected area was to be destroyed in the same place. Clothing and goods from the infected area were to be disinfected before they were carried away from the area.

A list of all inhabitants was to be drawn. Victims of plague were to be transferred to the isolation ward. One member of the family was allowed to keep company as long as the person observed rules of sanitation.

Houses had to be opened daily. Owners of a closed house who refused to do so could be ordered by the competent authority to open it. Houses with cases of plague had to be disinfected and the roofs opened. They had to be painted before they were used and the Health authorities informed about it. Destruction of rats was to be undertaken. Any person showing a dead rat to the competent authority would be paid 1 tanga per rat.

Physicians, heads of the families, storekeepers and others had to report immediately to the health authorities any cases of plague or dead rats. In the infected area vigorous inspection was to be carried out of godowns, pharmacies, drugstores and other places. In the infected area all temporary constructions were to be destroyed. Bonguis were to be employed to carry excreta for disposal in culverts opened for the purpose.

Rearing of pigs in Margão and Marmugoa was banned. Taluka administrators were instructed to appoint 40 labourers to help in the sanitation of the place. No animals could be kept around the house.
Source: *LREI, 1911,* Nova Goa, 1912, pp. 57 and 58.

Measures to improve the conditions of the natives

The Home Government issued a detailed decree to all its overseas colonies on 14 th October 1911. The purpose of this decree was to improve the health conditions of the colonies which were devastated by yellow fever, malaria and sleeping disease. The Health Services of the colonies were asked to introduce sanitary measures to prevent such diseases.
Source: *LREI, 1911*, Nova Goa, 1912, pp.737-742.

New price list of medicine

The local Government ordered in 1913 that the Health Services should fix the prices of medicine to be sold in all Government hospitals, pharmacies and dispensaries in Estado da India. This price was to be fixed in June of every year.
Source: *LREI 1913*, Nova Goa, 1913, pp. 329-332.

Burial of dead bodies

Taking into consideration the interest of public health the Governor General of Estado da India permitted the burial of dead bodies immediately after death in case they were victims of contagious disease of epidemic nature. This legislation was issued on 28th March 1914.
Source: *LREI 1914, Nova Goa, 1916, p. 110.*

Measures to control infectious diseases

Chicken pox, whooping cough. diphtheria broke out in 1916 in epidemic form in many parts of Goa.
    The need to prevent the entry in Goa of infectious diseases led the Government to issue a legislative order in 1916. By this order no ship crew could leave Goa without a medical certificate stating the name of the ship, date of sailing, the number of crew and the date of their vaccination. No boat could return to the point of departure unless it touched Marmugoa and Salcete. The crew were to be checked at this point, and vaccinated if necessary.
Source: *LREI 1916*, Nova Goa, 1917, pp. 182-183.

Syllabus for the nursing course

In 1916 the local Government approved a syllabus for the nursing course.

The course was of two years. Elementary anatomy, general idea about the genital organs and the changes they underwent during the pregnancy, problems of menstruation, symptoms of pregnancy, hygiene to be observed during pregnancy, diagnosis of normal delivery and other matter was to be taught in the first year. In the second year the students revised what was taught in the first year and studied more about complications during delivery, artificial respiration in the newly born, eclampsy, hemorrhoids in pregnancy, food and care of the new born and problems affecting the pregnant women. The duties of the nurse concerning the internal examination of the pregnant women and the rules of hygiene to be observed in this matter were discussed.

The practicals were to be carried out the at Hospital Regimental. Hindu girls with no knowledge of Portuguese were to be given a crash course in the same. Hindu girls without primary education possessing other requirements were allowed to join the midwifery course. They were to be trained in Marathi and Konkani.

Source: *LREI 1916,* Nova Goa, 1917, pp. 203-205; *LREI 1917,* Nova Goa, 1918, p. 170.

List of passengers from infected areas

The Government ordered in 1918 that a list of passengers entering Goa from infected regions should be maintained at the entry point.
Source: *LREI 1918,* Nova Goa, 1920, p. 478; *Boletim Oficial,* no.69, 27th August 1918.

Ban on panic creating Press reports

A ban was imposed on the press on 31st August 1918 by the Governor General of Estado da India Jose de Filipe Ribeiro. By this ban the press was forbidden to discuss or oppose measures adopted by the Government to control plague in Goa. Further the press was ordered to publish only information supplied by health authorities concerning plague.
Source: HAG: Ms. 10471 —*Corespondencia Diversa,* fl. 42.

Reorganisation of Health Services 1920

The existing health colonial decree had the sole aim of recruiting doctors for the overseas colonies who were trained in Tropical Medicine without considering the existing conditions and whether these doctors could practise what they learnt during their one year course at the Institute of Tropical Medicine. In the colonies these doctors had no opportunities to improve their conditions due to poor working arrangements.

The colonies did not have doctors specialized in radiology, venereal diseases, skin problems, pediatrics, ophthalmology, gynaecology, urology, abdominal surgery, etc. The lack of specialized doctors forced many colonists to seek medical care in Portugal even for minor surgery. Therefore a decree was passed on 4th October 1920 to provide facilities to doctors working in the colonies to specialize in Portugal and other countries for a period of no less then six months. Doctors eligible for study leave could make use of these facilities.

Source: *LREI 1920,* Nova Goa, 1921, pp. 412-420.

Benefits for doctors working in less developed colonies

In 1920 it was realized that Portuguese doctors often opted to work for colonies were salaries were higher. As a result there were no candidates for posts in colonies where salaries were low. Therefore, it was determined that a doctor from a colony transferred to another colony with the lower salaries was entitled to enjoy the benefits of the colony where he was working earlier.

Source: *LREI 1920,* Nova Goa, 1921, p. 361.

Admission for Tropical Medicine

Admission for the course of tropical medicine was to be carried out through interview held at the Health Services of Overseas Colonies once a year before the reopening of the course. They would be placed in grade II and were entitled to salary during their training period. Those who failed in the course or did not complete the course would be sent to Cabo Verde or Guine for a period of 18 months. Those who passed in the first instance had the right to acquire laboratory material required for their research work. These expenses were to be met by the respective colonies.

Source: *LREI 1920, Nova Goa, 1921, pp. 416-418.*

Nursing course in Margão

Dr. Inacio Manuel Miranda was granted permission by the Government to start a nursing course at Hospicio de Sagrado Coração, Margão. This was necessary due to high maternal mortality rate, acute shortage of nurses

and midwives.
Source: *LREI 1920,* Nova Goa, 1921, pp. 34-35; *Boletim Oficial,* no.13, 13th February 1920.

Activities of tooth pullers controlled

In 1922 the Government decided to control the activities of tooth pullers and quacks who practised as dentists.

Individuals desiring to practice dentistry had to obtain diploma in dentistry from Goa Medical School by appearing and passing dentistry examination. Individuals without diplomas were not allowed to practice. However, practising dentists who were medical doctors were exempted from acquiring such diplomas.

The Medical School Council prepared a plan for the diploma examination as per the Ministerial circular dated 13 July 1870.

Dentistry examinations were to be held in Goa Medical School. The candidates had to send together with their application form a fee of Rs.40 to the Director of the School and the necessary certificates. Any candidate failing in an oral examination could appear again only after 6 months. Diplomas were issued for Rs.50.
Source: *Boletim Oficial,* no.32, 21st April 1922.

Government nurses allowed private practice

In 1922 the Governor General permitted nurses working in the Health Services to render help to private individuals without upsetting their official duties. In addition to their salaries paid by the Government the nurses had to be compensated by individuals who required their services. The remuneration to be paid by private individuals was fixed by the Government. Those requiring the services of the nurses had to apply in writing to the Health Services giving their address, profession and other details. The remuneration had to be deposited at the Health Services who forwarded the same to the Government Treasury. The amount was later paid to the concerned nurse. This legislation would prevail for a period of two years until more nursing staff to work privately could be trained.
Source: *Boletim Oficial,* no. 54, 7th July 1922.

Nursing courses at Ribandar open to all

It appears that until 1922 the nursing course carried out at Hospital da

Misericordia at Ribandar was meant for the orphans of the institutions run by *Santa Casa da Misericordia* (Holy House of Mercy). On 31st July 1922 the Governor General of Estado da India granted permission for girls other than from the institutions run by Holy House of Mercy to join the nursing course held at Ribandar.
Source: *Boletim Oficial,* no. 62, 4th August 1922.

Control of medicinal drugs

Medicinal drugs were sold freely in Goa in commercial shops both wholesale as well on retail basis. This was against the existing rules. The practice was dangerous to public health. Only pharmacies had the right to sell medicine in retail and prepare medicine.

The Legislative Council and the Governor General approved a provisional decree by which only wholesale of drugs were allowed. They could not be sold in commercial shops. Retail sale of drugs and its preparation could be done only in pharmacies. However, commercial stores were permitted to sell foodstuff with prior permission of Health Services.
Source: *Boletim Oficial,* no.75, 19th September 1922.

Regulation for the Lazareto of Reis Magos

In 1925 the Government decided to bring together all the rules concerning Lazareto de Reis Magos established to isolate victims of epidemics, mainly passengers arriving from Bombay with the disease.
Source: *LREI 1925,* Nova Goa , 1926, p. 111.

Rules to be followed regarding the construction of houses

The Government of Goa issued detailed guidelines regarding the construction of houses so that proper rules of hygiene were observed.
Source: Supplement to *Boletim Oficial,* no. 89, 9th November 1925.

Measures against infectious diseases

Legislative measure issued on 4th March 1927 brought together all laws concerning the prevention and control of infectious diseases that broke out in Estado da India from time to time, namely smallpox, plague, cholera, typhoid, meningitis, dysentery, leprosy, pneumonic influenza, whooping

cough, chicken pox, diphtheria, mumps and others.
Source: *Boletim Oficial,* no. 18, 4th March 1927.

Permission granted to sponsor students for further studies

In 1934 the Central Government granted permission to the colonies to subsidize students desiring to study tropical medicine or to specialize further for a period of five months. Only doctors entitled to study leave could be selected.
Source: *Boletim Oficial,* no. 14, 16th February 1934; *LREI 1934,* Nova Goa, 1936, p. 88.

Admission to the nursing course

By legislation issued in 1935 the Government sought to regulate the admission of the students for the nursing courses at the Hospital Central, Hospital da Misericordia and Hospicio do Sagrado Coração. Only 20 students could be admitted for the first year course.
Source: *LREI 1935,* Nova Goa, 1938, p. 265.

Institute of Tropical Medicine in Lisbon

The Institute of Tropical Medicine was established in Lisbon by a decree dated 29th May 1935. The purpose was to train doctors in tropical medicine. The course was made compulsory to doctors who desired to work in the health cadre of overseas colonies.
 All the Portuguese overseas colonies were asked to contribute with one percent of their income towards the maintenance of Institute of Tropical Medicine.
Source: *LREI 1935,* Nova Goa, 1938, pp. 214-222.

Transfer of Health Staff

The Ministry for overseas colonies determined in 1936 that the staff belonging to the common health cadre should be transferred to another colony when promoted to the next higher grade. This was necessary so that the same person did not remain in a colony too long since hot climate and the standards of living differed in different Portuguese colonies.
Source: *LREI 1936,* Nova Goa, 1939, p.274.

Measures to improve the conditions of the natives

In 1948 the Portuguese Government decided to introduce some health measures to improve the conditions of the colonists and in particular to reduce the mortality rate among the natives.
Source: *Boletim Oficial*, no.43, 4th November 1948.

Vaccination facilities for colony-bound

In 1948 the Institute of Tropical Medicine at Lisbon made available vaccination against infectious diseases to all those who desired to go to the colonies.
Source: *Boletim Oficial*, no. 50, 23rd December 1948.

Facilities available to Government Servants

In 1948 the Government verified that the Government servants admitted in the Hospital Central were given greater discount than admissible. To end such practice the Government ordered on 23rd December 1948 that the discount given in the hospital to Government servants should not exceed the daily fees paid by private patients in the same category.
Source: *Boletim Oficial*, no. 50, 23rd December 1948.

Medical treatment at concessional rate

By a legislation dated 25th August 1949, Government servants earning upto Rs.85:11:05 and pensioners could avail of medical treatment for their families at concessional rate in Goa Medical School Hospital.
Source: *LREI 1949*, Nova Goa, 1950, p. 565.

Number of students for nursing course increased

Scarcity of trained nurses who could render assistance to the general public led the Government to raise the number of students who could be admitted to the first year of nursing course. The number was raised from 20 to 26 in Hospital da Misericordia and Hospicio do Sagrado Coração.
Source: *LREI 1949*, Nova Goa, 1950, pp. 718-719; *Boletim Oficial*, no. 42, 20th October 1949.

Permission granted to candidates with S.S.C. to join the nursing school

The legislative decree of 8th November 1956 had allowed candidates with Secondary School Certificate or elementary studies of a technical school to join the course of midwives. On twentieth March 1958 such facilities were granted to those wishing to join the nursing course.
Source: *LREI 1958*, Nova Goa, 1958, p. 427.

Subsidy for Government servants suffering from T.B.

The Government fixed a subsidy of Rs.125 for married and Rs.100 for unmarried Government servant suffering from T.B. To be eligible for such subsidy the concerned persons had to produce a certificate issued by Health Board stating that they suffered from contagious disease which posed danger to their families and colleagues.
Source: *LREI, 1958*, Nova Goa, 1958, pp. 89-90.

STATISTICAL AND DOCUMENTARY APPENDICES

Statistical and Documentary Appendices 251

APPENDIX 1-A

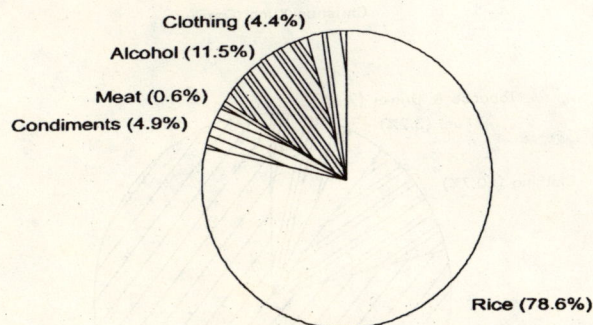

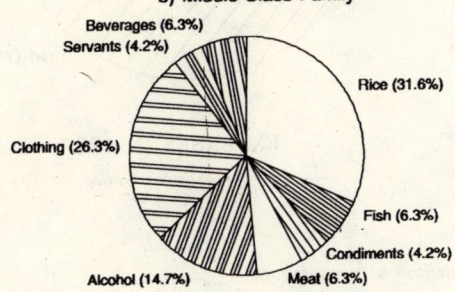

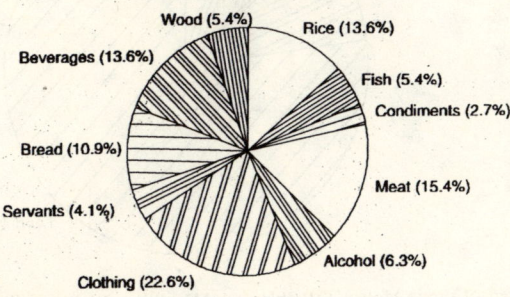

Source : J.N. da Fonsecás Customs and Manners at XCHR.

APPENDIX 1-B

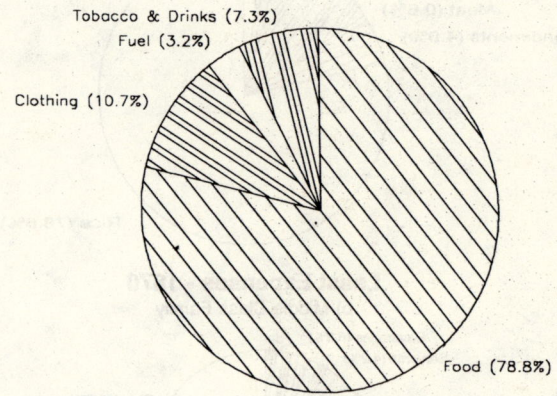

EXPENSES IN 1923
Christian Kunbi Family

EXPENSES IN 1923
Hindu Farmer Family

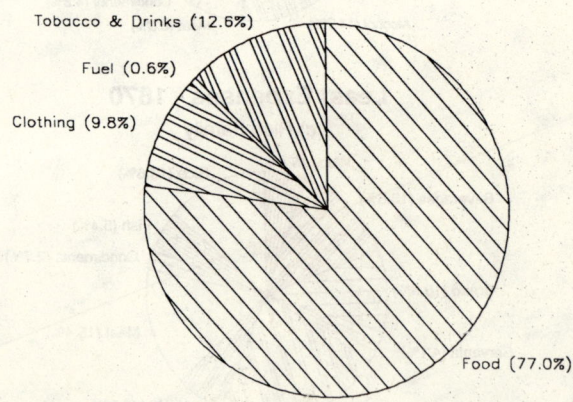

Source : Pedro Correia Afouso "O Problema da Mão d'Obra Agricola na India Porguguesa" *7° Concilio Provincial da India Portuguesa"*, Nova Goa, 1927, pp. 54-58.

Statistical and Documentary Appendices

APPENDIX 2-A

GROWTH OF POPULATION IN GOA 1600-1881

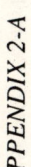

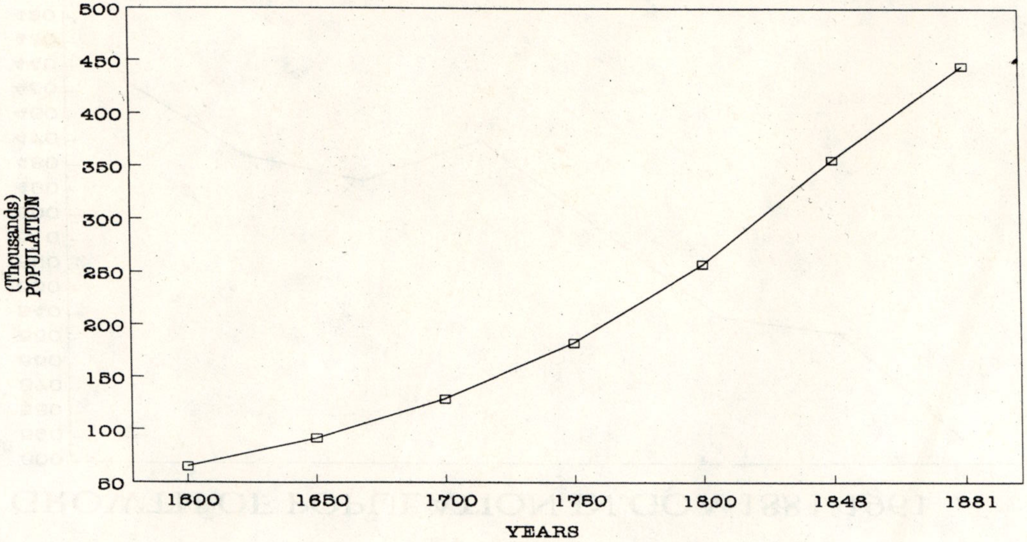

Source : Information compiled from the MSS. *Monções do Reino in Goa Historical Archives*

APPENDIX 2-B

GROWTH OF POPULATION IN GOA 1881-1961

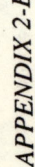

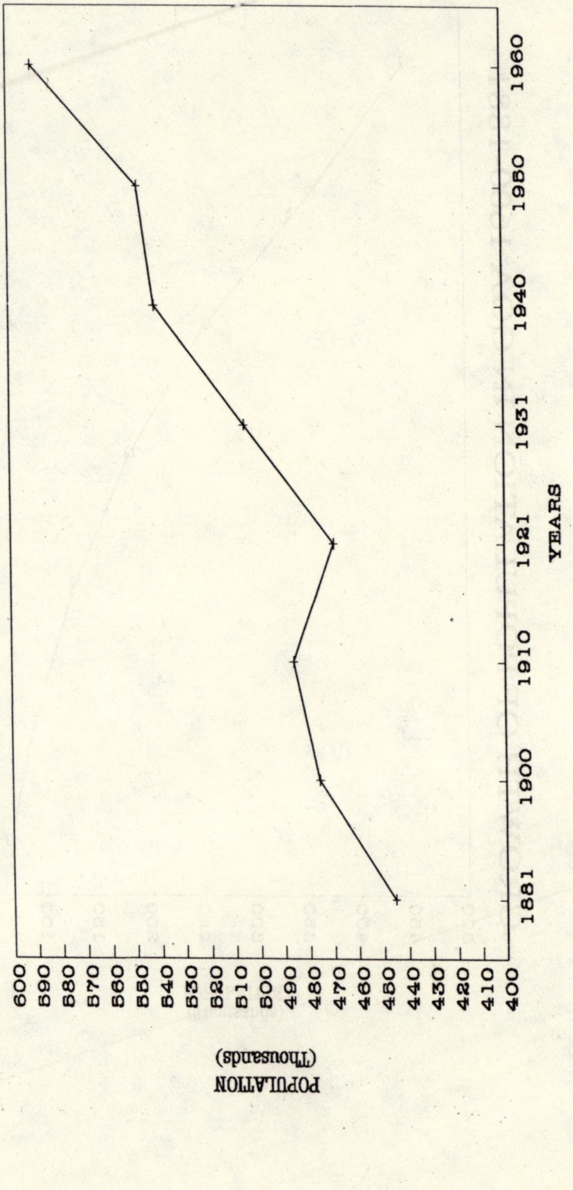

Source : 1881-1961 Census Reports.

APPENDIX 2-C

Density of Population in Goa 1881-1960
(Persons per Sq. Km.)

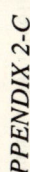

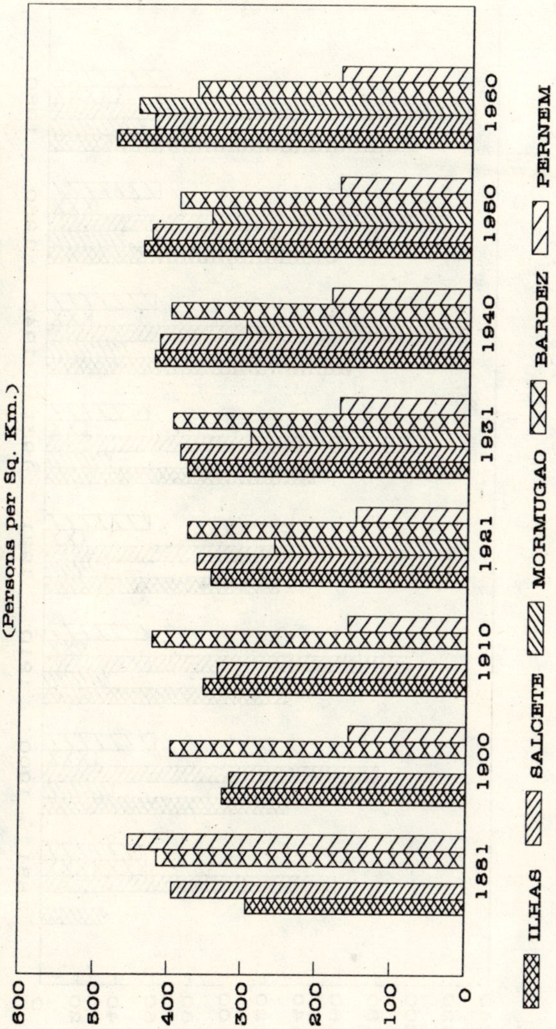

Source: 1881-1961 Census Reports.

APPENDIX 2-C (Contd.)

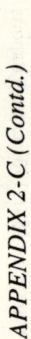

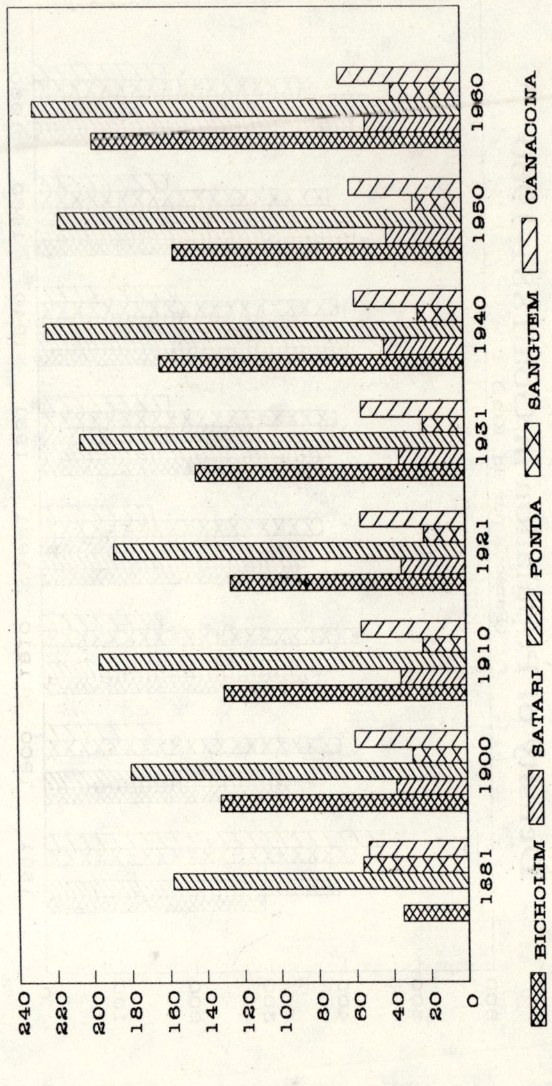

Source: 1881-1961 Census Reports.

APPENDIX 2-D

Percentage Distribution of Population
Religion-wise 1881–1960

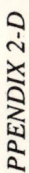

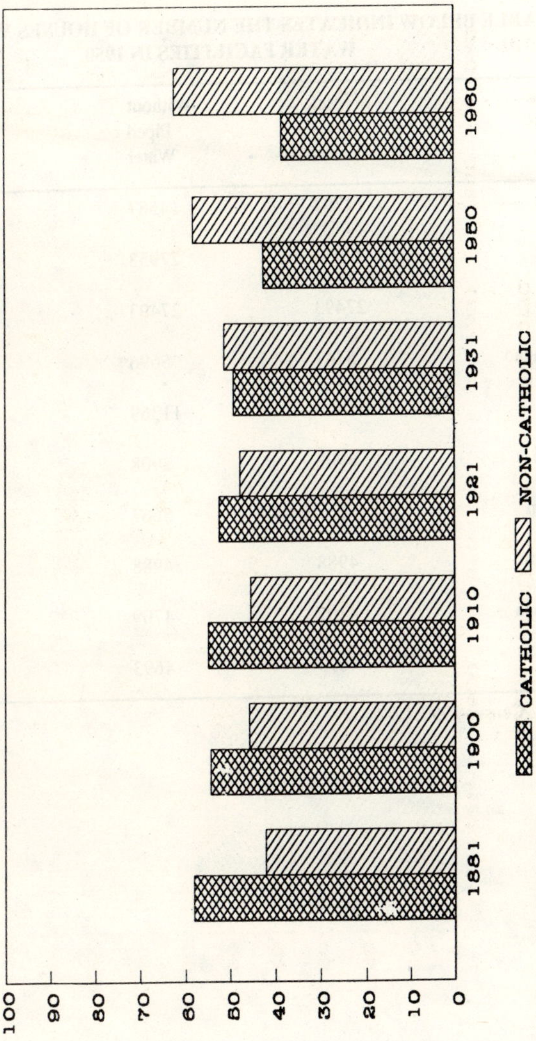

Source: 1881-1961 Census Reports.

APPENDIX 3-A

TABLE BELOW INDICATES THE NUMBER OF HOUSES WITH PIPED WATER FACILITIES IN 1950.

Talukas	Total Houses	Without Piped Water	With Piped Water
Ilhas	14793	14587	206
Bardez	27953	27953	51
Salcete	27493	27493	—
Mormagao	5747	5696	—
Ponda	11369	11369	—
Pernem	8908	8908	—
Quepem	5667	5667	—
Sanguem	4988	4988	—
Canacona	4709	4709	—
Satari	4693	4693	—

Source : Census 1950.

Statistical and Documentary Appendices

APPENDIX 3-B

On 12th February 1601 the captain of the city, the alderman, other officials of the Municipality and myself Antonio Monteiro, the Secretary of the Municipality of this noble city. Large number of Fidalgos, knights and other citizens connected with the administration were also present. The judge of the house of twenty four and majority of its members also attended the meeting.

The presiding councilor Nuno Velho de Macedo, told the assembly that the viceroy Ayres de Saldanha had requested the Senado (council) to consider the urgent need of water supply to the city, particularly in hot months of April, May and June, when most of the wells dried up. The viceroy had suggested that the Council must consider having water tanks and fountains such as were common in the towns and cities of Portugal and other parts of Europe. The presiding councilor explained that this could be undertaken with moderate expenditure by making use of the water of Timaya's tank which lay above Trindade and contained abundant water throughout the year. The undertaking would not fit within the bounds of the normal budget of the city, it would be necessary to finance it with funds from 1% additional Custom revenue.

There was difference of opinion among those present regarding the place to which the water from the reservoir should be directed. The justice of the peace then directed those present to take an oath and express their opinion in private through a secret ballot. It was decided by sixty-three votes to take the work and to finance it with 1% revenue. They also decided that the water should be directed to the old pillory which was considered as more central. A majority of fifty-three stood for this location. These resolutions were endorsed by the captain, the alderman, the other officials and by all the other present. The proceedings were recorded by Afonso Monteiro, the Secretary of the Council.

Signatures

Source: HAG: MS 7765 — Assentos da Camara, fls. 124v-126v.

APPENDIX 3-C

On 3rd November, 1601, the Captain of the city, the aldermen, and the other officials of the Municipality met in session. The attorney Francisco Serrão informed those present that the Viceroy had directed to bring to their notice that the streets and lanes were dirty. This was the cause of diseases and of descredit to the Municipality. Therefore, it was proposed to warn the town beadles to check the evil in the ward assigned to them with the penalty of losing their jobs or any other punishment which the Municipality may think appropriate. These beadles had to keep a watch and punish those who messed up the place.

The following beadles were called by the assembled: Francisco Dalgado, beadle of the High Court. Manoel Peixoto, beadle of the House of Accounts, Antonio Gonsalves, beadle of the Custom House, Aleixo Girão, town constanble, and Manoel Rodrigues da Costa, beadle assisting the market inspectors, and Francisco Gonsalves, town beadle. To all of them it was announced what the Viceroy wished to be conveyed. To each of them different wards and suburbs were assigned. The Secretary of the Municipality recorded the proceedings and the Captain, the alderman and other officials signed the act.

Signatures

Source: HAG: Ms. 7765—*Assentos da Camara*, fls.144- 144v.

APPENDIX 4-A

CHOLERA 1857

Place	No. of cases	Cured	Dead
Ilhas			
Goa Velha	34	28	06
Mandur	49	36	13
Chorão	55	32	23
Panjim	17	10	07
S. Estevão	67	61	06
S. Braz	14	14	–
Bardez			
Aldona	50	42	08
Assnora	13	07	06
Colvale	08	07	01
Salcete			
Margão	23	16	07
Benaulim	35	29	06
Mormugão	20	14	06
Aquem	11	07	04
Raçaim	09	06	03
Pernem	35	27	08
Ponda	55	42	13
Quepem	70	39	31
Canacona	08	03	05

Source: *Boletim de Governo do Estado da India*, no 1, de Janeiro de 1858, p. 4.

APPENDIX 4-B

CHOLERA CASES IN SEPTEMBER 1865

Place	Month	Days	Cases	Cured	Died
Panjim	Setembro	6-17	57	41	16
Ribandar	Setembro	–	9	6	3
Goa Velha	Setembro	–	9	6	3
Piedade	Setembro	–	6	3	3
Kumbarjua	Setembro	17-20	11	8	5
S. Matias	Setembro	–	6	3	3
S. Estevão	Setembro	–	11	9	2
Margão	Setembro	1-10	50	43	7
Margão	Setembro	10-16	100	87	13
S. J. Areal	Setembro	1-16	136	123	12
Colva	Setembro	10-16	16	13	3

Source: Germano Correia, *A colera-morbo na India Portuguesa, desde a sua conquista ata a actualidade-Estudo noso grafico*, ep [idemiologico e climato-sanitario, Nova Goa, 1919, p. 65.

APPENDIX 4-C

NUMBER OF PATIENTS TREATED FOR V.D. IN THE MILITARY HOSPITAL BETWEEN 1869-1880

Year	Patients treated for V.D.
1869	97
1870	86
1871	189
1872	204
1873	253
1874	218
1875	169
1876	212
1877	212
1878	272
1879	166
1880	135

Source : Alberto Germano Correia, *Prostituicão e Profilaxia Anti-venerea - Historia, Demografia, Etnografia, Higiene e Profilaxia, India Portuguesa Bastora*, 1938, p. 266.

APPENDIX 4-D

TABLE SHOWING NUMBER OF CASES AND DEATHS IN GOA DUE TO PLAGUE FROM 1901-1920

Year	Place	Cases	Deaths
1902	Ribander	33	17
1906	Mapuça	124	105
1910	Margão	64	50
1910-11	Mormugão	30	20
1912	Mormugão	06	03
1916	Margão	45	37
1916	Mormugão	06	06
1916	D. Paula	10	08
1917	Margão	46	36
1918	Margão	55	35
1919	Panjim	18	10
1920	Caranzalem	22	14

Source : *Arquivos da Escola Medico - Cirurgica de N. Goa*, Bastora, 1928, pp. 504 - 509.

APPENDIX 4-E

DEATHS DUE SYPHILIS IN GOA BETWEEN 1916-1935

Year	Male	Female	Total	1 year	1-19 years	20-39 years	40-59 years	Over 60 years
1916	18	11	29	–	4	14	11	–
1917	18	10	28	5	9	10	4	–
1918	10	11	21	2	5	10	4	–
1919	6	7	13	–	3	5	5	–
1921	14	9	23	1	1	13	8	–
1922	12	5	17	1	2	9	5	–
1923	11	4	15	–	–	4	10	1
1924	15	2	17	–	–	7	9	1
1925	12	3	15	1	2	2	10	–
1926	15	6	21	2	2	8	8	1
1927	8	2	10	1	–	3	5	1
1928	6	–	6	–	1	3	2	–
1929	17	4	21	1	–	11	7	2
1930	12	1	13	2	–	4	7	–
1931	10	5	15	2	–	9	4	–
1932	13	2	15	1	3	4	4	–
1933	15	1	16	3	1	5	5	2
1934	13	3	16	1	2	9	4	–
1935	14	1	15	–	1	10	2	2
Total:	239	79	326	9	28	140	114	10

Source: Germano Correia, India Portuguesa — *Prostituição e Profilaxia Anti-venerea Historia Demografia Etnografia Higiene e Profilaxia*, Bastora, 1938.

APPENDIX 4-F

IMPORTANT EPIDEMICS IN THE 16TH TO 20TH CENTURIES IN GOA

Epidemic	Year	Month	Place
Cholera	1543	Rainy season	City of Goa
Smallpox	1545	—	City of Goa
Smallpox & Cholera & Fevers & Plague (bubonic)	1570	—	City of Goa
Cholera	1618	—	City of Goa
Fevers	1619	—	City of Goa
Fevers	1635	—	City of Goa
Cholera	1670	—	Salcete
Smallpox	1705	—	Bardez
Cholera	1777	—	Salcete
Cholera	1789-92	—	Salcete
Cholera	1818	October-December	Ilhas
Smallpox	1825	April-June	—
Smallpox	1836	April	—
Cholera	1845	January-June	Ilhas, Bardez
Cholera	1849	Rainy season	Salcete
Cholera	1854	May-July	Ilhas, Bardez
Smallpox	1856	January	—
Cholera	1857	—	Bardez, Salcete Pernem, Ponda, Canacona
Cholera	1869	June-November	Whole of Goa
Cholera	1870	June-November	Ilhas, Bardez, Ponda, Salcete
Cholera	1878	July-November	Salcete, Bardez Bicholim, Quepem
Smallpox	1882 to 1883	December-June	—
Cholera	1882	April-July	Salcete, Sanguem
Cholera	1883	August-December	Quepem and nearby areas
Cholera	1884	4 months	Sanguem, Quepem, Salcete, Bardez
Cholera	1887	July	Salcete, Pernem
Smallpox	1888	February-July	—
Cholera	1892	May-July	Salcete, Quepem Ilhas
Smallpox	1893	February-July	—

Statistical and Documentary Appendices

Epidemic	Year	Month	Place
Cholera	1896	February-July	Canacona, Ponda Quepem
Cholera	1897	June-November	Salcete, Bardez Quepem
Cholera	1898	January-March	Whole of Goa
Cholera	1899	January-February	Ponda, Quepem
Plague	1899	November-December	Mormugao
Cholera	1900	July-November	Ilhas, Salcete Bardez, Pernem Bicholim
Smallpox	1900	January-June	—
Plague	1901-02	December	Ilhas, Bicholim Mormugão, Salcete
Cholera	1902	—	Ponda, Ilhas
Cholera	1904	July	—
Smallpox	1904	February-June	Bicholim, Satari
Cholera	1906	June-October	Bardez, Ilhas Ponda, Bicholim
Smallpox	1906	February-September	—
Plague	1906	March-May	Bardez
Plague	1907-09	December-May	Ilhas
Cholera	1907	September-December	Quepem, Salcete Bardez
Cholera	1907-08	December-Feburary	Sanguem, Quepem
Cholera	1909	January-September	Ilhas, Salcete Quepem
Smallpox	1909	February-September	Bardez
Plague	1910-11	November-April	Salcete, Mormugão
Cholera	1911	—	Ponda, Canacona
Cholera	1912	January-March	Bardez, Pernem
Plague	1912	February-March	Mormugão
Cholera	1913	July-September	Salcete, Ilhas .
Cholera	1914	July-October	Salcete, Ponda
Smallpox	1914	January-June	Quepem, Sanguem
Plague	1914-15	December-June	Mormugão
Cholera	1916-17	December-Feburary	Ilhas, Bardez, Salcete
Smallpox	1916	February-June	Ilhas, Salcete Pernem, Bardez, Sanquelim, Ponda
Plague	1915-16	December-May	Salcete, Ilhas
Plague	1917	March-November	Salcete
Plague	1918	February-October	Salcete
Cholera	1918	Whole year	Bardez, Ponda Quepem, Sanguem

Epidemic	Year	Month	Place
Influenza	1918	—	Bardez, Salcete and other places
Smallpox	1919	—	Ilhas, Bardez
Plague	1919	June-October	Mormugão, Ponda, Sanquelim, Salcete Panjim
Meningitis	1919	—	Salcete, Quepem
Plague	1920	February-April	Ilhas
Smallpox	1921	—	Ilhas, Bardez, Salcete, Satari, Sanquelim, Pernem
Cholera	1921-21	June-August	Satari, Sanquelim
Meningites	1921-27	—	Salcete
Cholera	1924	May-December	Sanguem, Sanquelim
Smallpox	1924	June-September	Salcete, Ilhas
Plague	1924	March-May	Panjim
Smallpox	1925-26	Whole Year	All over Goa
Plague	1927	September-November	Panjim
Smallpox	1927	—	Goa
Cholera	1928	—	Salcete
Influenza	1929	—	Salcete, Bardez Pernem
Plague	1930	—	Salcete
Dysentery	1930	—	Pernem
Meningitis	1930	—	Salcete
Dobo	1930	—	Bardez
Cholera	1933	—	Ilhas, Bardez, Ponda
Dysentery	1933	—	Ilhas
Smallpox	1933	—	Bardez
Typhoid	1933	—	Ilhas
Pempigus	1937	—	Bardez
Poliomelitis	1937-41	—	Bardez
Smallpox	1941	—	Bardez, Ilhas
Influenza	1950	—	Goa

Source : Data compiled from various sources mentioned in the text.

APPENDIX- 5

ORDINARY DIETS OF THE PATIENTS AT THE MILITARY HOSPITAL (1830)

Diet types (ordinary)

(1)   A – Canjee of one oitava boiled rice served for natives with fevers.
      B – Soup of one quarter chicken usually served to the Portuguese.

(2)   A – Canjee of one quarto boiled rice.
      B – 1/4 chicken with gravy and 2 ozs. bread for lunch and ½ chicken with 2 ozs. bread for dinner.

(3)   A – 3 ozs. toasted bread, 1 oz. sugar for lunch. Stewed chicken with one oitava rice and 3 ozs. bread for dinner.
      B – 4 ozs. of beef without gravy and 3 bread for lunch, 6 ozs. cooked beef with rice (pache-ril) and 3 ozs. bread for dinner.

(4)   A – 1\2 chicken without gravy, 4 ozs. bread for lunch. 1 chicken boiled with 1½ oitava rice and 4 ozs. bread for dinner.
      B – 8 ozs. beef without gravy with 4 ozs. bread for lunch and 12 ozs. cooked beef with oitava e meia of rice and 4 ozs. bread for dinner.

(5)   A – Canjee, fried fish for breakfast, one oitava rice, 4 ozs. fried fish for lunch. One quarter rice, 2 ozs. of fish curry, 2 ozs. fried fish.
      B – 4 ozs. of toast with 1 oz. sugar for breakfast, 3 oitavas boiled rice, 4 ozs. fish curry and 2 ozs. fried fish for lunch.
              One quarter rice, 2 ozs. fish curry, 2 ozs. fried fish.

Diet Types (Extraordinary)

(1) A – 2 ozs. bread soup, ½ oz. sugar.
     B – Soup of 1 oz. sago and sugar syrup.
     C – Soup of sago, mandõ of Cambay, 1 oz. sugar.

(2) A – 1 plate stewed vegetables and 4 ozs. bread.
     B – 4 ozs. toasted bread with 1 oz. sugar.
     C – One quarter boiled rice with 2 ozs. fish curry and 2 ozs. fish.

(3) A – Canjee of oitava boiled rice and one quarter chicken.
     B – 1½ oitava chicken, 2 ozs. fried rice.
     C – One quarter boiled rice, one quarter chicken curry.

Servants working in the hospital were served breakfast. Canjee and mango pickle, for lunch they were given rice curry and fish.

Ingredients used in preparation of various dishes in the Military Hospital 1830 :

For half roast chicken :-

Butter	3 oitavas
Pepper	6 grãos

For 1/2 stewed chicken :-

Onions	½ ozs.
Butter	3 oitavas
Pepper	3 grãos
Vinegar	6 oitavas

For another 1/2 chicken dish :-

Onion	½ oz.
Butter	3 oitavas
Pepper	6 grãos
Vinegar	½ oz.

For 2 ozs. fried fish :-

    Oil   2 oitavas

For 2 ozs. stewed fish :-

Oil 1	
Onion 1	oitava
Coconut 1	
Cumminseed	2 grãos
Chillies	10 grãos
Pepper	3 grãos
Tamarind	1½ oitava
Vinegar	1 oitava

For 2 ozs. roast beef :-

Butter	2 oitavas
Pepper	3 grãos

For beef steak (2 ozs.) :-

Onion	2 oitavas
Butter	2 oitavas
Pepper	4 grãos
Tamarind	1 oitavas
Vinegar	6 oitavas

For curry (fish or onion) :-

Saffron	1 gm.
Onions	18 gms.
Coconut	2 oitavas
Coriander	8 grãos
Chillies	10 grãos
Pepper	4 grãos
Tamarind	1½ oitava

Chicken curry :-

Onion	8 gms.
Garlic	1½ gms.
Coconut	2½ oitava
Cumminseeds	6 grãos
Coriander	8 grãos
Chillies	10 grãos
Pepper	8 grãos
Tamarind	2½ oitavas

For chicken or beef rice :-

Onions	1 oitava
Butter	1 oitava
Pepper	4 grãos
Vinegar	2 oitavas

Source : HAG: Ms 646 – Re gulamento do Hospital Real Militar, 1830, fls. 76-102

APPENDIX 6-A

LIST OF THE ACCUSED, TRIED AND SENTENCED BY INQUISIÇÃO DE GOA IN CHRONOLOGICAL ORDER FROM APRIL 1784 TO MARCH 1785.

Age		Punishment
30	Bartholameo Carvalho, Kunbi, farm labourer, married to Antonia from Cortalim, Salcete for seeking help of temples for the safe delivery of his wife. .aw off	Spiritual penance.
50	Miguel de Souza alias Babu Naique, married to Parciela Gomes from Cuncolim, Salcete for resorting to superstitious cure.	Spiritual penance. Exiled to Casa de Polvora for five years.
40	Feliciana, Kunbi, widow of André Rebelo, from Chinchinim, Salcete for resorting to superstitious cure.	Spiritual penance. Exiled for two years to Varca.
50	Manoel Fernandes, Kunbi, farm labourer, married to Paulina alias Francisca from Corlim, Ilhas for believing in non-Christian rituals.	Spiritual penance.
40	Antonio Gonsalves, married to Sabina, working at the Mint from Piedade, Ilhas for seeking help of temples to get cure for his sick relative.	Spiritual penance.
58	Manoel Duarte de Souza married to Micaela Serafina de Araujo, farm labourer from Nachinola, Bardez for seeking help of temples to find out if the disease he was suffering was due to witchcraft.	Spiritual penance.
60	Caetano Picardo, married to Angelina Pires, farm labourer from Piedade, Ilhas for attending certain rituals and taking a patient along with him.	Spitilual penance.
34	Nicolao Rebelo, farm labourer, married to Petronila de Almeida from Velção, Salcete for allowing a woman to perform superstitious rituals in his house for the cure of his son.	Spiritual penance.
48	Feliciana de Sequeira, widow of Antonio Miguel de Azavdo from Sancoale, Salcete for permitting a non-Christian to perform superstitious rituals for his cure.	Spiritual penance.

Source: Torre do Tombo: Conselho Geral do Santo Oficio, (Inquisição de Goa), Maço- 33, no.18

APPENDIX 6-B

LIST OF THE ACCUSED, TRIED AND SENTENCED BY INQUISIÇÃO DE GOA IN CHRONOLOGICAL ORDER FROM MARCH 1790 TO MARCH 1791

Age		Punishment
66	Catharina alias Boteli widow of João de Souza, midwife, from Nellur, Bardez for superstitious rituals at the time of the deliveries attended by her.	Repremanded and ordered not to practice her trade.
75	Anna Pinto widow of Bento Passanha, midwife from Chinchinim, Salcete for attributing the illness of a child to witchcraft and for advising superstitious remedies.	Exiled for two years to Rachol.
50	Domingos de Souza, married to Anna Pinto from Penha de França, Bardez farm labourer, caught at mid-day while making offerings at a temple on a hillock in the company of other Christians and non-Christians for the cure of a sick person.	Given instructions and asked to do spiritual penance of three years in Raia.
34	Salvador Magalhaes, married to Francisca Fernandes, tailor, from Nellur, Bardez province for eating meat on forbidden days and for making mockery of this ban.	Repremanded with spiritual penence.
70	Polpotto Naique, non-Christian, married to Deugui, from Porpangim, Bardez, sailor of a merchandise boat, accused of bringing to Goa another non-Christian from across the border to perform rituals at night in a temple for the health and happiness of some Christians who attended these rituals.	Lashings in the streets of the city and sent to Ponda for three years.

Source: Torre do Tombo: Conselho Geral do Santo Oficio (Inquisição de Goa), Maço -33, no.24.

APPENDIX 6-C

**LIST OF ACCUSED, TRIED AND BY INQUISIÇÃO
DE GOA IN MARCH 1795**

Rosa Fernandes widow of Manoel de Souza, from Combarjua, living at Chimbel-Ribandar, Ilhas, accused of offering a roaster, flour and rice to a non-Christian in order to seek cure of her son-in-law.

Francisco Barreto, married to Esperança de Souza, son-in-law of Rosa Fernandes, tailor from Velção, Salcete, living with his mother-in-law at Chimbel, accused of accepting şuperstitious cure and allowing non-Christian healer to kill the roaster for rituals that included wawing around the head little figures made of flour.

Source: Torre do Tombo: Conselho Geral do Santo Oficio,
          Maço- 38, no. 7.

APPENDIX 6-D

SOME COMMONLY USED GOAN PLANTS AND MINERALS IN GOA

Ambo (Mangifera Indica) is a well known seasonal fruit from Indian subcontinent. Goa has the best varieties. The plant was exported to Brazil by the Portuguese. The fruit contains Vitamins A and C. The unripe fruit is cooked in hot ashes and the pith mixed with water and sugar. The drink obtained is good for heat exhaustion and heat stroke. Kernel of the stone of mango fruit is prescribed for diarrhoea. The skin of the fruit is recommended for uterine, pulmonary and intestine disorders prepared in following manner: 10 gms. extract of the skin in 120 gms. water. One table spoon to be given every two hours. The gum of the tree mixed with lime is used for scabies and some other skin problems. Mango is laxative.

Ankli (Alanguim Lamarcki) is a large tree the fruit resembles a rose apple. It is antidote for opium. It is also remedy for infantile tuberculosis. Apa Rane, a well known quack of Goa used the bark of Ankli to control rheumatic pain and pneumonia.

Anjir (Ficus Carica). The fruit has many medicinal properties. Few figs taken after meals acts as laxative. Supposed to be good for cough. Hastens the appearance of rash in chicken pox and small pox. The plant was originally brought from Persia.

Bel(Aegle Marmalos). The pulp ground with sugar and rose water is used in diseases of the intestine, liver and dysentery. The pulp mixed with water forms a refreshing drink which offsets the effect of heat. Ripe fruit is sweet and laxative. The paste made of leaves of this tree helps inflamed eyes. The juice of the leaves mixed with honey is laxative.

Bavo (Cassia fistula). The plant is from Goa. This plant has smooth small branches. The leaves which are yellowish in colour fall in cold season. The fruit is laxative. The juice extracted from the leaves is used in skin disorders and harpies.

Banyan Tree (Ficus Bengalensis). Sap of the leaves is used in the cold season against cracked heels. Fibers hanging from its branches ground in water stop vomiting.

Candinni (Cassia Carandas) is found in the forests of Goa. The roots of this plant ground with water are prescribed two to three times a day against snake bite. Its leaves and fruits are used against scurvy.

Catecomer (Aloe Socotrina) This herb pounded with milk is given to those suffering from kidney and bladder problem.

(Source: Garcia D'Orta, Colloquios dos Simples e Drogas da India, Lisboa, 1895, pp. 83-84. Henceforth Garcia D'Orta).

Dakti Sutkant (Melia Azadirachta) or *Neem*. The leaves, skin and other products of Neem have medicinal value. Bitter leaves are used as antiseptic. Tender shoots ground into paste helps to relieve prickly heat. Crushed leaves made into a ball and applied on boils remove the pus specially in case of smallpox. Decoction of leaves with sesame oil is used to clean wounds and boils. Oil of the fruit is used in leprosy and rheumatism. Dry flowers prepared into a tonic is given to those recovering from fevers. A decoction of the bark is prescribed in case of a colic and uterine problems.

Dutro (Mactiel) grows wild in Goa. The plant resembles an egg plant and has thorny fruits. The sap and the seeds of this fruit have many interesting uses. In early period of Portuguese regime ladies from the upper strata used the sap to intoxicate their husbands. This was done so that they could have good time with their lovers while the husband remained in unconscious state for even longer than 24 hours. Dutro seeds are used to cure chronic colds, asthma, lack of sexual potency. The paste of dutro leaves mixed with salt is applied for mumps or in case of excessive sweating on palms. The fruit helps also to provide relief in asthma. The fruit is cut fine and dried. Next it is mixed with tobacco from Deccan. The mixture is then rolled on a banana leaf and smoked by asthama patient.

Doxim (Hibiscus rosa). A common shrub in Goa. The flowers have several colours. The most common are red, yellow and white. The roots of this shrub are used in the preparation of some kind of medicine. The roots of the shrub that produces white flowers are used mixed with milk, sugar and cumminseeds in case of blenorrhea. It is said that the flowers of this plant ground with papaya are taken to induce abortions.

(Source: Antonio de Piedade de Noronha, "Certos far- macos vegetais de Goa e a sua importancia na terapeutica, " Arquivos da Escola Medico-Cirurgica, Nova Goa, 1949, p.74).

Guava is a very nutritious fruit, good for digestion and helps in the normal evacuation of the bowels. A decoction made of leaves in used as a remedy to check vomiting and diarrhoea. The leaves are highly astringent. It is interesting to note that the leaves arrest diarrhoea but the fruit is a laxative.

Haldi (Curcuna Longa) or turmeric is used in cooking. It adds colour and prevents flatulence. Turmeric powder is used in fractures and to relieve pain. It prevents inflammation. Turmeric is used in the treatment of gonorrhoea. Turmeric mixed with hot milk is prescribed for cough.

Khair Champa (Plumeria Acutifolia) is also known as Portugalacho Champo. The plant is believed to be brought from Brazil by the Portuguese. It is usually grown in front of churches and temples. The bark of this tree is smooth with white flowers and yellow colour in the middle. There are others kinds with red flower and also white flowers with red border. The skin of the roots is used as laxative. Sap of the plant is used in rheumatic pain.

Karatim (Cucumis trigonus) These fruits are of two kinds. The fruit boiled and ground with snake milk was prescribed by quacks for mental problems. It is supposed to improve the memory.

Kant mogro (Achyrantes Aspera) is a common shrub in India. The plant is diuretic and is used in kidney disorders.

Kaner (Nerium Adorum) is a plant of medium height with white, yellow and red flowers. Bark of the root of this plants cures many skin disorders.

Limbu (Citrus Acida/Aurantifolia) has vitamin C. A fresh lime squeezed in a glass of warm water with four teaspoons of honey and a quarter teaspoon of salt is sipped in acute tonsillitis. A glassful of the same taken every night is natural preventive against cold. Fresh lime squeezed in tender coconut was prescribed in the treatment of typhoid, nausea and vomiting. It is also used as cosmetic, hair and stain remover.

Lasun (Allium Sativium) is used as ingredient in food. Garlic helps to lower the blood pressure and cholesterol. Paste of garlic provides relief from pain caused by a scorpion sting. It is believed that a clove of garlic eaten everyday increases longevity. Cloves of garlic boiled in milk are used against asthma.

Nervol (Capparis Trifolidata) was used in urinary problems. Leaves ground in vinegar are used in swellings and lut (a disease that causes burning of feet).

Methi (Trigonella Foenum Gareceum) helps to relieve constipation and lumbago. The leaves of fenugreek are used for healing ulcers in the mouth. An infusion of the leaves is used as a gargle for recurrent ulcers. A concoction of boiled seeds is a hair conditioner and good for hair growth.

Oddlo Gino (Leea Macrophylla). It grows wild in the hilly areas of Goa. The plant has large leaves, and produces numerous white flowers. The fruit resembles a cherry. The white gino has many medicinal properties and is widely used by herbalists. The powder applied on wounds helps to heal them. The roots ground with water is prescribed for acute and chronic liver problems twice a day for a period of seven days. During this period a strict diet has to be followed. The patient has to refrain from alcohol, chicken, fats, fatty fish, sour and salty foods.

Onions (Allium cepa). The bulb of the plant has many medicinal qualities: It is an excellent medicine against cholera and diarrhoea if mixed in vinegar. Onion juice is applied to the head to bring down high fever. Onion baked in hot ashes and applied to swollen piles is believed to give relief.

Pau de Cobra (Pauwolfia Serpentina) — a root used for rheumatism, smallpox, cholera and fevers. In case of fevers one ounce of powdered root was mixed with water and given to the patient to drink. It caused vomiting and helped to clear the bile.

(Source : Garcia D'Orta, *op. cit.,* pp.180-194)

Parbatic (Nyctanthes Arbor Tristies) or Night Jasmine. The flowers of the tree open only at night. The flowers mixed with water are applied for problems of the eyes, fevers, rheumatism. In case of intermittent fevers six to seven leaves ground with water and ginger are prescribed. The patient in such cases has to keep a diet. The seeds ground into powder are applied for scalp problems. The seeds and flowers are helpful in curing piles.

(Source: Lencastre Pereira d'Andrade, Plantas Medicinais de Goa, Part I, Bastora, 1899, p.26).

Papaya (*Carica papaya*) — Every part of the papaya tree is used as medicine. Raw papaya can lead to miscarriage. The fruit eaten with salt, cumminseeds and lime juice is used in the treatment of round worms and in constipation. Slices of raw of papaya cooked in meat makes the meat soft. Infusion of the fresh leaves is gargled to cure tonsillitis.

Pineapple (*Ananosa - sativa*) is originally brought from Brazil. Fresh juice of pineapple is soothing. The fruit which is rich in fibers acts a medicine for constipation.

Pomegranate (*Pumica granatum*) fruit diluted with water is prescribed to the patient having diarrhoea. Raw fruit is used in many digestive powders. Bark of the tree is used to get rid off intestinal worms. The dry infusion of flowers helpful in dysentery.

Peepal (*Ficus Religiosa*). A large tree. The decoction of the bark is used to clean ulcers and wounds.

Pitmari (*Naregamia Alata*) is a small shrub. The bark boiled with rice water is prescribed for dysentery. A concoction of boiled bark with a pinch of pepper and salt is given daily for common cold, piles, scurvy and anaemia.

Ricinus (*Ricinus Communis*) or castor plant grows wild in many parts of Goa. The fruit of the plant yields oil used mainly as purgative. The oil was prescribed for cholera patients. The oil mixed with some other ingredients is good against bed sores. The leaves of the tree mixed with sesame oil are applied against inflammation. Dry leaves of the plant smoked in a pipe tend to relieve hiccup.

Rhuibab imported from Macau or China was a good medicine for all kinds of liver problems and fevers.

(Source: HAG: Ms. 1325 —Macau, fl. 24.)

Ranudid (*Terammus labialis*). Seeds of this plant are used in cases of paralysis.

(Source: D.G. Dalgado, Flora de Goa e Savantvadi, Lisboa, 1898 .)

Statistical and Documentary Appendices

Sonth (Zingiber Officinale) or dried ginger is good remedy for headaches, specially migraines. It has to be ground with local feni (local alcoholic drink) to form poultice and applied on the forehead. Dried ginger is efficacious in rheumatism. Mixed with five times its quantity with jaggery, it gives protection against cold.

Sanvor (Bombax Malabaricum) bark is efficacious in dealing with abscesses. The root of the tree dried in the shade and made into a powder acts an aphrondisiac.

Savi Naravel (Viburnum foetidum) grows into a tree 5-10 feet high with smooth branches. The plant has many therapeutic values. A wine glass of the juice extracted from the leaves is taken everyday to prevent haemorrhage after delivery. Vaidyas and herbalists prescribe a concoction of the bark with some other ingredients in cases of fever. The juice of the leaves is applied to relieve cephalgia. In case of convulsions the juice of the leaves is applied on the head of the child.

Savo (Argemone Mexicana). Yellow Thistle or *Pila Datura.* Its roots are used as antidote for snake poison. Powder of the seeds is used to counteract the itch due to venereal disease. Oil of seeds helps to cure scabies and leprosy.

Salloc Kamallar (Nympheaceoe) or Lotus grows in water and is found in lakes and small ponds in Goa. The flowers are usually red or white. The juice extracted from the stem of these flowers is considered refreshing and a good tonic for hair ailments. The roots are used for relief from haemorrhoids.

Salsaparilha is used to purify blood. The bark of the tree was used for medical purpose in the Military Hospital of Goa. The roots are used to treat skin problems, syphilis, leucorrhoea, chronic cough, rheumatic pains and boils.

Sanders (Sercanda) are usually in three colours namely white, yellow and red. They came from the Portuguese island of Timor. They are like nut tree with fruits resembling cherries. The bark of this plant is ground and applied to the body for cooling and good smell. The Europeans in Goa used the fruit to stop headaches. Sanders were used in fevers.

Supari (Areca Catechu) or Betelnut is used as an ingredient of pan. Used as a dentifrice makes the teeth sparkle.

Tamarind (*Tamarindus Indica*). The fruit is used extensively in cooking. Its alkaline properties counteract hyper acidity, bilious fevers, nausea and thirst. Its an appetiser.

Tulsi (Ocimum Basilicum) plant is considered sacred and grown by the Hindus in pots and courtyard. If pustules of chicken pox delay their appearance. *Tulsi* leaves with saffron hastens the process. They are useful remedy for cough and fever. Taken with pepper in an infusion is reported to be a good remedy against malaria.

Turbit (Ipomoea Turpethum) is used as laxative.

Usky (Calycopteris Floribunda) grows widely in hilly areas of Goa. Many people chew the leaves to stop colic. Water boiled with the leaves is used for bath to cure skin eruptions.

Zambolli (Eugemia jambolona). The fruit of this tree has many medicinal properties. Fresh juice of the fruit is given to the children having diarrhoea. Curandeiros (quacks) often prescribe. the wine of the fruit for diabetes because of its effect on pancreas. About 46 to 56 gms. of the wine with 6-12 ounces of water is to be drunk daily for diabetes. The bark of the tree is astringent. Decoction of its bark deals effectively with swollen and bleeding gums.

Besoar Stones (Snake stone) a reddish yellow colour, there are also other colours. They are engendered in the paunch of he-goat on a very fine straw which is in the middle and so it goes on twisting and forming a rind like that of an onion. They are found in different sizes — found in Persia, and Malaca. It was used in Goa as antidote against poison, prickly heat, leprosy, itch and ringworm.

(Source: Garcia D'Orta, *op.cit.*, pp. 231-238).

Pedras Cordiais do Gaspar Antonio. These were made by Jesuit Gaspar Antonio at the college of St. Paul. After the death of Gaspar Antonio the secret was passed to Jorge Ungarate. It contained red and white corals, rubies, jacintos, topaz, sapphire, emerald, pedra bezoar, ambergris, almiscar and gold leaves. These pedras (stones) were of great demand in Europe, Asia and other places. The sale of these stones fetched the Jesuits an annual income of 50,000 xerafins. Pedras Cordiais had wide use to cure fevers, leprosy and anemias It helped to improve the eyesight.

(Source: John Freyer, *A New Account of East India and Persia*, vol. II, London, 1909, pp. 149-150).

BIBLIOGRAPHY

A. ARCHIVAL SOURCES:

1. Goa Historical Archives

Administração Civil Saude e Benificiencia (1914-1916).
Assentos da Camara (1535-1537).
Assentos do Conselho da Fazenda (1613-1808).
Botica do Convento Madre de Deus (1799-1835).
Botica do Convento do Santo Agostinho (1830-1837).
Cartas, Ordens, e Portarias (1858-1859).
Correspondencia diversa (1888-1927)
Correspondencia sobre reedificação da Cidade de Goa (1777-1778).
Custos dos artigos do Hospital de Misericordia (1780-1783).
Despezas do Convento da Graça (1747-1767).
Directorate of Accounts: collection of income and expenses of the Military Hospital (1811-1886).
Empregados do Hospital Militar (1886).
Estrangeiros (1815-1881).
Hospital da Misericordia (1612).
Hospital da Misericordia (1630).
Informações Annuais (1866).
Livro de Posturas (1808-1832).
Livro de Taxas de differentes industrias (1768).
Livro da receita e despesas de Medicamentos do Hospital do Convento de S. Jõao de Deus. (1733-1737).
Livro das Merces Gerais (1607-1883).
Macau (1693-1861).
Ordens aos Senadores (1777-1782).
Monções do Reino (1560-1914).
Papeis de Conventos Extintos (1612-1835).
Pessoal do Hospital Militar (1717).
Pessoal de Saude e Empregados do Hospital Militar (1886).

Portarias e Provisões (1785-1837).
Provisões, Alvaras e Regimentos (1515-1598).
Provisões a favor de Cristandade (1513-1843).
Receita e despeza dos Jesuitas (1686).
Registos Gerais do Senado de Goa (1570-1876).
Regulamento do Hospital Misericordia de Goa, (1612, 1630).
Regimentos e Regulamentos (1830-1839).
Regimentos de ordenados dos officias da Justica e Eccleziasticos (1626).
Vencimentos Civis (1771-1772).
Vencimentos dos diversos funcionarios (1775-1804).
Vencimentos Eclesiasticos (1770-1771).
Vencimentos dos diversos funcionarios (1775-1804).

2. Church Records at the Patriarchal Archives, Panjim:

Visitas Pastorais (1747-1927).
Rois de Christandade (1773-1941).
Parish Registers (1900-1961).

3. Xavier Centre of Historical Research, Goa

J.N. da Fonseca Collection: *Customs and Manners*.
J.N. da Fonseca Collection: *Questions and Responses*.
J.N. da Fonseca Collection: *Questions and Responses* — Regedor de Assolna.
J.N. da Fonseca Collection: *Administração Fiscal da 4ª Divisão de Novas Conquistas* .
Mhamai House Papers (1750-1825).

4. Arquivo Nacional da Torre do Tombo, Lisboa

Conselho Geral do Santo Oficio (17th and 18th centuries)
Documentos Remetidos da India - Livros 1-62
Chancelaria de D. Jose - Livro 66

B. PUBLISHED SOURCES:

1. Primary Sources

Abranches Garcia, J. I. de, *Archivo da Relação de Goa contendo varios*

Bibliography

documentos dos seculos 17, 18, 19, 2 vols, Nova Goa, Imprensa Nacional, 1872-1874.

Albuquerque Afonso de, *Cartas para el rei D. Manuel I*, ed. Antonio Baião, Lisboa, Livraria Sa da Costa, 1942.

Albuquerque, Afonso de, *Cartas, seguidas de documentos que as elucidam*, ed. Raymundo A. Bulhão Pato, 6 vols, Lisboa, Academia Real das Sciencias, 1884-1915.

Albuquerque, V. A.C.B.de, *Senado de Goa: Memoria Historico - Archaeologica*, Nova Goa, Imprensa Nacional, 1909.

Anais Franciscanos em Bardes, ed. Francisco Xavier Costa, Nova Goa, Shri Saraswati, 1926.

Anuario da Escola Medico Cirurgica de Nova Goa, 1910-1958.

Anuario do Estado da India Portuguesa, 1904, 1928, 1930, 1931, 1956, Goa, Imprensa Nacional.

Aragão, A. C. Teixeira de, *Descripção Geral e Historica das Moedas Cunhadas em nome dos Reis, Regentes e Governadores de Portugal*, III, Porto, Livraria Fernando Machado, 2nd edition, 1964.

Archivo Portuguez-Oriental, ed., J. H.da Cunha Rivara, 10 vols, Nova Goa, Imprensa Nacional, 1857-1876.

Archivo de Pharmacia e Sciencia Accessorias da India Portuguesa, Nova Goa, Imprensa National, 1864-1871.

Archivo Medico da India, Nova Goa, Imprensa National, 1894-1896.

Arquivos da Escola Medico Cirurgico de Nova Goa, 1927-1938, 1940, 1942, 1949, 1954, 1958, 1960, Bastora, Tipografia Rangel.

Arquivo Portugues Oriental, ed. A.B. de Braganza Pereira, 11 vols, Bastora, Tipografia Rangel, 1936-1940.

Asilo de N. Sra. dos Milagres de Mapuça: Relatorio e Contas 1921-1922, 1924-1925, Bastora, Tipografia Rangel, 1925.

Boletim de Filmoteca Ultramarina Portuguesa, 44 vols, Lisboa, Centro do Estudos Historicos Ultramarino, 1954-71.

Boletim Geral de Medicina e Farmacia, Bastora, Tipografia Rangel, (1929, 1931, 1933, 1934).

Boletim Geral de Medicina, Bastora, Tipografia Rangel, 1959.

Boletim do Governo do Estado da India, 1837-1880.

Boletim Oficial, Nova Goa, Imprensa National, 1880-1961.

Bullarium Patronatus in ecclesiis Africae, Asiae atque Oceaniae, ed. V. de Paiva Manso, 3 vols, Lisboa, Typographia Nacional, 1872.

Chagas Pinheiro, *Historia de Portugal Popular e ilustrada*, 1842-1895, Lisboa (third edition), Empresa da Historia de Portugal, 1899.

Census do Estado da India, 1881-1960.

Codigo das Posturas Municipais do Concelho de Ponda, 1903.
Codigo das Posturas do concelho das Ilhas de Goa de Setembro 1906, ed. Alvaro Paulo dos Remedios Furtado, Nova Goa, Tipografia R. M. Rau e Irmãos, 1928.
Collecção da Legislação Novissima do Ultramar, 1854-1867, Lisboa, Imprensa Nacional.
Documenta Indica, ed., Josef Wicki, 18 vols.(1540-1597), Rome, Monumenta Historica Societatis Iesu, 1948-1988.
Documentação para a Historia das Missões do Padroado Portugues do Oriente: India, ed. A. da Silva Rego, 12 vols, (1499-1582), Lisboa, Agencia Geral das Colonias, 1947-1958.
Documentação Ultramarina Portuguesa, ed. A. da Silva Rego, 5 vols, Lisboa, Centro de Estudos Historicos Ultramarinos, 1960-1970.
Documentos Remettidos da India, ed. Bulhão Pato, 5 vols, Lisboa, Academia Real das Sciencias, 1880-1935.
Estatistica Medica dos Hospitais das Provincias Ultramarinas referido ao ano 1869, 1871 and 1876, Lisboa, Imprensa Nacional, 1883.
Legislação do Estado da India, 1901-1961, Goa, Imprensa Nacional.
Livro do Pai dos Cristãos, ed. Josef Wicki, Lisboa, Centro de Estudos Historicos Ultramarinos, 1969.
Portugueses no Oriente, ed. E. A. de Sa Nogueira Pinto de Balsemão, 3 vols, Nova Goa, Imprensa Nacional, 1881-82.
Relatorio Annuario do Governo Geral do Estado da India - Administração do concelho das Ilhas de Goa, 1904, Nova Goa, Imprensa National, 1904.
Relatorio da Campanha Anti Pestosa em Margão e em varias aldeias de Salcete, Nova Goa, Imprensa National, 1918.
Relatorio dos Servicos de Saude do Estado da India (1889-1935), Nova Goa.
Revista Medico-Militar da India Portuguesa, 1862.
Summario Chronologico de Decretos Diocesanos desde 1775-1899 — Decretos do Arcebispo D. Francisco d'Assumpção e Brito, ed. Manuel João Socrates d'Albuquerque, Bastora, Tipografia Rangel, 1900.

2. Published Secondary Sources

Abreu, Miguel V. de, *O Governo do Vice-Rei Conde do Rio Pardo no Estado da India Portuguesa desde 1816-1821,* Nova Goa, Imprensa Nacional, 1869.

———, *Relação das alterações politicas de Goa desde 16 de Setembro de 1821 ate 18 de Outubro de 1822*, Nova Goa, Imprensa Nacional, 1862.

———, *Noção de alguns filhos distinctos da India Portuguesa*, Nova Goa, Imprensa Nacional, 1874.

Albuquerque, M. J.S. de, *Sumario Chronologico dos Decretos Diocesanos do Arcebispado de Goa desde 1775-1900*, Bastora, Tipografia Rangel, 1900.

———, *Hospicio do Clero - A Historia da sua Fundação e Contas*, Nova Goa, Tipografia Bragança, 1929.

Albuquerque, Tereza, *To Love Is To Serve — Catholics of Bombay*, Bombay, Heras Institute of Indian History and Culture, 1986.

Almeida, J. C., *Alguns aspectos Demograficos de Goa, Damão e Dio*, Goa, Governemnt Printing Press, 1965.

———, *Aspects of the Agricultural Activity in Goa, Daman and Diu*, Panjim, Manager of Publications, 1967.

Antão, Alfredo, "Algumas notas sobre mortalidade infantil no concelho de Sanguem", *Proceedings 1a. Conferencia Sanitaria de Goa, 1914*, Nova Goa, Imprensa National, 1917.

Andrade, Lencastre Pereira, *Plantas Medicinais de Goa*, Part I, Bastora, Tipografia Rangel, 1899.

Angle, Prabhakar S., *Goa: An Economic Review*, Panjim, The Goa Hindu Association Kala Vibhag, 1983.

Ayalla, Frederico Diniz de, *Goa antiga e moderna*, Nova Goa, Livraria Coelho, 1927.

A Escola Medico-Cirurgica de Goa — monografia, Goa, 1959.

Baião, Antonio, *A Inquisição de Goa*, 2 vols, Coimbra, Imprensa de Universidade, 1930-1945.

Bala, Poonam, *Imperialism and Medicine in Bengal — A socio-historical perspective*, New Delhi, Sage Publications, 1991.

Ballhatchet, K., *Race Sex and Class under the Raj*, New Delhi, Vikas Publishing House, 1969.

Barbosa, Duarte, *The Book of Duarte Barbosa*, 4 vols, London, Haklyyit Society, 1918-1921. Reprint, 1967.

Barreto Miranda, J. C., *Quadros Historicos de Goa*, III, Margão, Tipografia Ultramar, 1865.

Barreto, J. R. dos Remedios, *Plantas medicinais de Goa*, Bastora, Tipografia Rangel, 1959.

Barros, João de, *Decadas da Asia*, 4 vols, Lisboa, na Regia Officina Typografia, 1777 - 1778.

Bernier, François, *Travels in the Moghul Empire*, ed. Archibald Constable, New Delhi, S.Chand, 1927.

Bhattacharjee, P.J. and Shastri G.N., *Population in India*, New Delhi, 1976.

Bocarro, A., *Livro das Plantas de todos as Fortalezas Cidades e povoações do Estado da India Oriental*, in A.B. de Bragança Pereira (ed.), *Arquivo Portugues Oriental*, Vol II, Bastora, Tipografia Rangel, 1936-1940.

Bordalo, Francisco Maria, *Ensaio sobre a Estatisca do Estado da India*, in Jose Joaquim Lopes de Lima, *Ensaios sobre a estatisca das possessões Portuguesas na Africa, Asia, e na Oceania*, Lisboa, Imprensa Nacional, 1844-1862.

Botelho de Souza, Alfredo, *Subsidios para historia militar e maritima da India*, 4 vols, Lisboa, Agencia Geral das Colonias, 1940.

Boxer, C. R., *Race Relations in the Portuguese Colonial Empire 1415-1825*, London, Oxford University Press, 1963.

———,*The Portuguese Seaborne Empire 1415-1825*, Middlesex, Penguin Books, 1973.

Boxer, C. R., *Mary and Mysogymy: Women in Iberian Expansion Overseas* — Some facts, fancies and personality 1415-1815, London, G. Duckworth and Co, 1975.

———, *Portuguese India in the mid-seventeenth century*, Delhi, Oxford University Press, 1980.

Braganca Pereira, A. B., *Etnografia da India Portuguesa* 2 vols, Bastora, Tipografia Rangel, 1940.

———, ed. *Arquivo Portugues Oriental*, 11 vols, Bastora, Tipografia Rangel, 1936-1940.

Cabral e Sa, Mario, "Thresholds of Leisure", *Goa Cultural Patterns*, ed. S. V. Doshi, Bombay, Marg Publication, 1983.

Captain Kol, *Statistical Report on the Portuguese Settlements in India*, Bombay, Bombay Education Society Press, 1855.

Chronista de Tissuary, ed. J.H. da Cunha Rivara (monthly periodical), 4 vols, Nova Goa, Imprensa Nacional, 1866-68.

Conde de Linhares, *Diario do 3º Conde de Linhares*, 2 vols, LIsboa, Bibloteca Nacional, 1937- 1943.

Conde de Ficalho, *Garcia da Orta e o seu tempo*, Lisboa, Imprensa Nacional, 1886.

Constituições do Archebispado de Goa, ed. Dom Antonio Ta-veira de Neiva Brum, Lisboa, Imprensa Regia, 1910.

Correia-Afonso, John, *Jesuits Letters and Indian History 1542-1773*,

Bombay, Oxford University Press, 1969. First edition 1955.
———, ed. *Indo-Portuguese History: Sources and Problems*, Bombay, Oxford University Press, 1981.
Correia-Afonso, Pedro, *O Problema da Mão da Obra Agricola na India Portuguesa*, 7º *Congresso Provincial*, Nova Goa, 1927.
Correa, Gaspar, *Lendas da India*, 4 vols, Lisboa, Typographia da Academia Real das Sciencias, 1858-64.
Correia, A. C. Germano da Silva, *A cholera-morbo na India Portuguesa desde a sua conquista ate a actualidade - Estudo nosografico, epidemiologico e climato-sanitario Nova Goa*, Imprensa National, 1919.
———, *La vieille Goa*, Bastora, Tipografia Rangel, 1931.
———, *Historia do Ensino Medico na India Portuguesa nos seculos XVII, XVIII, XIX*, Bastora, Tipografia Rangel, 1941.
———, *Historia do ensino medico na India Portuguesa*, Nova Goa, Imprensa National, 1917.
———, *La Peste dans l'Inde Portugaise*, Nova Goa, Imprensa National, 1928.
———, *India Portuguesa - Prostituição e Profilaxia Anti-venerea - Historia Demografia Etnografia Hygiene e Profilaxia*, Bastora, Tipografia Rangel, 1938.
Correia, Filipe Neri, *Medicina Indigena*, Margão, Tipografia Nacional Editora, 1929.
Costa, Aleixo Manuel da, *Literatura Goesa — Apontamentos biobliograficos para sua historia*, Lisboa, Agencia Geral do Ultramar, 1967.
Costa, Constancio Roque da, *O tratado Anglo-Portuguez de 26 de Decembro de 1878*, Tipografia Ultramar, 1879.
Costa, Cristovam da, *Tratados das Drogas e medicina das Indias Orientais*, Lisboa, Junta da Investigacões do Ultramar, 1964.
Costa, A. Bruto da, *Goa sob a dominação Portuguesa*, Margão, Tipografia do Ultramar, 1897.
Coutinho, Fortunato, *Le regime paroissial des dioceses de rite latin de l'Inde des origines (XVIe siecle) a nous jours*, Louvain, Publications Universitaires, 1958.
Jean-Baptiste Tavernier's Travels in India, (ed.) Crooke William, 2 vols, Reprint Oriental Books Reprint Corporation, New Delhi, 1977.
Cruz, Antonio, *Men and Matters*, Ashok Printing Press, Vasco da Gama, 1974.
Congresso Provincial da India Portuguesa - Subsidios para sua Historia,

ed. Antonio Maria da Cunha, 6 vols, Nova Goa, Casa Luso Francesa, 1924-19331.

Cunha Gonsalves, L da, Usos e Costumes dos Habitantes não - Christãos da India Portuguesa", in *Estudos Coloniais*, 1, 1948-49, pp. 49-67.

Das, Sujit K., "Academic definations pointless prescriptions", *Economic and Political Weekly*, vol. XXVI, no. 14, April 6, 1991, Bombay, Sameeksha Trust Publication.

Dalgado, Daniel Gelasio, *Flora de Goa e Savantvadi*, Lisboa, Imprensa Nacional, 1898.

Dalgado, D.G., *Classificação botanica das plantas e das Drogas descriptas nos Coloquios da India de Garcia d' Orta*, Bombay, Nicol's Printing Work, 1894.

Dellon, François, *Narração da Inquisição de Goa*, Tr. M.V. Abreu, Nova Goa, Imprensa Nacional, 1866.

Dias Victor, *Velha Goa: seu saneamento*, Fasc I, Cidade de Goa, 1949.

Disney, A. "Smugglers and Smuggling in the West half of the Estado da India in the late sixteenth and early seventeenth centuries," *Indica*, XXVI, no. 1 and 2 March-September 1989.

Early Travels in India of Ralph Fitch, ed. William Foster, London, Oxford University Press, 1921.

Early Travels in India, ed. J. Talboys Wheeler, Calcutta, 1956.

Falcão, L. de F., *Livro em que se contem toda a Fazenda e Real patrimonio dos Reinos de Portugal, India e Ihas adjacentes e outras particularidades*, Lisboa, Imprensa Nacional, 1859.

Faria e Souza, Manuel de, *Asia Portuguesa*, (1590-1649), 6 vols, Lisboa, Livraria Civilizacão, 1666-75.

Felner, R. J. de Lima, *Subsidios para a historia da India Portuguesa*, Lisboa, Academia Real das Sciencias, 1868.

Fernandes, F.X.E., *India Portuguesa: Estudos Economicos Sociaes*, Bastora, Tipografia Rangel, 1905.

Fernandes, Avertano Correia, *A renovação economica da India Portuguesa*, Bastora, Tipografia Rangel, 1940.

Ferreira Martins, J. F., *Historia da Misericordia de Goa*, 3 vols, Nova Goa, Imprensa Nacional, 1910-1914.

Fonseca, J. N. da, *An Historical and Archaelogical Sketch of the City of Goa*, Bombay, Thacker and Co. Ltd, 1878, Reprint New Delhi, Asian Educational Service, 1986.

Forbes, James, *Oriental Memoirs*, 4 vols, New Delhi, Gian Publishers, 1988, (Reprint).

Foster, William, *Early Travels in India*, 1583-1619, Oxford, Oxford

University Press, 1921.
Fryer, John, *A New Account of East India and Persia*, 3 vols, London, 1909 - 1915. Reprint New Delhi, Asian Education.
Gaitonde, P. D., *Portuguese Pioneers in India* — Spolight on Medicine, Bombay, Popular Prakashan, 1983.
Goa Today: Pictorial Review of Goa, ed. L. D. Silva, Bombay, Western India House, 1952.
Garcia, Carlos, *A primeira mulher neurologista Portuguesa, Neurinoticias — Boletim da Sociedade Portuguesa de Neurologia,* no. 1, Lisboa, 1990.
Gracias, J.B.Amancio, *Historia Economico-Financeira da India Porutugesa* 1910-1947, Lisboa, Agencia Geral das Colonias, 1950.
———, *Medicos Europeus em Goa e nas Cortes Indianas nos seculos XVI a XVIII,* Bastora, Tipografia Rangel, 1939.
Gracias, Caetano F.X., *Flora sagrada da India*, Margão Typographia de Albergue,1912.
Gracias, Fatima, "Quality of Life in Colonial Goa: Its Hygienic Expression (19th-20th Centuries), *Essays in Goan History*, ed. Teotonio R. de Souza, New Delhi, Concept Publishing Company, 1989.
Grande Enciclopeadia Portuguesa Brasileira, 40 vols, Lisboa, (s.d.).
Gazeeter of India — Union Territory Goa, Daman and Diu, Part 1: Goa, ed. V.T. Gune, Bombay, Government Central Press, 1979.
Gonçalves, Sebastião, *Primeira Parte da Historia dos Religiosos da Companhia de Jesus*, ed. Josef Wicki, Coimbra, Atlantida, 1957-1962.
Guha Sumit, "Mortality decline in early twentieth century India : a preliminary inquiry", *The Indian Economic and Social History Review,* XXVIII, no.4 (October-December), 1991.
Habib, Irfan, *Caste and Money in Indian History*, Bombay, Bharat Printers, 1987.
Heredia, Rudolf, "Social Medicine for Hollistic Health — An Alternative Response to Present Crisis," *Economic and Political Weekly*, vol. XXV, nos. 48 and 49, December 1-8 1990, Bombay, Sameeksha Trust Publication.
———, "Unhelful Disappointments", *Economic and Political/Weekly*, vol. XXVI, nos. 31-32, August 3-10 1991.
Ifeka, Caroline, "The Image of Goa," *Indo -Portuguese History: Old Issues, New Questions,* ed. Teotonio R. de Souza, New Delhi, Concept Publishing Co, 1985.
Imperial Medicine and Indigenous Societies, ed. David Arnold, New

Delhi, Oxford University Press, 1989.
Indo-Portuguese Review, Calcutta, 1919-1928.
Issues in the Political Economy of the Health Care ed. John B. Mc Kinlay, New York, Tavistock Publications, 1984.
Jeffery, Roger, *The Politics of Health in India*, Berkeley, (USA) University of California Press, 1988.
Khana, Girija, *Herbal Remedies - A Handbook of Folk Medicine*, Vikas Publishing House, New Delhi, 1989.
Klein, Ira, "Population growth and mortality, Part I: The climacteric of death", *The Indian Economic and Social History Review*, 26-4-1989, New Delhi, Sage.
Klein, Ira, "Population growth and mortality in British India, Part II: The demographic revolution", *The Indian Economic and Social History Review*, 27-1-1990, New Delhi, Sage.
Kirk, Dudley, "Factors Affecting Moslem Natality," *Moslem Attitudes Towards Family Planning*, ed. Olivia Schiffelin, New York, The Population Council, 1967.
Kloguen, Dennis L. Cottineau de, *An Historical Sketch of Goa,* Madras, Gazette Press, 1831. Reprint Examiner Press, Bombay, 1910.
Kothari, Manu L, Mehta, Lopa A. "Violence in Modern Medicine", *Science, Hegemony and Violence,* ed. Ashis Nandy, New Delhi, Oxfprd University Press, 1990.
Lal, Vinay, "Politics of representing AIDS", *Economic and Political Weekly*, vol. XXVI, no. 47, November 23, 1991, Bombay, Sameesha Trust Publication.
Mandelslo's Travels in Western India, ed. M.S. Commissariat, London, Oxford University Press, 1931.
Manucci, Nicolau, *Storia do Mogor*, ed. W. Irwine, 4 vols, London, J. Murray, 1908. Reprint Calcutta, Editions Indian, 1965-1967.
Mascarenhas, Filipe de A., *Luta Antituberculosa em Bardez*, Nova Goa, Typografia Bragança and Co., 1925.
Mello, Alfredo Froilano Bachmann de,"Froilano de Mello" (A centenary tribute), *Boletim do Instituto Menezes Bragança*, no. 153, Bastora, Tipografia Rangel, 1987.
Mendes, A. Lopes, *A India Portuguesa,* 2 vols, New Delhi, Asian Educational Services, 1989 (Reprint).
Myrdal, Gunnar, *Asian Drama,* 3 vols, Middlesex, Penguin Books, 1968.
Nayar, K. R., "Changing international Gaze on Environment and Health Issues", *Social Action*, vol. 41, no. 1, January-March, 1991.
Noronha, Antonio de Piedade, "Certos farmacos vegetais de Goa e a sua

importancia na terapeutica," *Arquivos da Escola Medico-Cirurgica de Nova Goa*, Bastora, Tipografia Rangel, 1949.

Pacheco de Figueiredo, J. M., "Evolução do Ensino medico Cirurgico e Farmaceutico 1847-1945", offprint of *Arquivos da Escola Medico-Cirurgica de Goa*, Bastora, Tipografia Rangel, 1960.

———, "Contribuição de Portugal para a medicina no Oriente nos seculos XVI, XVII e XVIII", *Arquivos da Escola Medico-Cirurgica de Goa*, Bastora, Tipografia Rangel. 1960.

———, "Escola Medico-Cirurgica de Goa — Esboço Historico", *Arquivos da Escola Medico-Cirurgica de Goa,* Bastora, Tipografia Rangel, 1960.

Pearson, M. N., *The New Cambridge History of India: The Portuguese in India*, Cambridge, Cambridge University, 1987.

———, "Indigenous dominance in a colonial economy: The Goa Rendas, 1600-1670", *Mare Luso-Indicum*, 1973, II, 61-73.

Peregrino da Costa, P.J., *Medicos da Escola de Goa nos Quadros de Saude das Colonias* (1842-1942), Bastora, Tipografia Rangel, 1944.

———, *Contribuição dos medicos da Escola de Goa para o estudo de medicina tropical, para a sanidade das possesões ultramarinas, no combate da epidemias e nas campanhas colonias,* Bastora, Tipografia Rangel, 1954.

———, *A expansação do Goes pelo Mundo,* Cidade de Goa, Tipografia Sadananda, 1956.

———, *A Escola Medica de Goa e a sua projecção na India Portuguesa e no Ultramar*, Bastora, Tipografia Rangel, 1956.

Pina, Luis de, *Subsidios para Historia da Medicina Portuguesa Indiana do seculo XVII*, Porto, Araujo Sobrinho, 1931.

Pinto, Wiseman, "O Beriberi e' endemico em Goa", *Arquivo da Escola Medico-Cirurgico de Nova Goa,* Bastora, Tipografia Rangel, 1929.

Pombal, Armando, "Medicina Colonial — Os seus males e os seus problemas", offprint of *Jornal de Medico*, VI, (130): 253-257, July 1945. Primeira Conferencia Sanitaria 1914, Nova Goa, Imprensa Nacional, 1917.

Orta, Garcia, *Colloquios dos simples e drogas e cousas medicinaes da India e assim de algumas fructas achadas nella,* Lisboa, Imprensa Nacional, 1877.

Relação de Manuscritos e Obras Impressas Referente a Historia da Medicina Tropical no Ultramar Portugues e no Brasil (1740-1951), existentes no Arquivo Historico Ultramarino.

Rele, J.R., and Tara Kanitkar, *Fertility and Family Planning in Greater*

Bombay, Bombay, Popular Prakashan, 1980.

Sa, Aires F., *Hygiene de Panjim*, Nova Goa, Arthur e Viegas, 1908.

Sa, L. J. Bras de, "A epidemia de Pempigus numa aldea de Bardez" *Arquivos da Escola Medico-Cirurgica de Nova Goa*, Bastora, Tipografia Rangel, 1938.

―――, "Algumas notas epidemiologicas sobre a poliomielite em Goa", *Arquivos da Escola Medico-Cirurgica de Nova Goa*, Bastora, Tipografia Rangel, 1942.

Santa Maria, Agostinho de, *Historia da Fundacão do Real Convento de Santa Monica da Cidade de Goa*, Lisboa, A. Pedroso Galram, 1699.

Scammell, G. V., "The New World and Europe in the Sixteenth Century", *The Historical Journal*, XII, 3 (1989).

Schurhammer, Georg, *Francis Xavier: His life, His times, II*, Rome, Jesuit Historical Institute, 1977.

Sethi, P.K., "The Technology of Medicine", *Social Action*, Jan-March 1991, vol. 41, no. 1, New Delhi, Indian Social Institute.

Silva, F. A. Wolfango da, *Relatorio sobre a epidemia de peste Dezembro 1901 a Abril 1902*, Nova Goa, Imprensa National, 1902.

Silva, Francisco C.T. da, "Luta anti-sezonatica em Canacona 1950-1951", offprint of *Anais do Instituto da Medicina Tropical*, vol. IX, no. 2, June 1952, Lisboa.

Souza, B. G., de, *Goan Society in Transition*, Bombay, Popular Book Depot Printing Division, 1975.

Souza, Caetano Francisco de, *Instituições Portuguezas de Educação e Instrucção no Oriente*, Vol I, Bombay, Job Printing Press, 1890.

Souza, Francisco de, *Oriente Conquistado a Jesu Christo pelos Padres da Companhia de Jesus*, 2 vols, Bombay, Examiner Press, 1881-1886.

Souza, Teotonio R. de, "Xendi tax: A phase in the History of Luso-Hindu Relations in Goa (1704-1841 A.D.)", in *Studies in Foreign Relations of India*, ed. P.M. Joshi and M.A. Nayeem, Hyderabad, 1975.

―――, "Glimpses of Hindu Dominance of Goan Economy in the 17th century", *Indica*, XII, no. March 1975.

―――, "A Pious Hindu Commemarates in marble the actvities of the Paulists in Kumbarjua", *Goa Today*, February 1977.

Souza, Teotonio R. de, *Medieval Goa*, New Delhi, Concept Publishing Company, 1979.

―――, ed. *Indo-Portuguese History: Old Issues, New Questions*, New Delhi, Concept Publishing Company, 1985.

―――, "Spiritual Conquest of the East: A critique of the Church History of Portuguese Asia (16th and 17th centuries) in *Indian Church*

Review, vol. XIX, NI, June 1985.

———, "The Afro-Asian Church in the Portuguese Estado de India", in Ogbu U. Kalu (ed.), *African Church Histography: An Ecumenical Perspective* — Papers presented at a worshop on African Church History held at Nairobi, August 3-8, 1986, Berne, 1988.

———. "The Portuguese in Asia and their Church Patronage", *Western Colonialism in Asia and Christianity* ed. M. D. David, Bombay, Himalya Publishing House, 1988.

———, ed. *Essays on Goan History*, New Delhi, Concept Publishing Company, 1989.

———, ed. *Goa Through the Ages, II*, New Delhi, Concept Publishing Company, 1990.

Subrahmanyam, Sanjay, "The Portuguese, the port of Basrur, and the rice trade, 1600-1650," *The Indian Economic and Social History Review*, October-December 1984, vol. XXI, Delhi.

Subrahmanyam, Sanjay, "Precious Metal Flows and Prices in Western and Southern Asia, 1500-1750: Some Comparative and Conjunctural Aspects", *Studies in History*, 7-1-n.s (1991), New Delhi, Sage Publications.

The Voyage of John Huygen van Linschoten to the East Indies, ed. A. C. Burnell and P.A. Tiele, vol. 2, London, 1885. Reprint New Delhi, Asian Educational Services, 1988.

The Travels of Pietro Della Valle, ed. Edward Grey, London, 1892.

Thevenot and Careri, Indian Travels of Thevenot and Careri, ed. Surendranath Sen, New Delhi, Nacional Archives, 1949. (Reprint).

Viagem do Francisco Pyrard de Laval, ed. Magalhães Basto, 2 vols, Porto, Tipografia Domingos de Oliveira, 1944.

William, F. Rea, *The Economics of the Zambezi Missions*, 1580-1759, Roma, 1976.

Winnis, G. D., *The Black Legend of Portuguese India*, New Delhi, Concept Publishing Company, 1985.

Wheeler, J. T., *European Travellers in India*, Calcutta, 1956.

Xavier, F.N., *Colleccão das Leis Peculiares das Communidades*, 2 Parts, Nova Goa, 1852-55.

INDEX

Abortions, 61, 113
Acácio Gabriel Viegas, 198
Adelia Costa, 141, 195
Adeline de Souza, 142
Adil Shah, 88, 133
Agostinho de Souza, 198
Agostinho Vincente Lourenço, 186
Agriculture, 33
Aires de Sá, 188, 223
Albuquerque, 33, 91-92, 118
Alcoholism, 59, 105
Alfredo Costa, 197
Alorna, 93
Amulets, 162
Andre Paulo de Andrade, 197
Antonio Gracias, 142
Antonio Augusto do Rego, 189
Anuario da Escola Médico-Cirúrgica, 223
Arabia, 31
Archbishop, 26, 29
Archivo Medico da India, 222
Archivo de Pharmacia, 222
Archivo Portuguêz-Oriental, 220
Arquivos da Escola Médico-Cirúrgica, 222
Arroz preto, 36
Artisans, 23, 24, 25, 33
Asilo de S. Francisco Xavier, 138
Asilo dos Milagres, 137, 140
Asilo dos Alienados, 140-141
Asilo de N. Sra. de Piedade, 138
Augusto Carlos de Lemos, 187
Ayres de Saldanha, 73, 122

Bajus, 34
Bakers, 68, 77
Banguenim, 69-72, 125
Banianes, 27, 29
Baptism, 50
Barbers, 66
Baronio Monteiro, 66, 170
Barreto Moniz, 31, 91

Bassein, 29
Beggars, 26
Bengal, 31
Beriberi, 100
Bernado Bruto da Costa, 197
Bernier, 220
Birth registration, 50
Birth rate, 66, 75
Births, 37
Bleeding, 97, 125
Blockade, 50, 55
Bocarro, 27
Boia, 96
Boletim Oficial, 221
Boletim Geral de Medicina e Farmacia, 222
Boletim do Governo, 221
Boletim de Medicina e Farmacia, 223
Bongis, 68, 77
Bossuet Afonso, 195
Boticario, 118
Boyas, 31
Brahmin, 27
Bro. Afonso, 133
Bullarium Patronatus, 218

C. Matter, 126
Cabayas, 34, 66
Caetano Raimundo da Gama Pinto, 194
Caetano F.X. Gracias, 225
Calapur, 94
Camarte, 132-33
Canarins, 27, 59, 92
Canjee, 36
Capelo gratuito, 176
Careri, 91, 220
Carreira, 31, 39, 122
Cars, 31
Cartazes, 26
Casados, 24
Catholics, 47
Census, 48, 52-54, 55, 62, 220

Index 297

Chambasal, 36
Chappins, 32
Childbirth, 61
China, 26, 31, 36
Cholera, 56, 71, 80-81, 87-89, 93-96, 98-99, 109-110
Cholis, 34
Christian, 24, 28, 35, 36, 37, 53-54, 66, 132, 144, 164
Church, 27
Church Provincial Council, 26, 155
Church and Missionary reports, 217
Church Records, 214
City of Goa, 24, 70, 72, 75, 155
Cleanliness, 64, 65, 73, 121, 124, 129, 165
Clothes, 65, 66
College of St. Paul, 133
Communidades, 96
Conde de Linhares, 26, 28, 31, 70, 97, 136
Conferencia Sanitaria 1914, 224
Correspondência Diversa, 215
Cost of Living, 36, 38
Costa Portugal, 93, 177
Costas, 29
Cottineau, 36
Cristovão da Costa, 224
Cunha Rivara, 212, 220
Curandeiros, 152, 158-59
Curso Médico-Cirúrgico, 178
Customs House, 126
Cutlery, 30
Cyclonic storm, 90

D. G. Dalgado, 224
Dai, 60-61, 152, 155, 159, 167, 180
Deaths, 37
Defecate, 72, 78
Delegacias de Saúde, 146
Delegado de Saúde, 145
Deliveries, 60, 166, 167
Density, 55
Dentists, 159
Diapana, 160
Diarrheoa, 59
Diet, 124, 129
Diogo do Couto, 28
Directorate of Accounts collection, 214
Disease, 50, 65, 67, 74, 86-110
Disney, 29
Documenta Indica, 218

Dolim, 31
Domestic servants, 24
Dowry, 37
Drainage system, 65, 72, 78
Dress, 31, 34
Dutch, 27
Dutro, 171
Dysentery, 56-57, 59, 90, 170

Earthquake, 90
Eclampsy, 170
Economic blockade, 41
Emidio Afonso, 192
Emigration, 24, 33, 35, 38, 39, 51, 55, 101, 105-106
Endemic, 97
Entertainments, 32
Environment, 64-66, 68, 71-72, 82, 205, 206,
Epidemics, 48, 49, 57, 72, 81, 87-89, 92-96, 98-100, 104-105, 106-111
Escolastica Peres, 190
Europeans, 24

Famine, 48, 90
Feiticeiros, 152, 157
Feni, 36
Fernando Albuquerque, 190
Ferreira Martins, 225
Fertility, 53-54
Festivals, 37
Fevers, 57, 61, 90, 96-97, 101
Fidalgos, 25, 27, 29, 66, 134
Fish, 36, 73
Fitch, 31
Flora de Goa e Savantvadi, 225
Folk practitioners, 152
Folk Healers, 157
Fonseca Torrie, 180, 193
Fonseca's Collection, 215
Fontainhas, 75
Food, 30, 35, 80
Francis Xavier Teles da Silva, 164
Francisco Correia, 143
Francisco C. T. da Silva, 191
François Bernier, 154
Froilano de Mello, 101, 141, 184, 188
Fruits, 30, 36
Fryer, 68, 125
Furniture, 30

Ganvkars, 33
Garbage, 64-65, 72, 75, 76, 83
Garcia d'Orta, 88, 153, 193, 205, 223, 224
Gauda class, 53
Germano Correia, 184, 189, 225
Germany, 33
Ghadis, 152
Girasal, 35, 37
Goa Medical School, 178, 180-81, 184-85
Goan villages, 30, 33
Gorgoletas, 30
Great depression, 24
Gregorio Ribeiro, 176
Gujarat, 24
Gulam, 35

Hakims, 152-53
Health Services, 48, 78, 95, 137, 141, 145, 180, 184, 208
Health Board, 109
Herbolarios, 152
Hindus, 24, 27, 31, 34, 47, 53-55, 60, 65, 98
Horses, 29, 31
Hospice of O.L. of Health, 137
Hospicio do Clero, 138
Hospicio dos Desamparados, 137
Hospicio do Sagrado Coraço, 137, 139, 141
Hospitals, 116-144
Hospital Central, 131, 146
Hospital Militar, 98, 126
Hospital dos Pobres, 25, 132, 137
Hospital de Misericordia, 102, 117, 119, 130-36, 139-40
Hospital de N.Sra. de Piedade, 134
Hospital Abade Faria, 140
Hospital Regimental, 96, 101, 109, 117, 131
House, 28, 29, 30, 35, 38, 64, 66, 69, 70, 76, 78, 80-81
Hygiene, 64, 71, 72, 79, 81, 82

Ilha de Fogo, 92
Indigenous and Folk medicine, 152-72
Indigenous medicine, 153, 205
Infant mortality, 54, 57-60
Infectious diseases, 206
Influenza, 67, 103-104
Inquisiço de Goa, 217
Inquisition, 157, 205

Japan, 26

Jayakeshi I, 24
Jervis Pereira, 197
Jesuits, 25, 26, 46, 88, 121, 124-25, 127, 132-33
João Vicente Barreto, 187
João Costa Pereira, 142
John Fryer, 220
Jose Caetano Pereira, 196
Jose Antonio Valeriano Coutinho, 187
Jose Filipe Mesquita, 191
Jose Pedro Ismael Moniz, 187
Jose Camilo Lisboa, 196
Jua, 29

Kadambas, 24
King Phillip, 92
Klogen, 220
Kumbarjua, 94
Kunbi, 34, 36

Lady West, 137
Lake of Carambolim, 74
Landed gentry, 28, 34
Langoti, 34
Legislaço do Estado da India, 221
Lencastre Pereira, 225
Lepers, 25
Leprosaria Central, 141
Leprosy, 170
Lima Leito, 193
Linschoten, 59, 65, 86, 90-91, 124, 153, 219
Literacy, 55
Living standards, 23-46, 205
Lower class, 34, 36, 66
Luis Alvares, 142
Luis de Pina, 224
Luis Caetano Santana Alvares, 187, 197
Luis Cupertino Saldanha, 198

Machado, 142
Machila, 31, 39
Malaria, 49, 50, 53, 55-56, 59, 65, 68, 80, 97, 101, 106
Malnutrition, 58-59, 91, 206
Mandelslo, 30, 219
Mantras, 159
Manucci, 57, 86, 89, 220
Manuel Caetano Alvares, 176
Marital Status, 69-70
Marriages, 37, 38

Index

Martim Afonso, 88
Maternity deaths, 60-61
Mathias de Albuquerque, 123
Medical Board, 69
Medical School, 185
Meningitis, 104
Mental Asylum, 140
Merchants, 28
Mhamai House Papers, 215
Middle class, 27, 28, 33, 35, 67
Miguel Caetano Dias, 182, 194
Military Hospital, 57, 126, 128-31
Mine-owners, 28
Miracles, 163-65
Miranda Almeida, 177, 178, 193
Misericordia, 123
Mode of Transport, 30
Monções do Reino, 212
Morambas, 34
Mordomo, 120
Mortality, 46, 49, 56-57, 60, 61, 117
Mundkar, 32, 33
Municipal Council, 156
Municipality of Goa, 70
Munz, 34
Muslims, 47, 50, 54

Nachini, 30
Namasy, 34
Nautch girls, 92
New Conquests, 52, 60, 71, 81, 144-45
Night soil, 64, 68-69
Non-Christians, 24, 26, 28, 34-36, 132, 157, 178
Nursing homes, 116, 141

Old Conquests, 145
Opium, 105
Ornaments, 34

Pacheco de Figueiredo, 190
Padroado, 28
Palanquins, 30, 31, 92-93
Panditos, 155, 205
Panjim, 71, 72, 74-75, 76-78, 94
Papers of suppressed Convents, 215
Parish registers, 26, 46, 57, 217
Pastoral Visits, 27
Pauta das mezinhas, 119
Pedro Peregrino da Costa, 188

Pempigus, 105
Peres da Silva, 177
Persia, 31
Physicians, 94, 117, 156
Pietro della Valle, 219
Pinto do Rosario, 143
Plague, 77-78, 81, 90, 98-100
Plantas Medicinais de Goa, 225-26
Poliomyelitis, 105
Pollution, 82
Pondarinath S. Borcar, 191
Population, 46-61
Population density, 54
Portuguese, 25
Postura, 68, 76, 80-81
Practitioners, 88
Prazos, 26
Pregnancy, 165
Prostitution, 92, 102
Protected water, 64
Provises, alvaras e regimentos, 213
Provises a favor de Cristandade, 212
Pudvem, 34, 35
Pyrard, 25, 26, 27, 37, 69, 124, 219-20

Rachol, 94
Rafael Pereira, 193
Railways, 40, 101
Ramkrishna Lad, 198
Recolhimento de Serra, 135
Records of Goa Municipal Council, 213
Regedor, 80
Regulamento do Hospital de Misericordia, 214
Regulamentos, 214
Reinois, 24
Remedios Barreto's, 225
Revista Medico-Militar, 221
Rheumatism, 170
Rice, 35, 37, 38
Roberto Belarmino Frias, 194
Rodrigues Moacho, 193
Rois das Igrejas, 216
Royal Hospital, 56, 93, 117-120, 176-77
Rua Direita, 26, 73

S. Domingos, 69
S. José Areal, 95
S. Braz, 94
Samuel Purchas, 67

Sangradores, 152, 159
Sanitary Police, 78
Sanquelim, 94
Santa Maria Magdalena, 135
Santa Inez, 75
Santa Casa de Misericordia, 120, 132, 139-41, 205, 225
Sarvotta Gaddi, 31
Scurvy, 91, 93
Senado, 73
Sex ratio, 51
Silva Teles, 198
Sinays, 27
Skoda Afonso, 192
Slaves, 25-26, 32, 70
Smallpox, 80-81, 89-90, 92-93, 100, 107-109, 163-170
Smuggling, 29
Soldado Pratico, 28
Soldiers, 24-25, 27, 47, 57, 102, 131
Sombreiros, 154
Sotvi, 58, 106, 166
St. Francis Xavier, 25, 163-65
St. Lazarus, 132
State shipyard, 25
Still births, 50, 53
Superstitions, 161
Syphilis, 57, 60, 207

Tavernier, 125, 219
Teotonio de Souza, 33
Tetanus, 58
The mine owners, 41
The lower class, 71
Thevenot, 219
Tirtha, 71
Toilets, 64, 68-69, 74, 76-78, 80, 117
Tongas, 31, 39
Torre de Tombo, 217

Transport, 30, 39
Travellers Accounts, 219
Tuberculosis, 56, 101-102, 170, 206
Typhoid, 56, 65, 98, 103

Unani, 153
Unwed mothers, 54
Upper class, 28, 29-35, 40, 66, 68, 70
Urban poor, 24, 25, 27
Urban middle class, 27, 28
Utensils, 35

Vagrants, 25, 26
Vaidays, 27, 91, 152, 154, 155, 179, 205
Vatam, 35
Vedor de fazenda, 29
Vegetables, 30
Vencimentos Civis e Eclesiasticos, 213
Venereal disease, 91, 97, 102, 131
Viceroys, 29
Victor Dias, 195
Villages, 33, 37
Vincente Alvares, 182
Virgem Peregrina, 139
Visitas Pastorais, 216

Water, 30, 56, 69-72, 74, 76, 81, 131
Water supply, 64, 72
Wells, 70-72, 74, 76, 81
Western medicine, 206
Wine, 30
Wolfango da Silva, 187
Women, 32, 34, 51, 53, 54, 65-66, 91-92, 116, 157-58, 166, 180

Xenddy, 28

Zaddnim, 160